MEDICAL MASTERCLASS

EDITOR-IN-CHIEF

JOHN D FIRTH DM FRCP
Consultant Physician and Nephrologist
Addenbrooke's Hospital
Cambridge

NEUROLOGY, OPHTHALMOLOGY

ATRY

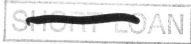
nd Neurosurgery and Institute of Neurology

ogist

ChB FCPsych(SA)

lth and Social Care NHS Trust

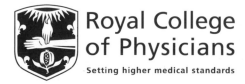
Royal College
of Physicians
Setting higher medical standards

Disclaimer

Although every effort has been made to ensure that drug doses and other information are presented accurately in this publication, the ultimate responsibility rests with the prescribing physician. Neither the publishers nor the authors can be held responsible for any consequences arising from the use of information contained herein. Any product mentioned in this publication should be used in accordance with the prescribing information prepared by the manufacturers.

The information presented in this publication reflects the opinions of its contributors and should not be taken to represent the policy and views of the Royal College of Physicians of London, unless this is specifically stated.

Every effort has been made by the contributors to contact holders of copyright to obtain permission to reproduce copyrighted material. However, if any have been inadvertently overlooked, the publisher will be pleased to make the necessary arrangements at the first opportunity.

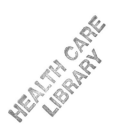

Dr LJ Coward MRCP(UK)
Specialist Registrar in Neurology
Barts and the London NHS Trust
London

Dr JD Firth DM FRCP
Consultant Physician and Nephrologist
Addenbrooke's Hospital
Cambridge

Dr V Kirchner MBChB FCPsych(SA)
Consultant Psychiatrist
Camden and Islington Mental Health and Social Care NHS Trust
London

Dr MS Lipsedge FRCP FRCPsych
Emeritus Consultant Psychiatrist
South London and Maudsley NHS Trust
London

Dr FJ Rugg-Gunn PhD MRCP(UK)
Consultant Neurologist
National Hospital for Neurology and Neurosurgery and
Institute of Neurology
University College London
London

Dr S Sathasivam PhD MRCP(UK)
Consultant Neurologist
The Walton Centre for Neurology and Neurosurgery NHS Trust
Liverpool

Dr C Turner MRCP(UK)
Locum Consultant Neurologist
Department of Neurology
National Hospital for Neurology and Neurosurgery
London

Dr NS Ward FRCP
Consultant Neurologist
National Hospital for Neurology and Neurosurgery and
Institute of Neurology
University College London
London

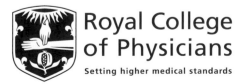

Royal College
of Physicians
Setting higher medical standards

Published by:
Royal College of Physicians of London
11 St. Andrews Place
Regent's Park
London NW1 4LE
United Kingdom

Set and printed by Graphicraft Limited, Hong Kong

First edition published 2001
Reprinted 2004
Second edition published 2008

ISBN: 978-1-86016-272-5 (this book)
ISBN: 978-1-86016-260-2 (set)

Distribution Information:
Jerwood Medical Education Resource Centre
Royal College of Physicians of London
11 St. Andrews Place
Regent's Park
London NW1 4LE
United Kingdom
Tel: +44 (0)207 935 1174 ext 422/490
Fax: +44 (0)207 486 6653
Email: merc@rcplondon.ac.uk
Web: http://www.rcplondon.ac.uk/

CONTENTS

CONTENTS

Since its initial publication in 2001, *Medical Masterclass* has been regarded as a key learning and teaching resource for physicians around the world. The resource was produced in part to meet the vision of the Royal College of Physicians: *'Doctors of the highest quality, serving patients well'*. This vision continues and, along with advances in clinical practice and changes in the format of the MRCP(UK) exam, has justified the publication of this second edition.

The MRCP(UK) is an international examination that seeks to advance the learning of and enhance the training process for physicians worldwide. On passing the exam physicians are recognised as having attained the required knowledge, skills and manner appropriate for training at a specialist level. However, passing the exam is a challenge. The pass rate at each sitting of the written papers is about 40%. Even the most prominent consultants have had to sit each part of the exam more than once in order to pass. With this challenge in mind, the College has produced *Medical Masterclass*, a comprehensive learning resource to help candidates with the preparation that is key to making the grade.

Medical Masterclass has been produced by the Education Department of the College. A work of this size represents a formidable amount of effort by the Editor-in-Chief – Dr John Firth – and his team of editors and authors. I would like to thank our colleagues for this wonderful educational product and wholeheartedly recommend it as an invaluable learning resource for all physicians preparing for their MRCP(UK) examination.

Professor Ian Gilmore MD PRCP
President of the Royal College of Physicians

PREFACE

The second edition of *Medical Masterclass* is produced and published by the Education Department of the Royal College of Physicians of London. It comprises 12 textbooks, a companion interactive website and two CD-ROMs. Its aim is to help doctors in their first few years of training to improve their medical knowledge and skills; and in particular to (a) learn how to deal with patients who are acutely ill, and (b) pass postgraduate examinations, such as the MRCP(UK) or European Diploma in Internal Medicine.

The 12 textbooks are divided as follows: two cover the scientific background to medicine, one is devoted to general clinical skills [including specific guidance on exam technique for PACES, the practical assessment of clinical examination skills that is the final part of the MRCP(UK) exam], one deals with acute medicine and the other eight cover the range of medical specialties.

The core material of each of the medical specialties is dealt with in seven sections:

- Case histories – you are presented with letters of referral commonly received in each specialty and led through the ways in which the patients' histories should be explored, and what should then follow in the way of investigation and/or treatment.

- Physical examination scenarios – these emphasise the logical analysis of physical signs and sensible clinical reasoning: 'having found this, what would you do?'

- Communication and ethical scenarios – what are the difficult issues that commonly arise in each specialty? What do you actually say to the 'frequently asked (but still very difficult) questions?'

- Acute presentations – what are the priorities if you are the doctor seeing the patient in the Emergency Department or the Medical Admissions Unit?

- Diseases and treatments – structured concise notes.

- Investigations and practical procedures – more short and to-the-point notes.

- Self assessment questions – in the form used in the MRCP(UK) Part 1 and Part 2 exams.

The companion website – which is continually updated – enables you to take mock MRCP(UK) Part 1 or Part 2 exams, or to be selective in the questions you tackle (if you want to do ten questions on cardiology, or any other specialty, you can do). For every question you complete you can see how your score compares with that of others who have logged onto the site and attempted it. The two CD-ROMs each contain 30 interactive cases requiring diagnosis and treatment.

I hope that you enjoy using *Medical Masterclass* to learn more about medicine, which – whatever is happening politically to primary care, hospitals and medical career structures – remains a wonderful occupation. It is sometimes intellectually and/or emotionally very challenging, and also sometimes extremely rewarding, particularly when reduced to the essential of a doctor trying to provide best care for a patient.

John Firth DM FRCP
Editor-in-Chief

ACKNOWLEDGEMENTS

Medical Masterclass has been produced by a team. The names of those who have written or edited material are clearly indicated elsewhere, but without the support of many other people it would not exist. Naming names is risky, but those worthy of particular note include: Sir Richard Thompson (College Treasurer) and Mrs Winnie Wade (Director of Education), who steered the project through committees that are traditionally described as labyrinthine, and which certainly seem so to me; and also Arthur Wadsworth (Project Co-ordinator) and Don Liu in the College Education Department office. Don is a veteran of the first edition of *Medical Masterclass*, and it would be fair to say that without his great efforts a second edition might not have seen the light of day.

John Firth DM FRCP
Editor-in-Chief

KEY FEATURES

We have created a range of icon boxes that sit among the text of the various *Medical Masterclass* modules. They are there to help you identify key information and to make learning easier and more enjoyable. Here is a brief explanation:

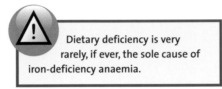

Iron-deficiency anaemia with a change in bowel habit in a middle-aged or older patient means colonic malignancy until proved otherwise.

This icon is used to highlight points of particular importance.

Dietary deficiency is very rarely, if ever, the sole cause of iron-deficiency anaemia.

This icon is used to indicate common or important drug interactions, pitfalls of practical procedures, or when to take symptoms or signs particularly seriously.

NEUROLOGY

Authors:

LJ Coward, FJ Rugg-Gunn, S Sathasivam, C Turner and NS Ward

Editor:

NS Ward

Editor-in-Chief:

JD Firth

1.1 History-taking

1.1.1 Episodic headache

Letter of referral to neurology outpatient clinic

Dear Doctor,

Re: Mrs Lucy Carter, aged 29 years

I would be grateful for your opinion regarding this woman who suffers frequent severe headaches. She is a teacher with no significant past medical history, but has had to take an unacceptable amount of time off work because of the pains since going back after maternity leave 4 months ago. I have prescribed her regular codeine phosphate, which she finds is of some benefit. Examination is normal, including BP.

Yours sincerely,

Introduction
The diagnosis of an episodic headache, as with facial pain (see Section 1.1.2), can virtually always be made on the history alone. It is certainly worth taking time over this: the commonest cause of an incorrect diagnosis is an incorrect history. It is important to note that the severity of pain does not indicate whether a headache is life-threatening or not. Your approach to the patient presenting with headache should be to establish the following.

- Are the headaches benign?

- If so, what is their cause?

In this patient there is a worry that the headaches are related to raised intracranial pressure secondary to a space-occupying lesion, hydrocephalus or idiopathic raised intracranial hypertension, or that they are caused by a systemic condition. However, it is much more likely that her headaches are benign. It is important to make the correct diagnosis in benign headaches to have the best chance of treating them effectively.

History of the presenting problem
It is useful to establish the following.

- How long has the patient had these headaches? Long-standing headaches (present for over 1 year) are almost always benign, so establish when the headaches truly began and not just when they got worse. In this case, did the headaches start during her pregnancy or after delivery?

- How often do they occur and for how long? Determine whether she is describing episodic discrete headaches or exacerbations with a constant background, which may also be described as recurrent. Ask specifically about the period between headaches (Fig. 1).

- Where does she get the pain? Is it bilateral, strictly unilateral, alternating unilateral, frontal, temporal or occipital? The use of a finger or hand to indicate the position will give some clue as to the quality of the pain (Fig. 2).

- What is the pain like? Is it throbbing (migraine); a deep, boring, intense unilateral pain (cluster headache); or band-like tightness/pressure around the head (tension-type headache)? The pain of a headache caused by raised intracranial pressure is non-specific.

- What does she do with herself during an attack? Most patients with severe headache prefer to remain still, but agitation during an attack is characteristic of cluster headache.

- Are there any precipitating or aggravating factors? Light, noise, movement and stress aggravate most headaches and so are not helpful in differentiating one type of headache from another. Exacerbation by coughing, sneezing or straining is also relatively non-specific. Alcohol can precipitate migraine and cluster headache (during a bout) but may alleviate tension-type headaches.

- Are there any associated features? 'Classical' migraine may be associated with visual phenomena such as seeing dazzling zigzag lines (fortification spectra). Many patients who experience this feel intensely nauseated. Additional features such as weakness, paraesthesiae, aphasia, diplopia and visual loss are often worrying

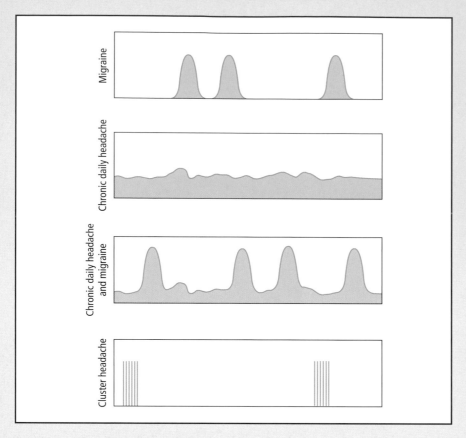

▲ **Fig. 1** Periodicity of pain in different headache symdromes.

but can all happen as part of migraine aura. Establish how closely these symptoms are associated with the headache. Any residual deficit should be taken seriously and investigated further. This young woman could not have giant-cell arteritis, but the diagnosis should be considered in anyone over the age of 60 years with severe headache: visual symptoms, jaw claudication, proximal muscle pain and constitutional symptoms would all support this diagnosis.

- What medication is she on now? Either it is not working and needs to be changed, or it is contributing significantly to the headache and so should be stopped. The codeine that has been prescribed is unlikely to be helping her and may be precipitating the headaches.

Warning symptoms or signs in the patient with headache

- Headaches of subacute onset with steady progression over days or weeks.
- A recent change in pattern or character of an established headache.
- Association with fever or other systemic features.
- Association with focal neurological signs, papilloedema, personality change or seizures could indicate a space-occupying lesion as the underlying cause.
- New onset of headache in people older than 50 years.

Other relevant history

Ask about the following.

- A previous history of depression, anxiety or neck trauma will be relevant if considering tension-type headache.

- Current or previous use of tetracyclines, corticosteroids or vitamin A derivatives may be associated with idiopathic intracranial hypertension.

- Recent weight gain or pregnancy in a woman of childbearing age (such as in this case) can precipitate idiopathic intracranial hypertension.

- Previous head injury, subarachnoid haemorrhage or meningitis may predispose to communicating hydrocephalus.

Plan for investigation and management

You should begin by explaining that under normal circumstances you need to confirm that her neurological examination is normal.

Investigations

Consider the following.

- Blood tests: erythrocyte sedimentation rate and C-reactive protein are important tests to carry out if giant-cell arteritis is suspected (see Section 1.1.2); otherwise blood tests are rarely helpful unless systemic disease is suspected.

- Brain imaging: it is often difficult to decide whether a patient with headache needs a brain scan. The yield will be very low and not infrequently an incidental finding will cause some difficulty. There is also increasing awareness of the exposure to radiation associated with CT scanning (equivalent to approximately 100–150 CXRs). However, if a clear diagnosis cannot be made and there are uncertainties as to whether the headache is benign, then it may be appropriate to perform a scan to exclude a space-occupying lesion or hydrocephalus. Imaging may

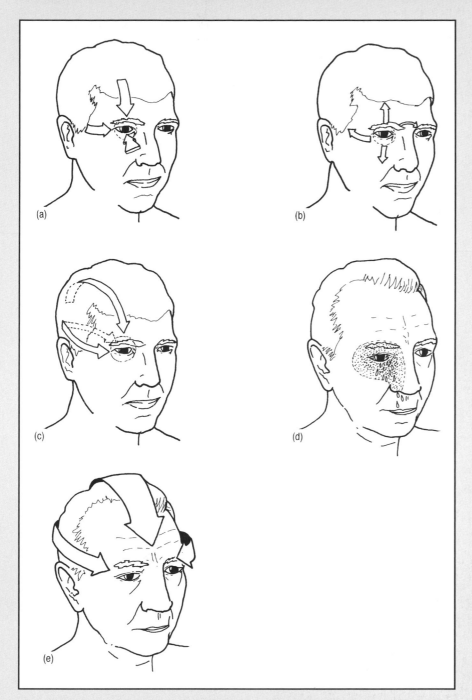

▲ **Fig. 2** Site of pain in different headache diagnoses. **(a)** Classical migraine. Pain is centred in and around the eye and the forehead on one or other side, and usually extends to involve the whole half-head. **(b)** Orbital onset migraine. The pain tends to start in and around the orbit and may extend across to the opposite eye and to the adjacent facial, frontal and temporal areas, but the main pain remains in the orbit itself. **(c)** Occipital onset migraine. The pain may start as a tightness in the occipital area, rather like tension headache, but will typically extend forward around the temporal area or over the top of the head. The ultimate location of the headache is in and around the eye. **(d)** Cluster headache. The pain is located in the eye and nostril. It is strictly unilateral and rarely changes side. Lacrimation, nasal blockage and discharge are common. **(e)** Tension headache. The pain has a quality like a tight band around the head, coming forwards to the forehead.

pressure on lumbar puncture (>25 cm H$_2$O) after normal brain imaging has been obtained.

Management

Management depends on the particular cause. For migraine, cluster headache and tension-type headache with exacerbations, see Section 2.6. For idiopathic intracranial hypertension:

- provide the patient with dietary advice to lose weight;

- repeat lumbar punctures;

- give the patient acetazolamide 750–1000 mg daily;

- be aware that deterioration in vision is likely to need optic nerve sheath fenestration.

Further discussion

In a young woman of childbearing age who has recently been pregnant or gained weight, idiopathic intracranial hypertension must be considered. Patients characteristically present with a gradual-onset headache associated with features of raised intracranial pressure. They may also complain of visual obscurations (transient bilateral visual loss occurring with changes in posture) and occasionally tinnitus. The headache itself has no specific features.

> ⚠ **Idiopathic intracranial hypertension** is no longer called 'benign' because of the danger of progressive visual loss associated with papilloedema. Sight must be monitored by regular formal visual field testing and intraocular pressure measurement, not simply by testing of acuity.

demonstrate slit-like ventricles in a patient with idiopathic intracranial hypertension, but may also be completely normal.

- Lumbar puncture: a diagnosis of idiopathic intracranial hypertension is confirmed by measuring an elevated opening

1.1.2 Facial pain

TABLE 1 CAUSES OF FACIAL PAIN

Type of facial pain	Causes
Intermittent	Trigeminal neuralgia
	Cluster headache
	Giant-cell arteritis
	Costen's syndrome
Constant	Postherpetic neuralgia
	Atypical facial pain
	Tolosa–Hunt syndrome

Introduction

The clinical history is the most important tool in reaching a diagnosis for the cause of facial pain (Table 1). Physical examination and investigations will often be normal. There are several causes of intermittent facial pain, but although the symptoms can be distressing it is usually possible to improve matters if the correct diagnosis is made. Constant facial pain is less common and often harder to treat than intermittent pain.

History of the presenting problem

Firstly, it is important to characterise the pain. Then you must identify the presence of any associated features that may give clues to the underlying diagnosis. Ask the patient to describe the pain as fully as possible and then, if not already volunteered, enquire specifically about the following.

- Where do you feel the pain? (Fig. 3.)

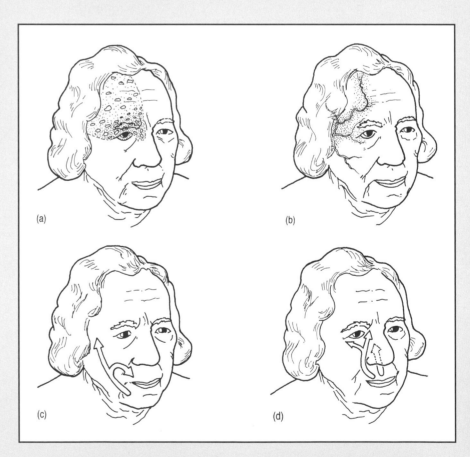

▲ **Fig. 3** Site of facial pain in different diagnoses. (**a**) Postherpetic neuralgia. The whole area of the first division of the fifth nerve may have been involved, but typically the most persistent and unpleasant pain is in the eye itself and the eyebrow. (**b**) Cranial arteritis. Although involvement of the superficial temporal artery has always been stressed, any artery in the head can be involved. There is a tendency for the pain to be worse nocturnally but still be present 24 hours a day and associated with systemic symptoms (weight loss and general ill-health). In most instances the patient's erythrocyte sedimentation rate (ESR) and C-reactive protein (CRP) will be markedly elevated. (**c**) Trigeminal neuralgia. The commonest pattern is pain radiating from the lower jaw, particularly the canine tooth, up to a position deep in front of the ear. The less common variant (**d**) involves pain starting in the incisors or canines of the upper jaw, and radiating up to and around the eye or, at its worst, up inside the nose.

- Is it intermittent or constant? (See Table 1.)
- How long have you had it for?
- Does anything make the pain better or worse?

As you obtain the answers to these questions, consider the diagnoses shown below.

Trigeminal neuralgia
A unilateral lancinating sharp pain that lasts for seconds, affecting the lower jaw and upper lip and set off by touch, chewing or talking (see Section 2.6).

Postherpetic neuralgia
The constant unilateral burning sensation (with occasional lancinating pains) comes on after herpes zoster ophthalmicus in 10% of cases. This usually affects the upper face, especially the eyebrow.

Cluster headache
An episodic deep boring pain situated on or around one eye (see Section 2.6).

Giant-cell arteritis
A diagnosis that should be considered in any patient over 60 years of age with recent-onset headache or facial pain. It may cause diffuse unilateral or bilateral headache, although the patient may concentrate on the symptom of temporal tenderness.

Costen's syndrome
Severe pain over the temperomandibular joint when eating.

Atypical facial pain
Described as a continuous unbearable pain, usually maxillary, and either unilateral or bilateral. This is a diagnosis of exclusion and is not to be made before other possibilities have been exhausted.

Tolosa–Hunt syndrome
An idiopathic granulomatous process in the anterior portion of the cavernous sinus or at the superior orbital fissure. Causes intraorbital and retro-orbital pain that may simulate cluster headache. Involvement of cranial nerves III, IV and VI leads to variable ophthalmoplegia.

Other relevant history
Are there any associated features? Consider the following points.

- Has there been any visual disturbance? This, together with jaw claudication, is an important clue to the diagnosis of giant-cell arteritis, as is the presence of constitutional symptoms.

- Has an eye gone red? Primary angle closure glaucoma often causes an intermittently painful red eye, but it may cause non-specific headaches. In milder, less acute cases coloured haloes seen around lights may be the main diagnostic clue. (See *Ophthalmology*, Section 1.2.1 for discussion of the patient presenting with a red eye.)

- Is there painful ophthalmoplegia? This would suggest ophthalmoplegic migraine (less likely to occur *de novo* at this age) or Tolosa–Hunt syndrome.

- Has there been a rash or any spots? Postherpetic neuralgia will have been preceded by herpes zoster ophthalmicus.

- Cluster headache has a number of associated features (see Section 2.6).

- Has there been discharge or bleeding from the nose? These would suggest a sinus problem in this context.

- If facial pain is associated with signs or symptoms suggestive of cerebral ischaemia, then look very closely for ipsilateral Horner's syndrome, as there may have been a carotid artery dissection.

- Paget's disease affecting the skull base may result in symptoms similar to trigeminal neuralgia.

- Atypical facial pain is said to be associated with depressive symptoms, but this may be a feature of any chronic pain syndrome.

Plan for investigation and management
You should explain to the patient that you would normally examine her face, throat, head and neck to confirm that there are no abnormalities as stated in the letter from her GP.

Investigations
These will be dictated by the likely diagnosis. In a woman of this age, the most important diagnosis to exclude is giant-cell arteritis, but the most likely diagnosis is trigeminal neuralgia. In general, if a confident clinical diagnosis cannot be made, the following tests or advice should be obtained.

- Inflammatory markers (CRP and ESR): it is best to check these yourself since they may not be part of the GP's 'routine blood tests'. If they are normal, then the diagnosis of giant-cell arteritis can be excluded with almost complete certainty.

- Temporal artery biopsy: if giant-cell arteritis is suspected.

- CT scan of head to rule out structural causes of pain,

particularly in the cavernous sinus.

- Ophthalmological opinion, especially if there is a red eye or ophthalmoplegia.

- Ear, nose and throat opinion.

Management

Management depends on the diagnosis.

- Trigeminal neuralgia: see Section 2.6.

- Postherpetic neuralgia: amitriptyline provides relief in 50% of cases; other useful drugs include gabapentin and pregabalin. Topical capsaicin cream may help. Transcutaneous electrical nerve stimulation (TENS) relieves pain in some patients.

- Giant-cell arteritis: the response to steroids is characteristic and often dramatic.

- Cluster headache: see Section 2.6.

- Atypical facial pain: there may be a limited response to amitriptyline, the dose of which may need to be titrated up according to response.

- Costen's syndrome: surgical correction of bite may be required.

- Tolosa–Hunt syndrome: usually responds to treatment with steroids.

Most cases of facial pain can be appropriately managed as an outpatient. Patients should be reviewed with the results of investigations as they become available and GPs must be informed of any new treatment that is to be prescribed, particularly high-dose steroids, so that regular monitoring for potential side effects can be arranged.

! Action must be taken on the same day in patients with suspected giant-cell arteritis. The results of inflammatory markers should be checked and, if raised, steroids started immediately. If a temporal artery biopsy is planned, it should not delay the initiation of steroids but should be arranged within 3 weeks of starting treatment to have the best chance of detecting any inflammation. A negative biopsy does not exclude the diagnosis since the inflammation can occur as 'skip lesions' with normal tissue in between.

1.1.3 Funny turns/blackouts

Letter of referral to general medical outpatient clinic

Dear Doctor,

Re: Mr Thomas Barnett, aged 76 years

Thank you for seeing this retired schoolteacher with a 6-month history of recurrent episodes of impaired consciousness. These seem to come on at any time and do not have any obvious distinguishing features, such that I am unable to tell whether they are cardiac or neurological in origin, or indeed are caused by something else. He has mild hypertension, for which he has taken bendroflumethiazide 2.5 mg od for some years, but has no other past medical history of note.

I would be grateful for your help with diagnosis and management.

Yours sincerely,

Introduction

'Funny turn' is a vague term that can be used to describe a multitude of different symptoms ranging from light-headedness to loss of consciousness. Making the diagnosis depends critically on the history. This can be difficult to obtain since the patient may have poor recollection of events, and ideally a witness account of at least one attack needs to be obtained (although this is clearly not possible in the PACES examination!). The key points to establish are whether or not the patient is experiencing vertigo, and whether there has been a loss of consciousness. The differential diagnosis will vary accordingly (Table 2).

History of the presenting problem

Is the patient describing vertigo?

It can sometimes be difficult to be certain. Ask about the following.

- A sensation of rotation of self or environment by definition is vertigo. However, many patients will not be this explicit and will describe to-and-fro or up-and-down movement of the body or head, or that the wall/floor moves, or that they veer to one side during symptoms 'as if being pulled down by a magnet'. These symptoms, which merge into the very non-specific complaint of 'unsteadiness', are difficult to sort out. Further probing is required.

- Are the symptoms aggravated by moving, closing the eyes or riding in a car? Is he disinclined to walk during an attack? All suggest that the symptom should be regarded as vertigo.

- The duration of attacks is crucial: benign positional vertigo lasts only minutes, whereas the vertigo of Ménière's disease can last for hours.

TABLE 2 COMMON OR IMPORTANT CAUSES OF RECURRENT 'FUNNY TURNS'

Symptom	Common causes	Other causes
Vertigo	Ménière's disease Benign positional vertigo Cerebellopontine angle lesion	Vertebrobasilar TIA (rare) Drugs, eg aminoglycosides
Giddy/dizzy/unsteady	Anxiety Drugs (various) Multiple deficits of sensory input	Cervical spondylosis TIA Anaemia or polycythaemia Hypoglycaemia
Presyncope or syncope	Postural hypotension Cardiac arrhythmia Vasovagal Ventricular outflow obstruction, eg aortic stenosis or hypertrophic obstructive cardiomyopathy Specific precipitant, eg carotid sinus syncope	Specific precipitant, eg cough or micturition syncope Myocardial ischaemia
Transient loss of awareness/consciousness	Epilepsy Causes of syncope Non-epileptic (psychogenic) attacks	Transient global amnesia

TIA, transient ischaemic attack.

• The role of posture in the generation of vertiginous symptoms is often overplayed: most cases of vertigo will be worse on movement. If movement of the neck, eg twisting to look when reversing the car, precipitates vertigo, then vertebrobasilar ischaemia is possible. However, this is an exceedingly rare cause of vertigo and should be considered only if other symptoms suggesting brain ischaemia also occur.

> A peripheral vestibular disorder is strongly suggested by a history of the symptoms being provoked by rolling over in bed.

It is not uncommon for patients to be unable to describe their symptoms in any more detail than light-headedness, giddiness, dizziness or intermittent unsteadiness. In these cases the wide differential diagnoses listed in Table 2 need to be considered.

Is the patient describing presyncope?

Does he describe early visual symptoms, muffled sounds, feelings of hot or cold, or feeling light-headed? These features would be suggestive of a transient fall in cerebral blood flow. Symptoms on standing suggest postural hypotension, while those associated with effort, chest pain, shortness of breath or palpitations are more likely to have a cardiac cause. Was it preceded by coughing vigorously or by micturition, suggesting a specific syncopal syndrome?

New-onset vasovagal presyncope or syncope would not be expected to occur in a patient aged 76 years, but when they do, such episodes typically occur when a patient has been standing up in hot and stuffy rooms, have quite a long prodrome of 'feeling faint' and culminate in a dizzy feeling where noises seem to become loud before the patient collapses. Consciousness is restored almost as soon as the patient falls to the ground or is encouraged to lie down by someone who recognises what is happening. In those susceptible, vasovagal syncope can also be induced by painful or unpleasant stimuli. Vasovagal syncope is frequently accompanied by brief myoclonic limb movements, which are commonly misinterpreted as epileptic.

Was there loss of consciousness in these attacks (syncope)?

If syncope has occurred, was it preceded by presyncopal symptoms that could give a clue to the diagnosis? A witness account of pallor followed by flushing would be very suggestive of a Stokes–Adams attack (due to the intermittent development of complete heart block), but this does not occur in all patients.

Could the cause be epilepsy?

> ⚠ The presence of jerking limbs and incontinence does not prove epilepsy as the primary cause. Anoxic fits can occur following prolonged cerebral anoxia, such as when an individual is propped up after passing out. A helpful differentiating factor can be the length of time taken to come round after an episode, which may be prolonged in a postictal state and short after an anoxic event.

If the patient was awake but unresponsive during an attack, ask specifically about any warnings that he or any witness may have noticed. Features such as lip smacking, fiddling with clothes or stereotyped movements would be suggestive of a complex partial seizure.

Are there any additional features in the history to help?

Consider the following points.

- A history of tinnitus and deafness in the context of episodic vertigo points towards Ménière's disease or even a cerebellopontine angle lesion (acoustic neuroma), particularly if ataxia and/or facial weakness is also present.

- Do other neurological symptoms occur? In their absence, transient ischaemic attacks of either the anterior or posterior circulation are unlikely.

- If the patient mentions feeling unsteady, then ask about how he finds walking, particularly over uneven ground, or if he has tripped on paving stones; also ask about numbness in the feet and hands. Those with peripheral neuropathy may be susceptible to bouts of unsteadiness, especially when other sensory modalities such as vision are simultaneously impaired, eg getting out of bed at night in the dark.

- Does he have any biological features of depression? It is not uncommon for depression to present with somatic symptoms.

- Do not forget alcohol. Many are familiar with the 'funny turns' that can be precipitated by drinking.

Could the cause of a funny turn be transient global amnesia?

Did the patient have an episode of amnesia and confusion lasting for several hours? If so consider the diagnosis of transient global amnesia, in which self-identity is preserved. The degree of retrograde amnesia shrinks significantly after the attack. The significance of recognising this not-uncommon condition is that it is benign, recurs only very infrequently, and does not require investigation.

Other relevant history

Has the patient ever suffered from stroke, myocardial infarction, angina, heart valve disease, cardiac dysrhythmia or epilepsy? A full history of current and recently prescribed drugs is clearly important, especially those likely to cause or exacerbate postural hypotension, eg diuretics (as in this case) and antihypertensives. Ask about risk factors for atheromatous vascular disease: smoking, hypertension, diabetes mellitus, family history of stroke, ischaemic heart disease and hyperlipidaemia.

Plan for investigation and management

Investigations

In many cases a diagnosis can be made on the basis of the history, when selected confirmatory investigations may be required. When no clear diagnosis can be made, then consider the following.

- Are the 'funny turns' a marker of ill-health? Check the patient's FBC, electrolytes, renal and liver function tests, glucose, inflammatory markers and CXR. In some cases other tests, eg thyroid function or vitamin B_{12} levels, may be indicated.

- Are the episodes cardiac? Check resting 12-lead ECG, 24-hour ambulatory ECG and echocardiogram (if there is clinical suspicion of valvular or other structural abnormality). In the patient with frequent, troublesome and potentially life-threatening syncope, repeated monitoring or even inpatient observation may be required.

- Are the episodes neurological? Any patient with focal neurological features or new-onset seizures must have a CT scan of the brain. An MRI scan of the brain and internal auditory meati is indicated if an acoustic neuroma is suspected. An electroencephalogram is usually unhelpful and is unnecessary unless a seizure disorder is strongly suspected.

- If there is vertigo, then specialist otological referral should be considered.

Management

Management will depend on the precise diagnosis, but note in particular the following.

- Vestibular retraining may be useful for those with benign positional vertigo.

- Vestibular suppressants can help in other forms of vertigo.

- Cardiac arrhythmias may require permanent pacemakers and/or drug therapy, and structural cardiac lesions (eg aortic stenosis) may warrant surgery.

- A clear history of seizures warrants treatment with antiepileptic medications, but these should not be given as a 'therapeutic trial'.

In many patients, particularly the elderly, it is likely that several factors will be identified without any one of them being clearly responsible for the 'funny turns'. It is always difficult to know how far to pursue investigation, the severity of symptoms and the patient's wishes being important considerations. In any case of 'funny turns, cause unknown' it is important to adopt a sensible approach to symptomatic treatment, eg giving advice regarding postural symptoms, provision of a stick to provide extra sensory input, and control of hypertension and diabetes.

Further discussion

There are specific guidelines issued by the UK Driver and Vehicle Licensing Agency (DVLA) regarding driving restrictions for patients who have episodes of loss of awareness. A clear history of a vasovagal episode carries no restrictions, whereas an attack with seizure markers results in a 1-year driving licence suspension. Episodes with no aetiological basis are stratified according to their perceived chance of recurrence and range from a 4-week to 6-month suspension. Further details are available from the DVLA website (www.dvla.gov.uk).

1.1.4 Increasing seizure frequency

Letter of referral to neurology outpatient clinic

Dear Doctor,

Re: Mrs Sally-Anne Cooke, aged 30 years

This woman with previously well-controlled idiopathic epilepsy for many years has experienced worsening seizure control over the last 3 months. Her medication (sodium valproate 600 mg bd) has not changed and she seems otherwise fit and well, so I am at a loss as to an explanation. What do you think has happened and how can we improve things?

Yours sincerely,

Introduction

The most important points to establish are the level of previous seizure control, whether this has been achieved easily and by what means. A full and careful drug history is required. In the case described, the first question is whether the increased seizure frequency has occurred despite an adequate blood concentration of antiepileptic. Causes of deterioration in seizure control can be divided into those secondary to a fall in level of available drug and those that occur despite adequate drug levels (Table 3).

History of the presenting problem

Is this due to a fall in blood concentration of antiepileptic?

- Is the patient's compliance good, or does she forget to take her tablets from time to time?

- Has she started taking new medication that would alter the metabolism of existing antiepileptics? Many drugs antagonise or potentiate

antiepileptic effect. If in any doubt, always refer to the *British National Formulary*.

- Has there been any diarrhoea or vomiting to cause reduced absorption?

- Is the patient using an inactive outdated preparation or has the prescription been incorrectly dispensed? Ask if the patient has noticed any change in the tablets that she has been given.

- Is the patient pregnant?

Are there new factors exacerbating epilepsy?

Is the patient getting sufficient sleep? Has she started working on a night shift or is she being kept awake by a young child? Is there a possibility of excessive consumption of alcohol/abuse of drugs?

Any cause of acute illness, eg chest or urinary tract infection, can lead to a deterioration in epileptic control, in which case the appropriate history would need to be explored. There is no suggestion in the letter of referral that intercurrent

TABLE 3 CAUSES OF DETERIORATION IN SEIZURE CONTROL[1]

Drug level	Causes to consider
Reduced drug level	Poor compliance Poor absorption Drug interactions Pregnancy Outdated or erroneous drug preparations
Increased seizure frequency despite stable drug levels	Poor sleep Excessive alcohol/illicit drugs Non-epileptic seizures Progression of aetiological basis of seizure disorder, ie cerebral tumour Reduced efficacy of, or development of tolerance to, antiepileptic medication, ie with benzodiazepines

1. Any cause of acute illness or metabolic disturbance can cause a temporary deterioration in seizure control.

acute illness is the cause of the increased seizure frequency in this woman.

Are the new attacks epileptic?

Non-organic, 'functional' or non-epileptic attacks may occur in patients with concurrent true epilepsy. This can be a very difficult diagnosis to make, and some pointers to pseudo-seizures include:

- change in the nature of attack;
- patient is experiencing social or financial gain;
- attacks occur in the presence of observers, often in emotional situations;
- a specific pattern of injuries including carpet burns or biting of the tip rather than the sides of the tongue;
- tremulous or flailing limb movements, or pelvic thrusting;
- unusually rapid postictal recovery.

Could there be a new or expanding lesion?

This is a particular concern in patients in whom a structural lesion is known to be responsible for the attacks: it is essential to exclude expansion of the lesion. Warning symptoms include:

- recent headache, nausea or vomiting;
- new focal neurological symptoms.

Other relevant history

Increased seizure frequency is seen in about one-third of pregnant epileptic patients, usually in the later stages of pregnancy and related to expansion of the blood volume and changes in plasma protein binding and metabolism. Some patients will require an increase in drug dosage.

> **!** Addition of new antiepileptic drugs can worsen as well as improve seizure control. This is especially likely to happen if inappropriate medication is used for particular epileptic syndromes, eg carbamazepine may aggravate myoclonic jerks and absence seizures in juvenile myoclonic epilepsy.

Plan for investigation and management

Investigations

In this case, with no suggestion on history or examination of intercurrent acute illness and no change in neurological examination, then unless the reason for loss of epileptic control is apparent from the history (see Table 3) perform the following investigations.

- Check FBC; electrolytes; renal, liver and thyroid function tests; serum calcium and inflammatory markers as a 'screen'. Check pregnancy test if appropriate.
- Check serum levels of antiepileptic medication. Therapeutic ranges are known for a number of antiepileptic drugs, although these should be used as a guide rather than as the sole basis for altering drug dosages.
- Imaging may be required if a new or expanding lesion is considered likely, but otherwise a brain scan is not necessary.
- If non-epileptic attacks are suspected, measurement of serum prolactin within 30 minutes of an attack can be helpful; this may be elevated following genuine seizures (convulsive) but not following functional seizures.

Management

Management includes the following and will depend on the cause of increased seizure frequency:

- improve compliance;
- increase dose or consider additional antiepileptic medication;
- more sleep, less alcohol.

If seizure frequency remains increased despite appropriate drug levels and lifestyle, then revisit the possibility of non-epileptic seizures. Ambulatory electroencephalography during an attack may help to make this diagnosis. Remember, however, that patients can become tolerant to drugs, particularly benzodiazepines, and it may be necessary to introduce new antiepileptic medication.

Further discussion

In patients with focal lesions, eg hippocampal sclerosis, there is a higher chance that seizures may remain drug resistant, in which case it may be appropriate to refer them for consideration of surgical treatment.

1.1.5 Numb toes

Letter of referral to neurology outpatient clinic

Dear Doctor,

Re: Mr Nigel Thomas, aged 50 years

I would be grateful if you could see this man who has developed numbness and tingling in his toes and feet, and more recently his fingertips. He also complains that he trips up occasionally. He works as a publican, smokes 10–20 cigarettes per day and drinks about 25 units of alcohol per week. He has no significant past medical history but takes omeprazole occasionally for symptoms of reflux. Examination was normal, except that I could not elicit tendon reflexes in his legs.

I would value your help with diagnosis and management.

Yours sincerely,

Introduction

The combination of distal sensory symptoms and absent or depressed deep tendon reflexes makes peripheral neuropathy (polyneuropathy or mononeuritis multiplex) very likely in this case. It is essential to determine if the patient has any motor involvement, eg foot drop, as neuropathies can be predominantly motor or sensory, or most commonly both. Focal and multifocal neuropathies may also occur (see Section 2.1.1)

> 🔑 Particular care needs to be taken to look for a treatable or reversible cause of neuropathy.

History of the presenting problem

> 🔑 Does this case require urgent attention or not? This will be determined by how acute the symptoms are: could this be Guillain–Barré syndrome?

Important points in the history are to establish:

- duration of symptoms;
- rate of progression;
- presence of any worrying associated symptoms, eg difficulty in breathing.

Symptoms of short duration that are progressing rapidly clearly need more rapid assessment than those that are long-standing and gradually worsening.

What are the characteristics of a peripheral nerve dysfunction?

Although the examination will be the most useful aid in answering this question, some features of the history will also be helpful. Peripheral nervous system dysfunction would be suggested by description of:

- tingling, numbness and burning in the feet (Fig. 4), together with a description of feeling as if walking on cotton wool (peripheral neuropathy);

- numb fingertips (peripheral neuropathy);

- catching the feet on uneven ground (foot drop/distal weakness) or difficulty in rising from a chair and going up and down stairs (proximal weakness).

What type of neuropathy is it?

The duration of symptoms and the rate of progression give clues.

- If acute, consider Guillain–Barré syndrome.

- Subacute symptoms may also indicate a neuropathy associated with vasculitis, systemic inflammatory disorders or malignancy.

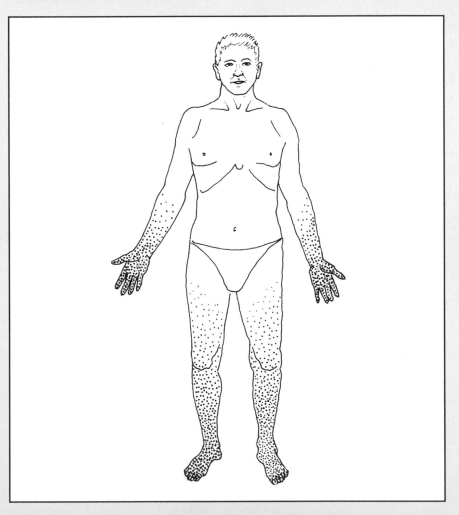

▲ **Fig. 4** Sensory loss in periperal neuropathy. All modalities should be equally affected, but the transition phase to light touch, pain and temperature sensation is not a sharp cut-off – it gradually fades.

- Very long-standing symptoms may be hereditary.

- Painful neuropathies may also indicate a serious underlying pathology.

For further information see Section 2.1.

Other relevant history

Ask specifically about the following, which may give clues to the cause of neuropathy.

- Diabetes mellitus.

- Alcohol intake: does this man really drink 25 units a week, and has he drunk more heavily in the past? He may have cut down when he noticed the symptoms in his feet.

- Current medication: check all drugs in the *British National Formulary*. Is neuropathy listed as a side effect? (Not for omeprazole.)

- Dietary history: is he vegetarian or vegan?

- Pernicious anaemia.

- Hypothyroidism.

- Weight loss: consider paraneoplastic neuropathy.

- Smoking: again consider paraneoplastic condition.

Plan for investigation and management

In routine clinical practice you would obviously examine the patient to confirm the presence of a peripheral neuropathy. It is important to try to determine if this is a large-fibre or small-fibre neuropathy (see Section 2.1).

Investigations

History and examination may enable focused investigations. For fuller details, see Section 2.1, but if there are no clear clinical leads then the following would be appropriate.

Blood tests In all cases perform FBC, erythrocyte sedimentation rate, vitamin B_{12}/folate, urea and electrolytes, glucose, liver function tests, thyroid funtion tests and C-reactive protein. As indicated conduct antinuclear antibodies, extractable nuclear antigen, antineutrophil cytoplasmic antibodies, antineuronal antibodies, heavy metals, porphyrins and genetic testing.

Nerve conduction studies and electromyography These will establish if the neuropathy is generalised or multifocal, motor and/or sensory, and axonal or demyelinating. However, note that standard nerve conduction studies only detect abnormalities of large fibres, hence a patient presenting with distal reduction in pain and temperature, and preserved proprioception and reflexes may have normal nerve conduction studies. A more specialised test (detection of thermal thresholds) is required to detect an isolated small-fibre neuropathy. Limited nerve conduction studies of affected family members may be appropriate.

Cerebrospinal fluid examination This is not usually required for diagnosis, but may be helpful in inflammatory neuropathies with proximal involvement (elevated protein) and paraneoplastic neuropathies (elevated protein).

Nerve biopsy The superficial radial or sural nerve is most commonly biopsied. These are readily accessible pure sensory nerves, so another nerve must be used if the problem is exclusively motor. It is best if the chosen nerve is involved clinically but not severely affected, in which case only end-stage disease processes may be seen. Biopsies may show diagnostic abnormalities in vasculitis or amyloidosis, but in general the diagnostic yield is low.

Other investigations A hunt for underlying malignancy is often unrewarding, but should be pursued if there are suggestive symptoms, eg in chest or abdomen, or if routine tests reveal clues.

Management

If the condition is acute or subacute, the patient may need to be admitted to hospital for investigation. If it is a chronic condition, then outpatient investigations followed by a review in clinic is appropriate.

Management depends on the underlying cause (Section 2.1). Remove any insult or correct any metabolic/endocrine abnormality as appropriate. While this may prevent further nerve damage, axonal recovery in particular is slow.

Inflammatory Chronic inflammatory demyelinating polyradiculopolyneuropathy may respond to steroids. Both plasma exchange and intravenous immunoglobulin (IVIG) have equal efficacy. Some clinicians will try a 6–8 week course of high-dose oral prednisolone and reserve IVIG for cases not responsive to steroids; others use IVIG as first-line treatment. Treatment courses may need to be repeated if the condition relapses and some patients become treatment dependent, requiring regular IVIG to maintain well-being.

Vasculitic neuropathy Initial treatment is with high-dose oral prednisolone or, if severe, a short course of intravenous methylprednisolone followed by maintenance oral steroids. The use of IVIG is anecdotal, but it would appear sensible and is becoming more widely used. Systemic necrotising vasculitides may require cyclophosphamide.

Further discussion

Painful neuropathies (see Section 2.1) can be extremely difficult to treat. Drugs such as pregabalin, gabapentin, carbamazepine, lamotrigine and amitriptyline may be helpful in symptom control. The role of opioids in neuropathic pain is less clear. If all other medications fail, then a trial of opioid therapy is justified.

Meralgia paraesthetica is an entrapment neuropathy of the lateral cutaneous nerve of the thigh. The nerve is entrapped in the lateral end of the inguinal ligament. It causes sensory changes only, with no motor or deep tendon reflex changes. Symptoms include numbness or tingling, and occasionally a burning sensation, on the lateral aspect of the thigh down to, but not below, the knee. The lateral cutaneous nerve is vulnerable to focal compression (eg from a seatbelt), may be damaged during abdominal, pelvic or inguinal operations, or can be stretched by pelvic masses (eg pregnancy).

1.1.6 Tremor

Letter of referral to neurology outpatient clinic

Dear Doctor,

Re: Mr Alan Barnes, aged 60 years

Thank you for reviewing this accountant who has recently noticed a tremor in his right hand. He is especially worried as it is affecting his writing. His uncle developed Parkinson's disease in his seventies. He has no significant past medical history, does not smoke and drinks 20 units of alcohol per week. Please could you advise

TABLE 4 COMMON CAUSES OF TREMOR	
Tremor type	Diagnosis
Resting	Parkinson's disease (3–6 Hz)
Action/intention	Cerebellar (3 Hz)
Postural	BET (5–8 Hz): sporadic or familial Enhanced physiological: exacerbated by anxiety

BET, benign essential tremor.

as to whether you feel he has Parkinson's disease and what treatments we should offer him?

Yours sincerely,

Introduction

The main differential diagnoses of tremor are shown in Table 4. It is important to differentiate tremors that are most severe at rest, suggesting idiopathic Parkinson's disease (IPD), from tremors that are worst when the patient performs an action, suggesting benign essential tremor (BET).

Whether a tremor is maximal at rest or on action is diagnostically important.

History of the presenting problem

In routine clinical practice, but not in PACES, it may be possible to make the diagnosis before or as the patient enters the consulting room. If the tremor is part of Parkinson's disease or a cerebellar disorder, the patient's gait may also be affected. Observation will enable focused history-taking.

Is this Parkinson's disease?

Ask specifically about the following.

- Do his movements feel slow and stiff?

- Has his handwriting changed? A presenting feature in this case, the writing typically becomes smaller and fatigues in those who have IPD.

- Is the tremor most marked at rest?

- Is there asymmetry of symptoms? Parkinson's disease is almost always asymmetrical at onset.

- Has the patient's gait changed? Is his posture more stooped? Are his steps shorter? All of these are typical of Parkinson's disease.

- Does the patient feel that he 'hurries to catch up with himself' (festinant gait)?

- Does he have difficulty turning over in bed?

IPD can only be diagnosed if upper-limb bradykinesia is present.

Is this benign essential tremor?

BET is a fine tremor that often starts in childhood or adolescence, but presents only later when it becomes functionally debilitating. Some older patients may present with a tremor similar to BET that is due to discrete vascular lesions.

Ask specifically about the following.

- Is the tremor worse on using the affected limb? Typically it affects the arms during activities such as using a knife and fork or holding a cup, ie an action tremor.

- Is there a family history? BET can be sporadic or can occur in the context of a family history that is autosomal dominant with variable penetrance.

- Does alcohol improve the symptoms? BET often gets better with alcohol and may lead to dependence in severe cases.

Is this cerebellar disease?

Tremor is rarely the only symptom or sign of cerebellar disease. The patient will more often have a broad-based staggering gait if the tremor is due to cerebellar disease.

Is this physiological tremor?

Physiological tremor is a small-amplitude, higher-frequency tremor that is enhanced by fear or anxiety. It may be pathologically enhanced by:

- thyrotoxicosis;

- hypoglycaemia;

- alcohol withdrawal;

- drugs (β_2 agonists, caffeine and amphetamine).

Other causes of tremor

Consider these rare causes of tremor.

- Some 'Parkinson-plus' syndromes such as progressive supranuclear palsy (Steele–Richardson–Olszewski syndrome) or multiple system atrophy may present with tremor, but this is not usually typical of IPD.

- Wilson's disease: tremor may be an early feature in 30% of cases.

- Peripheral neuropathies: fine distal tremor is occasionally seen as part of a peripheral neuropathy. Ask about numbness or tingling of hands and feet.

- Dystonic tremor: often patients with dystonia may appear to have a tremor in the dystonic limb due to intermittent contraction and relaxation of the affected muscles, eg side-to-side tremor of craniocervical dystonia or 'torticollis'.

Other relevant history

The risk factors for Parkinson's disease and essential tremor are poorly understood and a positive family history is only helpful if the relative was affected at a young age (<50 years), suggesting a possible genetic cause.

However, if cerebellar disease is suspected, then past neurological and vascular history are important, with an empahsis on vascular risk factors and possible demyelinating episodes, eg optic neuritis, complex intermittent sensory symptoms and paraplegia. The cerebellum is a common site for some metastases, such as bronchogenic and breast carcinoma, and therefore relevant aspects of the history should be taken to exclude possible underlying malignancy.

Plan for investigation and management

After explaining to the patient that under normal clinical circumstances you would perform a neurological examination in order to elucidate the type of tremor he was suffering from (see Section 1.2.10), you would plan as follows.

Investigations

Parkinson's disease and essential tremor are clinical diagnoses and no investigations are required in the context of a typical history and examination. If the parkinsonian picture is atypical, eg symmetrical bradykinesia mostly affecting the lower limbs with a frontal apraxic

gait, then brain imaging can be performed to exclude structural or ischaemic disease.

Management

Management depends on the precise diagnosis.

- Parkinson's disease: see Section 2.3.

- BET: often reassurance that this is not something more serious is sufficient. If medication is desired, beta-blockers, primidone, anticholinergics and clonazepam are the drugs of choice.

- Cerebellar disease: this will depend on the nature of the insult. See separate sections on demyelinating (Section 2.5), malignant (Section 2.9) and vascular (Section 2.8) conditions.

Further discussion

Patients with BET and IPD will have difficulty writing: patients with IPD will complain that their writing fatigues and becomes smaller ('micrographia'), whereas patients with BET will complain that their writing has become illegible and 'scrawly'. Patients with IPD often only notice their tremor on one side, whereas those with BET will often notice it affecting both sides, although one side is usually more severely affected. Both groups of patients will notice that their tremor is worse with stress. In general, the 'benign' tremors such as BET are faster than the 'pathological' tremors such as IPD. Despite a thorough history and examination there is sometimes still doubt about the differentiation of the tremor of BET from that of IPD, in which case the patient is monitored over time until the diagnosis becomes clearer. A radioactive dopamine transporter (DAT) scan can also be performed. This indirectly assesses the density of presynaptic dopaminergic terminals and in IPD there is often gross asymmetrical loss in the basal ganglia.

1.1.7 Memory problems

Letter of referral to neurology outpatient clinic

Dear Doctor,

Re: Mr Jack Shaw, aged 60 years

I'd be grateful if you could review this 60-year-old retired schoolteacher who has had episodes of forgetfulness for the past 2 months. His elderly mother, who he cared for, died 6 months ago from probable Alzheimer's disease. Please could you advise me as to whether you feel his memory problems are the early stages of dementia as he is especially concerned about this. His past medical history is pretty unremarkable. He was diagnosed as having hypertension about 5 years ago and has been on amlodipine and bisoprolol since then, with BP 140/78 mmHg when last checked.

Yours sincerely,

Introduction

Dementia is the impairment of cognitive function affecting the content, but not the level, of consciousness. It is essential to obtain an independent description, eg from a relative, since a 'forgetful' patient's history may be unreliable (this will not be possible in PACES, although details may be given in the letter of referral). There are many causes of dementia (Table 5), but it is particularly important to rule out those that are potentially reversible.

TABLE 5 DIFFERENTIAL DIAGNOSIS OF DEMENTIA

Common	Uncommon
Alzheimer's disease	Alcohol-related
Multi-infarct dementia/subcortical	Hydrocephalus
ischaemic leucoencephalopathy	Parkinson's disease
Dementia with Lewy bodies (DLB)	Huntington's disease
	Creutzfeldt–Jakob disease (CJD)
	Frontotemporal dementia
	Tumours
	Drug toxicity
	Hypothyroidism
	Chronic subdural haematoma
	Vitamin B_{12} deficiency
	Neurosyphilis
	AIDS dementia complex

The commonest and most important condition to distinguish from dementia is depressive pseudodementia, which is eminently treatable.

History of the presenting problem

What are the characteristics of the memory impairment?

After a general enquiry along the lines 'Give me some examples of the problems you've been having with your memory', ask the following questions if the relevant details do not emerge spontaneously.

- Was the onset of memory difficulties associated with a precipitating cause, eg a head injury causing a subdural haematoma?

- Was the onset of the dementia subacute (eg in normal-pressure hydrocephalus or CJD) or chronic (eg in Alzheimer's disease or vascular dementia)?

- Is the course of the dementia gradual or stepwise in progression? The latter is seen in multi-infarct vascular dementia. Is there fluctuating cognitive impairment affecting both memory and higher cortical functions (eg language and visuospatial ability) suggesting DLB?

- Does the patient seem slow, with disturbance of attention and motivation? This is more suggestive of so-called 'subcortical' dementia. As the name implies, there is less cortical dysfunction and more disturbance of structures such as the basal ganglia and basal forebrain. Subcortical features are less likely to be seen in Alzheimer's disease but may be seen in a wide variety of pathological processes affecting these deeper subcortical structures, including vascular dementia due to small-vessel disease or 'subcortical ischaemic leucoencephalopathy'.

- Is there prominent behavioural disinhibition, loss of social skills, emotional blunting and language dysfunction? These features, together with personality change, are seen in frontotemporal dementia.

Associated features

- Are there any neuropsychiatric symptoms (eg depression, apathy or irritability) or motor abnormalities (eg extrapyramidal features)? These are more common in subcortical than cortical dementias.

- Are there delusions, visual hallucinations or the disturbances of sleep pattern associated with the motor features of parkinsonism, suggesting DLB?

- Is there any gait disturbance or urinary incontinence, suggesting normal-pressure hydrocephalus?

- Is there associated headache with features suggesting raised intracranial pressure, eg it is worse on awakening, stooping or coughing?

Other relevant history

- Are there atheromatous vascular risk factors [eg smoking, hypertension (as in this case) or diabetes], cerebrovascular events (eg strokes) or signs of heart disease (eg atrial fibrillation).

- Could there be hypothyroidism?

- There is a family history of dementia in this case, but always pursue this possibility in every patient, not only because there may be a genetic cause of the condition (eg familial Alzheimer's disease or Huntington's disease) but also because it is very likely to explain why a patient is so concerned about the possibility, even if there is very little evidence to support it.

- A detailed drug history is essential, but drugs tend to cause confusion rather than dementia.

- Take a detailed sexual history (neurosyphilis is now extremely rare) and assess alcohol intake. As always, adopt a tactful approach, explaining why you need the information before embarking on direct questions that some might

find intrusive and objectionable: 'Sometimes alcohol can cause problems like this. Are you a heavy drinker now? Have you ever been a heavy drinker in the past? Some infections of the brain can rarely cause this sort of problem – the sort of infections that can be spread by sexual contact. Who have you had sexual contact with in the past?'

- Could this be depression, perhaps precipitated in this patient's case by the death of his mother? How is his mood? Does he enjoy anything? Has he lost interest in things he used to do? Is he tearful at times? What time does he wake in the mornings? Has he felt depressed or thought of his death/suicide since the death of his mother?

Plan for investigation and management

Investigations

Any clinical clue to the conditions listed in Table 5 should be followed, but controversy surrounds what constitutes a cost-effective series of investigations because of different estimates of the incidence of reversible dementias. Many physicians would consider the following.

Blood tests Check FBC; electrolytes; renal, liver and thyroid function tests; inflammatory markers (erythrocyte sedimentation rate or C-reactive protein); serum vitamin B_{12} level; and syphilis serology. Genetic testing may be useful in familial Alzheimer's disease.

> ⚠ Genetic testing raises complex ethical issues. The consequences of genetic testing must be carefully considered as significant harm can result from inadequate counselling (see Section 1.3.2).

Neuroimaging This is used to rule out structural and sometimes treatable causes of dementia such as tumours, normal-pressure hydrocephalus or chronic subdural haematoma. In cases of Alzheimer's disease, CT or MRI scans of the brain show cerebral atrophy, especially in the medial temporal lobes, whereas single-photon emission CT (SPECT) shows temporoparietal hypoperfusion. MRI may play a role in the early diagnosis of Alzheimer's disease, which will be crucial if and when treatments that are effective in slowing progression of the disease become available.

Cerebrospinal fluid Testing of the cerebrospinal fluid (CSF) is rarely warranted unless there are atypical clinical features such as systemic symptoms, rapid progression or unusual signs. The CSF cell count, protein and glucose are normal in patients with Alzheimer's disease. S100 and 14-3-3 are two proteins that can be measured in the CSF, and may be raised in any condition where there is rapid neuronal loss and gliosis such as sporadic CJD. If neurosyphilis is suspected, then treponemal serology should be performed on the CSF (and empirical treatment commenced if there is doubt).

Electroencephalography This is not particularly useful because of the overlap in electroencephalogram patterns in different forms of dementia. In Alzheimer's disease there is a loss of alpha activity and an increase in diffuse slow waves. In sporadic CJD there may be 'periodic sharp waves'.

Management

Management will depend on the precise diagnosis. For Alzheimer's disease, see Section 2.4. Patients should be reviewed after their investigations and trial of treatment where appropriate.

> If a depressive element is suspected to be contributing to some or all of the clinical picture, then a trial of antidepressants is warranted.

TABLE 6 CAUSES OF CHOREA

Common	Uncommon
Levodopa-induced dyskinesias Huntington's disease Basal ganglia strokes	Systemic lupus erythematosus (SLE)/primary antiphospholipid syndrome Carbon monoxide poisoning Pregnancy Sydenham's chorea (post streptococcal) Genetic (neuroacanthocytosis, Wilson's disease, benign hereditary chorea) Hyperthyroidism Polycythaemia rubra vera Drugs, especially neuroleptics and oral contraceptives Cerebral palsy 'Senile chorea'

Further discussion

It is very common in patients with depressive pseudo-dementia to have a high degree of insight into their memory disturbance, whereas in cases of Alzheimer's disease (after the initial stages) patients often have very little awareness of their memory problems and are often not distressed by their difficulties. A close friend or relative is therefore essential for accurate history-taking, and in PACES you would emphasise that you wished to talk to a relative/close friend to supplement your history from the patient.

1.1.8 Chorea

Letter of referral to a neurology outpatient clinic

Dear Doctor,

Re: Mrs Ethel Lane, aged 72 years

I would be grateful for your urgent review of this woman who is known to you with Parkinson's disease. She has started to develop writhing and jerky spontaneous movements over the past few weeks, which have become very disabling and tiring. I have been gradually increasing her parkinsonian medications since you commenced them 5 years ago. Please could you advise as to the cause of these movements and their management.

Yours sincerely,

Introduction

Chorea is a continuous or intermittent flow of irregular, jerky and sometimes explosive movements that move from one part of the body to another. Each movement is brief and often appears as a fragment of what might have been a normal movement. Causes of chorea are shown in Table 6, the commonest being in the context of chronic L-dopa treatment in Parkinson's disease, clearly the presumptive diagnosis in this case, or as part of Huntington's disease (HD).

History of the presenting problem

Which parts of the body are affected?

Chorea often affects movement and speech and can be extremely disabling for some patients. A useful trick in routine practice (but not in PACES) that highlights any minor degree of chorea is to ask the patient to perform a repetitive task or to walk.

When did the condition begin?

Patients who present with chorea as young adults often have a different cause from that in the elderly, although there is significant overlap. A young adult with chorea should

raise suspicions of HD, Wilson's disease and other rare genetic disorders. Young adults are also more likely to present with post-Sydenham's chorea, especially in women who are pregnant or taking the oral contraceptive pill. Antiphospholipid syndrome, SLE and thyrotoxicosis are also commoner in young adults.

The elderly patient with chorea often has a history of at least 2 years' treatment with L-dopa, usually for Parkinson's disease, as in this case.

How fast was the onset?

If the onset is acute, then the commonest cause of chorea in the elderly is in association with a stroke in the basal ganglia, which often affects the contralateral side of the body. When the stroke involves the contralateral subthalamic nucleus, patients develop severe chorea or 'hemiballismus'.

> 'Senile chorea' is a controversial diagnosis where no cause can be found in the elderly. However, many of these patients probably have chorea that is drug-induced or associated with basal ganglia strokes, and some have been found to have late-onset HD.

Other relevant history

The most important aspects of the history to elucidate in a patient with chorea are:

- a full drug history;

- family history;

- vascular risk factors.

Relatives of the patient may be helpful in clarifying these events.

Plan for investigation and management

Investigations

- Blood tests should include FBC (particularly noting the haematocrit); fresh blood film for acanthocytes (look in three samples for cells with many thorn-like projections from the surface membrane in an extremely rare condition called amyotrophic chorea-acanthocytosis); clotting (prolonged activated partial thromboplastin time in lupus anticoagulant); and erythrocyte sedimentation rate.

- Urea and electrolytes, glucose, liver function test, thyroid function test, copper, caeruloplasmin, antinuclear antibody, anticardiolipin antibodies and antistreptolysin O titres.

- Imaging: CT scans may demonstrate multiple infarcts in the elderly or atrophy of the caudate nucleus in those with HD. MRI is more sensitive at detecting subcortical infarcts and caudate nucleus atrophy in HD.

- Genetic tests for HD (see Section 1.3.1).

Management

Any underlying disorder, eg Wilson's disease, should be treated. Some forms of chorea are self-limiting, eg Sydenham's and post-stroke. Some

patients with HD do not find their chorea troublesome. If the patient becomes significantly symptomatic, then pharmacological therapies to reduce chorea are available, including tetrabenazine (although this can cause depression) and neuroleptics, eg risperidone, sulpiride and olanzapine. Patients with Parkinson's disease should have a thorough drug and 'on/off' history taken. Some patients can convert part of their L-dopa therapy to smaller doses in conjunction with a dopamine agonist. In older patients who are sensitive to the neuropsychiatric side effects of agonists, total L-dopa dose reduction is often required, resulting in poor mobility.

⚠️ **Genetic causes of chorea**

The pattern of inheritance may help, although the family history, especially in patients with HD, may be missing or incomplete because of a high incidence of early mortality in affected relatives.

Further discussion

Genetic testing for HD is now readily available in genetic reference laboratories. This needs to be undertaken sensitively and with the help of trained geneticists. Presymptomatic testing is a difficult

issue and many patients at risk of developing HD choose not to be tested (see Section 1.3.1).

1.1.9 Muscle weakness and pain

Letter of referral to neurology outpatient clinic

Dear Doctor,

Re: Mr Mark Perrin, aged 25 years

I would be grateful if you could see this man who complains of pain in his muscles and weakness on exercise that has been getting worse for the last few months and is now preventing him from playing football. He has no significant past medical history, except for mild asthma for which he occasionally uses a salbutamol inhaler. I cannot find anything abnormal on neurological examination. Is there anything going on?

Yours sincerely,

Introduction

The list of causes of muscle pain is extensive, but pain or muscle cramps occurring on exercise limits the differential diagnosis (Table 7).

TABLE 7 CAUSES OF MUSCLE PAIN ON EXERCISE

Cause	Diagnoses
Metabolic	Carnitine palmitoyltransferase (CPT) deficiency and other disorders of fatty acid metabolism McArdle's disease and other disorders of glycogen metabolism Mitochondrial myopathy
Other	Hypothyroidism
Ischaemia	Lumbar canal stenosis[1] Claudication[1]

1. Muscular pain restricted to the legs, excepting rare cases of arm claudication.

> Examination may be normal between attacks in cases of McArdle's disease or CPT deficiency, although some cases develop a myopathy following recurrent episodes.

History of the presenting problem

In a young, otherwise fit, man the important differential is between a disorder of lipid or carbohydrate metabolism. These conditions are described in Section 2.2, which explains the significance of the questions below.

Is this a disorder of energy production?

- How much exercise is possible before the onset of pain?

- Is a 'second wind' phenomenon experienced?

- Are there associated painful muscle cramps?

- Have there been episodes of dark urine (indicating rhabdomyolysis)?

- Is there a family history? Autosomal recessive inheritance is seen in CPT deficiency and McArdle's disease, maternal inheritance in mitochondrial disorders.

Is this hypothyroidism?

Ask about weight gain, lethargy, cold intolerance and other symptoms of hypothyroidism.

Is this mechanical (lumbar canal stenosis)?

Find out if the symptoms are:

- confined to the legs;

- improved by bending over.

Lumbar canal stenosis would be unusual in a young man. It is usually caused by progressive hypertrophy of the facet joints and disc degeneration leading to narrowing of the lumbar canal. Lumbar claudication (pain and heaviness of the legs, often proximal) is experienced on standing or walking. Flexion improves the diameter of the canal and therefore the symptoms, hence patients often report no problems with cycling, in which the lumbar spine is often flexed.

Is this muscle ischaemia?

Unlikely in a young man, but in other cases check if the patient is an arteriopath with multiple vascular risk factors.

Other relevant history

Was the patient sporty as a child/teenager? If so, this suggests an 'acquired' illness rather than a metabolic myopathy, which is a lifelong condition.

Plan for investigation and management

You should explain to the patient that under normal circumstances you would examine him to confirm that there are no abnormalities, as stated in the letter from the GP. If the condition is acute or subacute, the patient may need to be admitted for investigations. If it is a chronic condition, then outpatient investigations followed by review in clinic is appropriate.

Blood tests

- FBC.

- Erythrocyte sedimentation rate/C-reactive protein (if raised, suggests inflammatory cause).

- Electrolytes, renal, liver and bone function (routine screen).

- Thyroid function.

- Creatine kinase.

Other tests

Electromyography may show spontaneous activity or myopathic features; a muscle biopsy is most likely to reveal the specific diagnosis. MRI can show patterns of wasting, which may assist in diagnosis. For a fuller discussion, see Section 2.2. Lumbar canal stenosis is diagnosed by imaging (MRI) and treated by surgical decompression.

Further discussion

It is important to counsel patients with metabolic myopathy about the need to avoid situations likely to precipitate myoglobinuria, which may lead to acute renal failure. Patients with disorders of carbohydrate metabolism should be advised to slow down exercise if they begin to recognise the first onset of symptoms of muscle pain and weakness, and then only resume exercise in small increments. In contrast, patients with disorders of lipid metabolism are prone to more severe attacks of myoglobinuria, which usually develop after prolonged exercise and are worse in a fasting state, and they should be advised to avoid any situation that provokes muscle pain or cramps.

1.1.10 Sleep disorders

Letter of referral to neurology outpatient clinic

Dear Doctor,

Re: Mr Frank Richards, aged 60 years

Thank you for seeing this self-employed businessman with excessive daytime sleepiness, which is now interfering with his work and social life. Most recently he fell asleep whilst driving and is understandably concerned. He has a past history of ischaemic heart disease, with a myocardial infarction 5 years ago followed by coronary artery grafting. He is now free of cardiac symptoms. His regular medications consist of bisoprolol, enalapril, atorvastatin and aspirin. He is obese (weight 113 kg, BMI 35.7).

Yours sincerely,

Introduction
'This patient complains of daytime sleepiness' is not an infrequent referral, but the narcoleptic syndrome is much less common and even if patients tell you that they have 'narcolepsy', other causes should be considered (see below and Table 8).

Differential diagnosis of excessive daytime sleepiness

- Insomnia (insufficient sleep).
- Non-restorative sleep.
- Narcolepsy.

History of the presenting problem
A sleep history is required: what time does the patient go to bed, when does he wake up in the morning, how often does he wake during the night and what does he do when he wakes? Exactly what does 'excessive daytime sleepiness' mean? How often does he actually fall asleep and has he ever fallen asleep when trying to stay awake, eg when driving, as in this case? The answers to these questions will help to place the problem into one of two categories.

TABLE 8 CAUSES OF INSOMNIA

Cause	Diagnosis
Wrong environment	Noisy Too light/cold/hot Disturbed by partner Antisocial conditions: shift-work, etc.
Psychophysiological	Anxiety/depression Bipolar affective disorders
Endocrine	Thyrotoxicosis
Physical	Pain Nocturia Restless legs syndrome Parkinson's disease
Drugs	Alcohol Coffee Prescription: steroids, beta-blockers, phenytoin, bronchodilators, diuretics, stimulants
Hereditary	Fatal familial insomnia

- Insomnia: Table 8 lists the most common causes for an inability to obtain sufficient sleep; further questioning should be designed to address these issues.

- Non-restorative sleep: the patient appears to spend a sufficient time asleep but does not awake refreshed. The main causes of this are shown in Table 9.

Could the patient have any of the conditions listed in Tables 8 and 9, or narcolepsy? Further history should be directed to looking for evidence of the following conditions in particular.

Obstructive sleep apnoea
Does the patient have a morning headache? Patients with obstructive sleep apnoea retain carbon dioxide, resulting in headache. The observations of a partner are essential: these will not be directly available in PACES but may be recorded in the referral letter. The important issues include the following.

- Does he snore loudly?

- Does he sometimes appear to stop breathing?

- Does he resume breathing with a large gasp?

Central sleep apnoea
There will usually be a history of a brainstem event or of other symptoms to suggest more widespread neurodegenerative disease.

TABLE 9 CAUSES OF NON-RESTORATIVE SLEEP

Aetiology	Causes
Obstructive sleep apnoea	Associated with obesity
Central	Brainstem lesions Degenerative brain conditions
Mixed	Seen in myotonic dystrophy

Parasomnias

These are a group of disorders that usually start in childhood and can be linked to particular stages of sleep. They can be disorders of movement, including hypnic jerks, periodic movements of sleep, sleep paralysis and sleep-walking; disorders of autonomic function with symptoms of sympathetic overdrive; or more complex abnormalities such as sleep terrors.

> Parasomnias are rare in an adult population and can only be diagnosed by a witness account.

Narcoleptic syndrome

This is classically defined as the triad of narcolepsy, cataplexy and hypnogogic hallucinations (and other parasomnias, especially sleep paralysis) although not all patients will have all the symptoms.

- Narcolepsy: daytime sleep attacks often occur without warning, at times of emotion and after a carbohydrate load. Typically patients feel refreshed after each episode of sleep.

- Cataplexy: these are episodes of partial (often face or jaw) or complete loss of muscle tone that result in the patient falling to the ground. They are often triggered by strong emotional stimuli, usually laughter.

- Hypnogogic hallucinations: presleep dreams associated with sleep-onset rapid eye movement (REM) activity. In sleep paralysis, which is not restricted to the narcoleptic syndrome, the patient feels completely paralysed at sleep onset (less commonly on waking), and this feeling is often associated with terror, anxiety and fear. Recovery is spontaneous.

Other relevant history

This is important in the case of central sleep apnoea. Adults with parasomnias may have been sleep-walkers or tooth-grinders as children.

The family history may be relevant in some rare diseases. Familial fatal insomnia is a hereditary disease caused by an Asp→Asn mutation at codon 178 of the human prion protein gene in the presence of a methionine at codon 129. The same mutation at codon 178 but with a valine at codon 129 results in familial Creutzfeldt–Jakob disease. Fatal familial insomnia is a rapidly fatal disease characterised by insomnia and dysautonomia, and also more widespread neurological involvement including pyramidal, cerebellar and cognitive signs.

Plan for investigation and management

The approach to investigations and management will be determined by findings in the history. It may be that nothing more than simple advice is required.

Insomnia

It is often sufficient to improve sleep hygiene, whether that means sleeping with ear plugs, lining the curtains or not drinking coffee after 6 p.m. Psychiatric and physical disorders that are felt to be contributing must be addressed.

Sleep apnoea

Patients who might have sleep apnoea should be referred to a respiratory specialist with an interest in sleep disorders for further investigation and/or treatment. The initial test will be to monitor arterial oxygen tension overnight using a pulse oximeter, looking for characteristic drops in oxygen saturations at frequent intervals. Treatment involves weight loss and non-invasive ventilatory support at night.

Narcoleptic syndrome

This diagnosis should be confirmed with a multiple sleep latency test, which is performed in a specialist sleep centre. During this test, five episodes of sleep are permitted during the day; a rapid onset of sleep and REM sleep within 15 minutes of onset in the absence of sleep deprivation are both features indicative of narcolepsy. The excessive sleepiness of narcolepsy can be treated with modafinil or dexamfetamine. The cataplexy, sleep paralysis and hypnagogic/hypnopompic hallucinations respond to antidepressants; fluoxetine or clomipramine are the most frequently prescribed.

Further discussion

The Epworth Sleepiness Scale provides a quantitative measure of the patient's general level of sleepiness (Fig. 5). Patients rate the chance that they would fall asleep during different routine daytime situations during the previous week. Answers to the questions are rated from 0 to 3, with 0 meaning they would never fall asleep in a given situation and 3 representing a high chance. A score of 10 or more suggests the need for further evaluation.

Approximately 90% of all narcoleptic patients with definite cataplexy have the human leucocyte antigen (HLA) allele DQB1 0602, compared with approximately 25% of the general population. The sensitivity of testing for DQB1 0602 is decreased to 70% if cataplexy is absent. There is some evidence that hypocretin levels in the cerebrospinal fluid are reduced in patients with narcolepsy, which is consistent with a loss of hypocretin-containing neurons in the hypothalamus.

The Epworth Sleepiness Scale

Score

0 = would never doze
1 = slight chance
2 = moderate chance
3 = high chance

Situation	Chance of Dozing or Sleeping (Score 0–3)
Sitting and reading	☐
Watching television	☐
Sitting inactive in a public place, eg theatre, meeting	☐
As a passenger in a car for an hour without a break	☐
Lying down to rest in the afternoon	☐
Sitting and talking to someone	☐
Sitting quietly after lunch (no alcohol)	☐
In a car, while stopped in traffic	☐
TOTAL SCORE	☐

▲**Fig. 5** The Epworth Sleepiness Scale.

1.1.11 Dysphagia

Letter of referral to neurology outpatient clinic

Dear Doctor,

Re: Mr Dennis Blair, aged 66 years

I would be grateful if you could see this man who has an 18-month history of gradually progressive dysphagia. I initially thought that this was due to a hiatus hernia, but an upper gastrointestinal endoscopy only showed very mild oesophagitis and he was not helped by a trial of ranitidine. He has no significant past medical history apart from migraine, takes no regular medication, has not smoked for many years and drinks very little alcohol.

I am at a loss to explain his symptoms and would be grateful for your opinion.

Yours sincerely,

Introduction

> Dysphagia (difficulty in swallowing) must be distinguished from odynophagia (painful swallowing) and the globus sensation (a feeling of a lump in the throat).

It is necessary to determine if the patient's symptoms are due to an oropharyngeal or an oesophageal cause, and whether this is attributable to a mechanical, motility, neurological or muscular problem (Table 10).

History of the presenting problem

In many cases of dysphagia there are clear indications that the problem is likely to be mechanical, eg the patient has a long history of acid reflux or other digestive problems, is known to have a hiatus hernia or reflux oesophagitis, and oesophageal stricture is likely. The approach to such a case is discussed in detail in *Gastroenterology and Hepatology*, Section 1.1.2, and this diagnosis was clearly considered and excluded by the GP in this case. When there is no such history, the wide differential diagnosis of dysphagia must be considered. Think about the conditions listed in Table 10 when taking the history of the dysphagia itself, as well as of associated features.

What are the characteristics of the dysphagia?

- Is there choking or coughing due to aspiration? This is more likely to occur in those with

TABLE 10 COMMON CAUSES OF DYSPHAGIA

Type of disorder	Oropharyngeal	Oesophageal
Mechanical	Tumour Zenker's diverticulum Neck surgery Goitre Retropharyngeal mass	Tumour Schatzki's ring Posterior mediastinal mass Peptic stricture
Motility	Achalasia Scleroderma	Achalasia Scleroderma
Neurological	Pseudobulbar palsy (eg stroke or MND) Bulbar palsy (eg poliomyelitis or MND) Myasthenia gravis	Idiopathic autonomic dysfunction Vagal neuropathy due to diabetes
Muscular	Polymyositis Myotonic dystrophy	Polymyositis

MND, motor neuron disease.

neurological or muscular disorders than with mechanical problems.

- Is swallowing worse with liquids than with solids? Patients with neuromuscular disorders usually complain of difficulties with liquids first, whereas those with mechanical disorders tend to complain that solid food sticks.

- Is there nasal regurgitation? This is more common in neuromuscular disorders affecting the oropharynx.

What are the associated features?

- Is the dysphagia causing weight loss? This may arise because dysphagia is preventing adequate food intake, but may also indicate a malignant cause.

- Is the course of the symptoms progressive? This might indicate a worsening mechanical lesion, but if the problem is neuromuscular then the time course can also give important diagnostic clues, eg inexorable progression in MND, fluctuating course in myasthenia gravis or a static situation following a stroke.

- Are there muscle cramps, which are common in MND, or muscle weakness?

- Does the patient complain of respiratory difficulties? These might indicate MND or myasthenia gravis, but might also be attributable to aspiration.

- Is speech affected? If so, how? This is likely to indicate a neuromuscular cause.

- Are there any sensory, sphincter or visual disturbances? If the problem is neuromuscular and yet these systems are not involved, then MND is more likely.

- Are there clues to any of the other diagnoses listed in Table 10? For instance, a history of Raynaud's

phenomenon may indicate scleroderma with associated oesophageal motility disorder.

Other relevant history

A careful 'gastrointestinal' past medical history is clearly required. In this case the GP has clearly explored the issues. If not, then ask 'Do you get indigestion? Do you take any treatments for indigestion? Have you ever done so? Have you ever had a barium meal or an endoscopy test?' As regards neurological causes, is the patient at increased risk of stroke? Is there a family history of neurological problems?

Plan for investigation and management

You should mention to the patient that under normal clinical circumstances you would do a full neurological examination, including an assessment of swallowing (see Section 1.2.16). You would then plan to proceed as follows.

Investigations

Aside from FBC (for anaemia), electrolytes (for hypokalaemia if vomiting), and renal, liver and bone function tests (for hypoalbuminaemia as nutritional marker), checking the following may be helpful if certain conditions are suspected:

- autoimmune screen (connective tissue diseases);

- serum immunoglobulins and electrophoresis (lymphoproliferative diseases) and thyroid function tests (thyrotoxicosis) to exclude diseases that may mimic MND;

- anti-acetylcholine receptor antibody (myasthenia gravis);

- creatine kinase, erythrocyte sedimentation rate and C-reactive protein (inflammatory muscle disease).

A full nutritional assessment is required for any patient whose main problem is dysphagia, and many will require investigation (barium swallow or endoscopy) for a mechanical cause.

MRI is needed to exclude the presence of lesions in the brainstem if there is evidence of other cranial nerve dysfunction that suggests a structural cause.

Electrophysiological studies help diagnose MND, myasthenia gravis and inflammatory muscle disease (eg polymyositis).

Management

Management will depend on the specific diagnosis. Poor nutrition itself may require symptomatic treatment, eg nasogastric feeding in the short term or percutaneous endoscopic gastrostomy (PEG) tube feeding in the long term. This can raise difficult ethical problems: should the patient with a progressive and irreversible neurological condition be started on PEG feeding? See *Gastroenterology and Hepatology*, Section 1.3.1 for consideration of this issue.

If the condition is acute or subacute, the patient may need to be admitted to hospital for the investigations. If it is a chronic condition, then outpatient investigations followed by review in clinic is appropriate.

Further discussion

There are three phases of normal swallowing.

Oral phase

This is divided into preparatory and propulsive phases.

- Preparatory phase: bolus of food is processed to make it swallowable.

• Propulsive phase: bolus is propelled from the oral cavity into the oropharynx.

Contractions of the tongue and striated muscles of mastication mix the bolus of food with saliva, and then propel it from the anterior oral cavity into the oropharynx.

Pharyngeal phase

This involves a rapid sequence of events: the soft palate rises, the hyoid bone and larynx move upwards and forwards, the vocal folds move to the midline, and the epiglottis folds backwards to protect the airway. The tongue pushes backwards and downwards into the pharynx to propel the bolus down. The pharyngeal walls contract from top to bottom, helping propel the bolus downwards. The upper oesophageal sphincter relaxes during this phase and closes after passage of the food.

Oesophageal phase

The bolus of food is propelled downwards by peristaltic movement from the cervical oesophagus to the lower oesophageal sphincter. The lower oesophageal sphincter relaxes at initiation of the swallow; this relaxation persists until the food bolus enters the stomach.

1.1.12 Visual hallucinations

Letter of referral to neurology outpatient clinic

Dear Doctor,

Re: Mrs Christina Churchill, aged 63 years

I would be grateful for your opinion regarding this woman who has begun to experience visual hallucinations over the last 2 months. She has a history of depression in the past and takes amitriptyline 100 mg on, which she has done for many years, but is otherwise well. Physical examination is unremarkable.

Yours sincerely,

Introduction

There are many causes of visual hallucinations, which can usefully be classified as described in Table 11. Some cases present in the context of identifiable pre-existing disease (eg dementia, Parkinson's disease or diffuse Lewy body disease, psychoses and migraine) but in those occurring *de novo* you must decide which patients are likely to have an intracranial structural lesion.

History of the presenting problem

Keep the working classification shown in Table 11 in mind as you establish the features of the hallucination.

• Does the patient think it is real or not?

• What form does it take, simple or complex?

• Does it affect the whole visual field or just a hemifield?

• Is it affected by closing or moving the eye(s)?

TABLE 11 WORKING CLASSIFICATION OF VISUAL HALLUCINATIONS	
Type of hallucination	**Associated conditions**
Perceived by the patient as real	Psychiatric disorders Dementia Parkinson's disease: usually associated with antiparkinsonian drugs Acute confusional states: occur in addition to systemic features Delirium tremens: typically small moving objects or animals Some epileptic phenomena (see below) Drugs
Recognised as unreal by the patient (pseudo-hallucinations)	*Purely visual* Visual hallucinations secondary to eye disease, occurring in the whole visual field and disappearing with eye closure. Causes may be simple or complex (cataracts, macular degeneration, glaucoma, choroidal neovascularisation) Hemianopic hallucinations, ie occipital lobe lesions (infarct, haemorrhage or tumour) causing unilateral (usually complex) visual hallucinations, which disappear with saccadic eye movements *May involve hallucinations in other sensory modalities* Associated with epileptic aura or seizures, stereotyped and usually short-lived (<30 seconds), may be simple or complex occurring in a hemifield and not affected by saccadic eye movements. May be perceived as real by some patients Associated with migraine aura; usually simple images, lines, fortification spectra and flashing lights Peduncular hallucinosis: a rare syndrome of often complex visual hallucinations, sleep disturbance and agitation that is secondary to a lesion in the midbrain or thalamus Drugs

- How long does it last?

- If the patient has experienced more than one, are they always the same?

- Are any other senses involved?

A full drug history is essential, including prescribed and non-prescribed drugs, as is a careful history of alcohol consumption .

> Medication for Parkinson's disease is particularly likely to induce visual hallucinations.

Other relevant history
Is the patient known to have a history of any of the following:

- stroke;

- Parkinson's disease;

- dementia;

- psychiatric disease;

- visual disturbance;

- epilepsy;

- alcohol abuse;

- drug abuse.

Plan for investigation and management
You should begin by explaining that under normal circumstances you need to confirm that her neurological examination is normal.

Investigations

> Any patient with complex visual hallucinations in the absence of a known neurological disease (Parkinson's disease, dementia, delirium tremens or acute confusional state) should have a brain scan.

In addition, simple visual hallucinations that are stereotyped may well be ictal and patients with these should also be scanned.

The following may also be appropriate.

- 'Screening tests': FBC, electrolytes, renal and liver function tests (including γ-glutamyl transpeptidase), glucose, inflammatory markers and CXR.

- Electroencephalogram only if frequent suspected ictal events.

Management
This will depend on the diagnosis.

- Epileptic visual hallucinations usually respond to antiepileptics.

- Occipital lobe lesions: the hallucinations are often self-limiting and the outcome will depend on the nature of the lesion, eg stroke or tumour.

- Parkinson's disease: reduce anticholinergic therapy and then dopamine agonists if the patient is disturbed by the hallucinations. You may need to reduce the dose of levodopa, but unfortunately patients do not tolerate this well.

- Delirium tremens: this is an unlikely diagnosis in a patient who is not acutely unwell.

Further discussion

How would examination help distinguish the cause of the hallucinations?

- Visual system: the presence of severely impaired visual acuity may be the cause. Visual field defects will be extremely useful in alerting you to the presence of a space-occupying lesion and its likely location.

- Other neurological signs, particularly brainstem signs ('peduncular hallucinosis') or evidence of Parkinson's disease, will also direct towards a particular cause.

1.2 Clinical examination

1.2.1 Numb toes and foot drop

Instruction

This 50-year-old man complains of numbness and tingling in his toes. He also says that he trips up frequently when walking. Please examine his legs.

General features
Although it might appear that these symptoms are most likely the result of peripheral nerve pathology, do not immediately exclude the possibility of central nervous system or combined (peripheral and central nervous system) pathology. In addition, the symptoms may be part of a more generalised disorder. Is the patient systemically well? Are there indications of any of the conditions discussed in Section 2.1? Look in particular for the following.

- Cachexia: may suggest malignancy or alcoholism.

- Evidence of alcoholism/chronic liver disease.

- Vasculitic rash: probably indicating systemic vasculitis in this context.

- Signs of hypothyroidism, which can produce mild neuropathy.

- Postural hypotension (evidence of this is not likely to be available in PACES, but it is an issue that could be mentioned in discussion): likely to indicate an autonomic component.

Neurological examination

Is this a peripheral or central nervous system disorder?

Look for the following patterns as you examine the legs.

Peripheral nervous system Typical findings include:

- distal weakness;
- absent ankle reflexes (with or without knee reflexes);
- stocking distribution sensory loss;
- wasting (if the problem is severe).

If there is a loss of sensation to temperature, but preservation of proprioception, power and reflexes, then consider a small-fibre neuropathy (see Section 2.1).

Central nervous system Typical findings include:

- spastic tone;
- weakness both proximally and distally, but predominantly in leg flexors;
- brisk reflexes;
- extensor plantars;
- possible sensory level on abdomen or higher.

The arms may also provide useful information.

- Distal blunting to pinprick with absent reflexes indicates a peripheral neuropathy.
- Loss of dexterity, absent biceps and supinator reflexes, and brisk triceps reflexes (inverted supinator/biceps reflex pattern) suggests a lesion at C5/6 leading to cervical cord compression below

this level, as well as compression of the C6 root.

Are the signs symmetrical?

In this case, asymmetry in the context of an upper motor neuron syndrome would represent Brown–Séquard syndrome, with loss of proprioception ipsilateral to the weak leg, and loss of pain and temperature sensation contralateral to the weak leg. Asymmetric lower motor neuron findings suggest mononeuritis multiplex or entrapment neuropathies (for a discussion of peripheral nerve lesions, see Section 1.2.2).

Further discussion

Hereditary motor and sensory neuropathy

This is common in PACES. Note the following.

- It is divided into type I (demyelinating), type II (axonal), type III (Dejerine–Sottas) and some other subtypes.
- Previously called Charcot–Marie–Tooth disease and peroneal muscular atrophy.
- Inverted champagne-bottle legs (and similar process in arms/ hands).
- Sensory abnormalities are much less prominent than motor ones.
- Lateral popliteal nerves are sometimes palpable.

Subacute degeneration of the spinal cord

- Vitamin B_{12} deficiency may cause a peripheral neuropathy but can also result in additional corticospinal tract and dorsal column degeneration, which leads to combined upper and lower motor neuron features.

- Either the peripheral nervous system or spinal cord may be affected first in the early stages, but objective sensory abnormalities usually result from posterior column involvement and less often from peripheral neuropathy.
- Early in the course impaired joint position and vibration sense predominate.
- Typically the legs are affected before the arms.
- At presentation, 50% of patients have absent ankle jerks but are hyperreflexic at the knees; their plantars may be flexor initially, but eventually become extensor.

The clinical picture can be variable, but remember that this is a treatable condition and must not be missed.

1.2.2 Weakness in one leg

Instruction

This 46-year-old woman complains of weakness in her right leg. Please examine her legs.

General features

Is it painful for the patient to move about? In the presence of coexistent back and leg pain, a radiculopathy or plexopathy/sciatic nerve lesion should be suspected (Figs 6 and 7). More distal symptoms in the absence of back pain would indicate a more peripheral nerve lesion, eg common peroneal nerve palsy.

Neurological examination

The back
Check the following.

- Local tenderness: consider vertebral collapse or fracture.

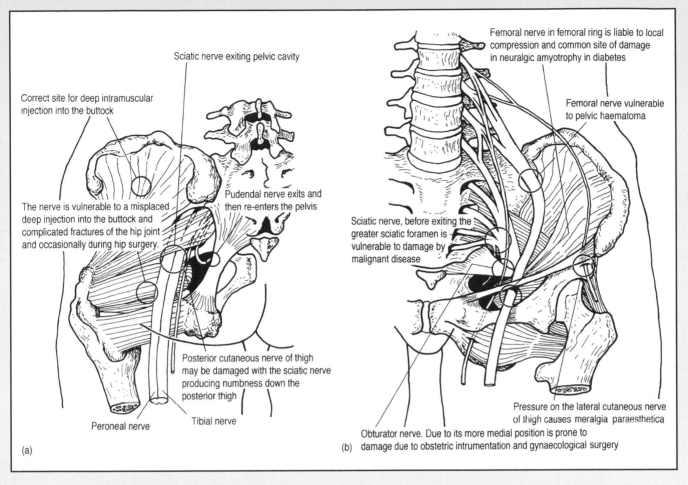

Correct site for deep intramuscular injection into the buttock

Sciatic nerve exiting pelvic cavity

Pudendal nerve exits and then re-enters the pelvis

The nerve is vulnerable to a misplaced deep injection into the buttock and complicated fractures of the hip joint and occasionally during hip surgery.

Posterior cutaneous nerve of thigh may be damaged with the sciatic nerve producing numbness down the posterior thigh

Peroneal nerve

Tibial nerve

(a)

Femoral nerve in femoral ring is liable to local compression and common site of damage in neuralgic amyotrophy in diabetes

Femoral nerve vulnerable to pelvic haematoma

Sciatic nerve, before exiting the greater sciatic foramen is vulnerable to damage by malignant disease

Pressure on the lateral cutaneous nerve of thigh causes meralgia paraesthetica

Obturator nerve. Due to its more medial position is prone to damage due to obstetric intrumentation and gynaecological surgery

(b)

▲**Fig. 6** Posterior (**a**) and anterior (**b**) nerve supply to the leg.

- Paraspinal muscular spasm (in response to pain).

- Restricted movement.

- Radiation of pain (Table 12).

Straight leg raising

Unilateral restriction may signify sciatic tension, but may also be limited by pain in the absence of nerve or root compression.

Legs

Check carefully for the following.

1. Is there any wasting or fasciculation?

2. Is there any weakness? If so, what is the distribution? Specifically check for lesions of the following roots:

   (a) L2 weakness of hip flexion and thigh adduction;

   (b) L3 weakness of thigh adduction and knee extension;

   (c) L4 weakness of knee extension and ankle inversion;

   (d) L5 weakness of ankle dorsiflexion, inversion and

TABLE 12 PAIN RADIATION IN RADICULAR LESIONS	
Nerve	**Pain radiation**
L2 and L3	Pain radiates to anterior thigh
L4	Pain radiates through the knee and down the medial side of the calf to the medial malleolus
L5	Pain radiates through the buttock, down the posterolateral aspect of the thigh, through the lateral aspect of calf and across the dorsum of the foot to the big toe
S1	Pain radiates through the inner buttock to the posterior aspect of the thigh, then through the posterolateral aspect of calf to the lateral border of the foot

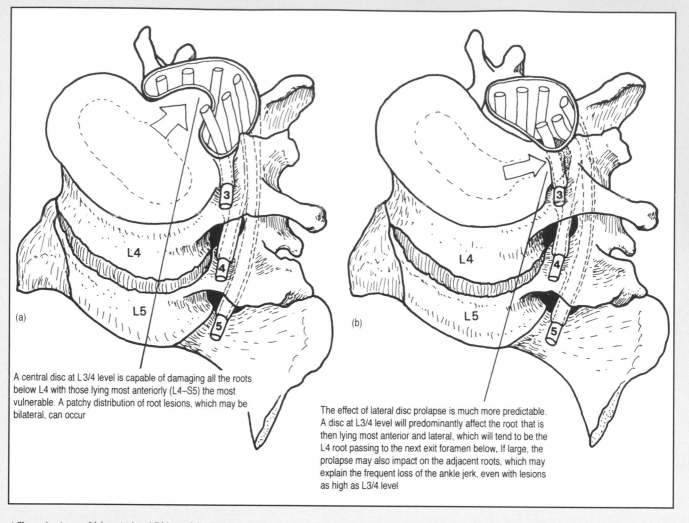

A central disc at L 3/4 level is capable of damaging all the roots below L4 with those lying most anteriorly (L4–S5) the most vulnerable. A patchy distribution of root lesions, which may be bilateral, can occur

The effect of lateral disc prolapse is much more predictable. A disc at L3/4 level will predominantly affect the root that is then lying most anterior and lateral, which will tend to be the L4 root passing to the next exit foramen below. If large, the prolapse may also impact on the adjacent roots, which may explain the frequent loss of the ankle jerk, even with lesions as high as L3/4 level

▲**Fig. 7** Anatomy of **(a)** central and **(b)** lateral disc protrusion.

eversion and dorsiflexion of the great toe;

(e) S1 weakness of plantar flexion, eversion and knee flexion.

3. Are reflexes normal? Hyporeflexia or areflexia is only seen with lesions of the following roots:

(a) L3 and L 4 (knee jerk);

(b) S1 (ankle jerk).

4. Sensory abnormalities in a well-defined distribution will help with localisation (Fig. 8).

Peripheral nerve lesions

Common peroneal (or fibular) nerve palsy Look for evidence of the following.

- Causes foot drop with loss of ankle and toe dorsiflexion, and ankle eversion.

- Causes numbness over the lateral aspect of the lower leg and dorsum of the foot.

- Is usually due to pressure over the fibular head.

> 🔑 Differentiation between a common peroneal nerve lesion and an L5 root lesion is a common clinical dilemma: a common peroneal nerve lesion will cause weakness of ankle dorsiflexion and eversion, but will not affect inversion.

Posterior tibial nerve palsy (tarsal tunnel syndrome) Look for evidence of the following.

- Wasting may occur in the intrinsic muscles of the foot, leading to weakness of toe flexion.

- Causes a burning sensation in the toes and sole of the foot, with reduced sensation on the sole.

- Entrapment usually occurs behind and below the medial malleolus.

Femoral nerve lesion Look for evidence of the following.

- Causes wasting and weakness of knee extensors.

- Results in a depressed or absent knee jerk.

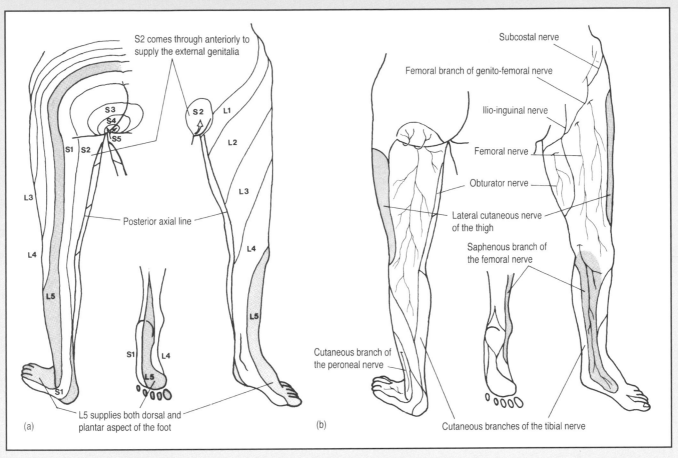

▲**Fig. 8** (a) Cutaneous nerve root supply of the leg (note that the sensory areas spiral round the leg as shown). (b) Cutaneous nerve supply of the leg (the sensory areas are vertically distributed).

- Causes sensory loss in the anterior thigh and medial part of knee.

- May be compressed by a psoas abscess or haematoma, or damaged by fractures of the pelvis, traction during surgery or thrombotic lesions of the vasa nervorum, eg in diabetes mellitus.

Sciatic nerve lesion Look for evidence of the following.

- The sciatic nerve splits to form the common peroneal nerve and posterior tibial nerve, so damage to the sciatic nerve encompasses both of the above.

- Causes weakness in all muscles below the knee, as well as knee flexors.

- Causes sensory loss over the lateral border of the lower leg and entire foot, except the medial malleolus which is supplied by the saphenous nerve.

> 🔑 Because muscle groups receive innervation from more than one root, weakness may be minimal in someone with a single root lesion. Thus, in the case of severe weakness, eg complete foot drop, a peripheral nerve lesion or multilevel radiculopathy must be implicated. Furthermore, weakness that fails to conform to a simple pattern may be due to a lumbosacral plexus lesion.

> ⚠️ A common clinical mistake is to expect loss of the ankle jerk with foot drop. If this is the case, it suggests involvement of both L5 and S1.

Further discussion

What are the causes of back and unilateral leg pain?

There are many causes of back pain. Radiation to a leg implies involvement of nerve root or lumbosacral plexus and limits the differential diagnosis (Table 13). L5 and S1 are the most commonly affected nerves in degenerative disease; L4 is involved occasionally, but L2 and L3 rarely, and if they are the diagnosis is not likely to be simple degeneration.

> 🔑 If weakness, eg foot drop, is associated with pain and only comes on with exercise, then consider lumbar canal stenosis. In the outpatient clinic, the patient with this history but no physical signs should be asked to walk until the symptoms come on, as this may reveal abnormal signs.

TABLE 13 CAUSES OF BACK AND LEG PAIN

Site of lesion	Diagnoses

Radiculopathy	Disc disease
	Degenerative spinal disease
	Infective spinal disease (pyogenic abscess, tuberculosis)
	Malignant spinal disease (secondary tumour, myeloma)
	    Intrinsic, eg secondary tumour, myeloma
	    Extrinsic, eg extramedullary, nerve sheath tumour, meningeal
	    infiltration

Plexopathy/sciatic nerve lesion	Pelvic retroperitoneal mass
	    Tumour
	    Haematoma
	    Abscess
	Hip fracture
	Misplaced deep muscular injection

1.2.3 Spastic legs

Instruction

This man complains of stiffness and heaviness in his legs and has difficulty walking. Please examine his legs

General features

Stiffness or heaviness is more suggestive of upper rather than lower motor neuron weakness, ie spastic paraparesis rather than peripheral neuropathy. The causes of a spastic paraparesis are listed in Table 14. Patients with weak legs will often have walking aids or wheelchairs next to the bed. There is often coincidental sphincter involvement so a catheter bag may be present.

> ⚠ Beware bladder dysfunction as this implies interruption of S2–S4, either centrally (spinal cord compression or conus lesion) (Fig. 9) or peripherally (cauda equina lesion, pelvic pathology or autonomic dysfunction).

Take note of the patient's speech during introductions: if it is slurred, then the patient may have multiple sclerosis, cerebral palsy, one of the rare genetic conditions or motor neuron disease. While you are shaking the patient's hand, also have a look to see if there is wasting (motor neuron disease) or ataxia (multiple sclerosis or genetic conditions) in the hands. Look for signs of surgical or traumatic injury along the whole of the spine.

Neurological examination

Motor

Tone will be increased in the leg muscles, particularly the extensors. This results in an increase in tone on rapid flexion at the knee (a 'spastic catch'). There may be clonus at the ankles, which is best tested with the knee flexed. Power will be reduced in a 'pyramidal pattern', ie extensors less affected than flexors in the legs; indeed the extensors may be strong. Deep tendon reflexes will be brisk. If the weakness is severe, then coordination will be difficult to assess. Plantar responses will be extensor, unless there is concurrent peripheral neuropathy (eg subacute combined degeneration of the cord).

> 🔑 Vitamin B$_{12}$ deficiency may cause a peripheral neuropathy but may also result in additional corticospinal tract and dorsal column degeneration, leading to combined upper and lower motor neuron features. The clinical picture can be variable, but remember that this is a treatable condition and must not be missed.

Sensory

There may be a 'sensory level' if the sensory tracts are also involved, but they may also be spared (eg motor neuron disease).

> ⚠ Although demonstrating a sensory level points to the spinal cord, it is notoriously inaccurate at localising the level of the pathology. You should therefore use all possible

TABLE 14 CAUSES OF SPASTIC PARAPARESIS

Common	Uncommon
Multiple sclerosis Cerebral palsy Spinal injury Cord compression, eg cervical spondylosis, tumours, abscess, vertebral fracture/dislocation	Genetic conditions, eg hereditary spastic paraplegia, Friedreich's ataxia, spinocerebellar ataxias Vitamin B$_{12}$ and E deficiencies Vascular malformations Syphilis/HIV/human T-cell lymphotrophic virus-1 Syringomyelia Anterior spinal artery occlusion Motor neuron disease

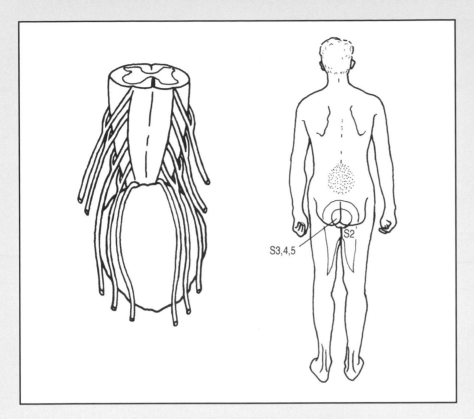

▲Fig. 9 Conus lesion of the spinal cord. A lesion of the conus will affect the sacral roots from the inside outwards, hence the perianal and perineal areas are involved first, with progressive numbness and often surprisingly little pain.

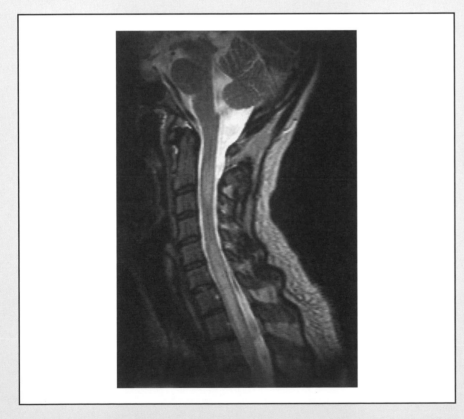

▲Fig. 10 Increased signal on a T2-weighted sagittal MRI of the cervical cord, indicative of an intrinsic lesion and probably inflammatory.

clinical signs to help you. For example, a patient with a sensory level at the umbilicus (T10) who also has brisk arm reflexes is likely to have a lesion in the cervical cord above C5 rather than at T10. The significance of this is that it is the cervical cord that requires imaging, not the thoracic cord. It is generally much better to start imaging at the top (cervical) and work down, rather than the other way round (Fig. 10).

Gait

In routine clinical practice and in PACES always ask the patient to walk, giving whatever assistance is necessary (the examiners will stop you if there isn't time and they want to start asking questions). The patient may walk with a spastic gait which, if severe, becomes 'scissoring', ie legs crossing over each other as the patient walks.

Further discussion

An acute onset or an acute deterioration on a background of a chronic progressive story is a medical emergency and should prompt urgent imaging of the spine. A more slowly progressive onset can be investigated less urgently.

Remember that bilateral cortical lesions affecting the leg areas of both primary motor cortices can cause a spastic paraplegia: this is classically associated with a parasagittal meningioma.

1.2.4 Gait disturbance

Instruction

This woman has unsteadiness and difficulty in walking. Please examine her gait and proceed with your neurological examination to establish the diagnosis.

Station 3: Central Nervous System Examination

TABLE 15 COMMONLY ENCOUNTERED ABNORMAL GAITS

Diagnosis	Main characteristic
PD	Shuffling/stooped
Cerebellar	Wide based
Peripheral neuropathy	High stepping
Diffuse cerebrovascular disease	*Marche à petit pas*
Proximal myopathy	Waddling
Pyramidal tract involvement	
Unilateral	Circumduction
Bilateral	Scissor gait

PD, Parkinson's disease.

General features

The common causes of gait disturbance together with their main characteristics are shown in Table 15. General observation on introduction to the patient may yield some clues to the diagnosis.

- Parkinson's disease (PD) is suggested by the patient looking hypomimic (paucity of facial expression), blinking infrequently and having difficulty holding saliva in the mouth due to a poor swallow frequency. Careful observation of the hands may reveal an asymmetrical 3–6 Hz resting 'pill-rolling' tremor.

- The patient with cerebellar ataxia may infrequently have a head tremor or 'titubation' and an intention tremor in the arms on shaking hands, and may also have a slurring dysarthria.

- The patient with peripheral neuropathy may have wasting in the hands and be wearing bilateral splints or ankle–foot orthoses.

- Diffuse cerebrovascular disease is often associated with a dementia when severe enough to cause gait impairment and the patient may have a pseudobulbar palsy with dysarthria.

Neurological examination

The patient should be asked to walk a distance of at least 10 m as normally as possible. Make sure that you walk alongside the patient if he or she appears to be very imbalanced. Based on this inspection the most probable diagnosis should be made and then corroborating signs sought on examination.

Is it Parkinson's disease?

Look specifically for these features, remembering that many of them may be asymmetrical:

- Gait is typically short-stepped, shuffling and festinant, with reduced or absent arm swing. In early disease, a slight reduction in arm swing on one side may be the only abnormality. Freezing of gait occurs later in the disease. The patient will often have problems initiating walking, but once started has difficulty stopping.

- Posture is flexed, stooped and when severe is referred to as 'simian'.

- Hypomimia, ie paucity of facial expression with 'mask-like' facies and a reduced blink rate.

- The rest tremor of the hands is classically pill-rolling and most marked at rest. It is best seen with the hands resting, palms facing inwards, on the lap or over the edge of an armchair. The tremor may be intermittent and if not seen can be elicited by mental distraction, such as counting backwards from 20, or it often comes on with walking. It is typically asymmetrical. Tremor seen in the legs is highly suggestive of PD. Tremor may also occur in the chin, neck and tongue.

- Bradykinesia, ie slowness and fatiguability of rapid movements. Ask the patient to open and close each hand as widely and as rapidly as possible, or to tap the thumb of one hand with each finger of the same hand in rapid succession with the widest amplitude possible. If not obviously slow, then continue this exercise at least 10 times to demonstrate decrement in rate and amplitude. An extrapyramidal syndrome cannot be diagnosed without this feature.

- Extrapyramidal rigidity with 'cogwheeling', ie the combination of rigidity and tremor, is best demonstrated by slow and gentle rotation of the wrist.

- Ask the patient to write a phrase such as 'Mary had a little lamb' several times, looking for the development of micrographia. Ask the patient to draw a spiral, which may demonstrate tremor as well as micrographia.

- Note that the glabellar tap (which involves tapping the glabella and observing whether the patient blinks) is a non-specific test that is not clinically useful, although it used to be said that failure of this response due to fatigue (ie blinking stops with repeated taps) indicated PD, especially in younger patients.

- Drug-induced parkinsonism may appear clinically identical, although it tends to be more symmetrical. Wilson's disease may present with parkinsonism and is associated with Kayser–Fleischer rings (usually only visible with a slit lamp).

Is it cerebellar disease?

The following are features of cerebellar disease.

- Titubation (head tremor) is uncommon.

- Dysarthria (scanning speech).

- Nystagmus (horizontal and jerky) and jerky pursuit eye movements.

- Limb ataxia: upper limb (failure of rapid alternating movements, intention tremor and dysmetria with past pointing) and lower limb (heel–shin ataxia, wide-based gait and inability to perform heel–toe walking).

Is it peripheral neuropathy?

See Section 1.2.1 for further details on peripheral neuropathy. The neuropathy may be a polyneuropathy, which will lead to symmetrical signs in a 'glove and stocking' distribution, or less commonly is due to bilateral mononeuropathies affecting the common peroneal or sciatic nerves, which are more likely to be asymmetrical. The patient's gait is often 'high-stepping' as a consequence of both bilateral foot drop and sensory loss. The main findings include:

- wasting distally in the legs, feet and hands;

- possible fasciculations if there is axonal loss;

- atrophic changes in the skin (oedematous, purple, hairless and pigmented) due to loss of autonomic and sensory fibres;

- ulcers associated with pressure points (heel, between toes and sacrum);

- reduced tone, although this is often difficult to differentiate from normal;

- distal weakness (foot drop and hand weakness);

- reduced or absent reflexes;

- glove and stocking sensory loss.

Is it diffuse cerebrovascular disease?

Patients with either bilateral large-vessel frontal infarcts or subcortical ischaemic leucoencephalopathy may have a 'frontal apraxic' gait, which characteristically leads to a *marche à petit pas* appearance and is commonly mistaken for the gait of PD. In *marche à petit pas*, the steps are small, broad-based, 'stuck to the floor' and shuffling. Turning requires several steps and there may (in contrast to PD) be excessive arm swing. The stance is upright with the centre of gravity being normal, as opposed to shifted forwards as in PD. There is often poor gait initiation, but this is also seen in PD.

In the patient with diffuse cerebrovascular disease there are often symmetrical extrapyramidal signs that are more severe in the legs than the arms or face. *Marche à petit pas* is therefore sometimes termed 'lower-body parkinsonism'. There is no resting tremor and the bradykinesia is symmetrical. The rigidity seen with frontal lobe disease (sometimes called *Gegenhalten*) is often due to poor attention and not due to a true increase in tone. Other diseases that can cause a frontal apraxic gait include hydrocephalus and subdural haematomas: these should be considered in any patient, especially if the gait disorder is isolated.

Is it myopathic?

Look for the following features.

- The patient may have 'myopathic facies' with wasting of temporalis and muscles of mastication.

- Waddling gait: failure to stabilise the pelvis caused by predominant involvement of pelvic girdle and proximal leg muscles.

- Wasting of affected muscle groups.

- Usually more prominent proximal weakness: distal myopathies are rare apart from myotonic dystrophy.

- Reflexes are preserved until there is severe muscle wasting.

- No sensory signs.

Is it a spastic gait?

In unilateral upper motor neuron syndromes, the gait is stiff with circumduction and toe dragging of the affected leg. When bilateral upper motor neuron lesions occur, both legs are stiff and patients develop a scissoring gait (see Section 1.2.3). The common signs are:

- spastic tone, pyramidal weakness, brisk reflexes and extensor plantar responses, all upper motor neuron signs;

- there may be a sensory level when there is spinal cord disease.

> ⚠️ In routine clinical practice, do not forget to look beyond the neurological system for important diagnostic clues.
>
> - Does the patient look as though he or she has lost weight? Is there lymphadenopathy? Are there masses in the breast, or on abdominal and rectal examination? Is the chest examination normal? If metastatic disease is suspected, which may apply to some cases of cerebellar, neuropathic, spastic or myopathic gait disturbance, then a full systemic examination should be performed.
> - If vascular disease is suspected, then a full cardiovascular assessment is required, including heart rhythm, murmurs, bruits and evidence of hypercholesterolaemia and chronic smoking.

Further discussion

The differentiation of frontal gait apraxia and idiopathic PD can sometimes be difficult, especially in the elderly where the two diseases may coexist. Patients who have PD and have been treated for it can sometimes be difficult to assess blindly without the history, but the presence of only extrapyramidal signs and the predominance of upper limb and face involvement should make the diagnosis of idiopathic PD clearer.

1.2.5 Cerebellar syndrome

Instruction

This women presents with a 2-month history of progressive imbalance and slurred speech. Please examine her gait/cranial nerves/arms (instruction could be to focus on any one of these).

General features

Multiple sclerosis, common in routine clinical practice and in PACES, would be high on the list of differential diagnoses. It is quite likely that her imbalance is due to cerebellar involvement, but you should also consider a spastic paraparesis (see Section 1.2.3). The common causes of a cerebellar syndrome are given in Table 16. The patient with cerebellar ataxia may have a head tremor or 'titubation'

and an intention tremor in the arms when shaking hands. The patient may also have a slurring dysarthria and use walking aids or a wheelchair.

Neurological examination

Gait ataxia

If you have not yet observed the gait, ask the patient to walk a distance of at least 10 m as normally as possible. Make sure that you walk alongside the patient if he or she appears to be very imbalanced. A broad-based (to improve stability) ataxic gait is characteristic of cerebellar disease, but in mild cases the unsteadiness may be apparent only when walking heel to toe (tandem walking). In a unilateral cerebellar hemisphere lesion, there is unsteadiness towards the side of the lesion. In truncal ataxia there is difficulty sitting or standing without support. For discussion of other gait abnormalities, see Section 1.2.4.

Subsequent examination should focus on the cerebellar system and then go on to examine other features to delineate the cause.

In midline or generalised cerebellar disease, an abnormal gait is likely to be the most prominent physical sign and coordination of the arms may appear normal.

Incoordination of movement

Cerebellar dysfunction causes impairment of the process of controlling movements once they have been initiated. This gives rise to ataxia (incoordination) with the following signs.

- Intention tremor: there is no tremor at rest, but when the patient moves a limb an oscillating tremor develops that increases in amplitude as the limb moves towards the target.

- Dysdiadochokinesia: inability to carry out rapid alternating movements with regularity.

- Dysmetria: inability to control smooth and accurate targeted movements. The movements are jerky with overshooting of the target, as manifested in the finger–nose and heel–shin tests.

Ataxic dysarthric speech

Speech can be slow, slurred and scanning in quality. In scanning speech, there is loss of variation of intonation and the words may be broken up into syllables. Ask the patient to say words with several consonants such as 'baby hippopotamus' and 'British constitution'.

Abnormal eye movements

- 'Jerky' pursuits: pursuit movements are slow, with catch-up saccadic movements on attempting to maintain fixation on the moving target.

- Dysmetria of saccades: on attempting to fixate on a target, the eyes overshoot and oscillate several times before fixation is achieved.

- Nystagmus: this is maximal on gaze towards the side of the lesion and is jerky, ie it has a slow and a fast phase. Nystagmus results

TABLE 16 CAUSES OF A CEREBELLAR SYNDROME	
Common	**Uncommon**
Multiple sclerosis	Genetic syndromes including spinocerebellar ataxias,
Drugs: alcohol, phenytoin,	Friedreich's ataxia, ataxia telangiectasia
carbamazepine	Prion disease
Neoplasms	Infections, eg tuberculosis, meningitis
Infarction/haemorrhage	Arnold–Chiari malformation
Paraneoplastic syndrome	Vitamin B_{12} and E deficiencies

from damage to the vestibular connections of the cerebellum.

Titubation

Nodding tremor of the head may occur, mainly in the anterior–posterior (nodding) plane.

Altered posture

A unilateral cerebellar lesion may cause the head (and when the lesion is recent and severe, also the body) to tilt towards the side of the lesion.

Hypotonia

Hypotonia is a relatively minor feature of cerebellar disease, resulting from depression of α and γ motor neuron activity. Hypotonia can sometimes be demonstrated clinically by decreased resistance to passive movement (eg extension of a limb), by 'pendular' reflexes or by the rebound phenomenon. This occurs when the patient's outstretched arms are pressed down for a few seconds and then abruptly released by the examiner. The arms may rebound upwards and continue to oscillate for longer than expected.

Other features

Once it has been determined that the patient has a cerebellar syndrome, neurological and general examinations should be conducted to try to delineate the cause.

- If the patient has multiple sclerosis, then there may be a spastic tetraparesis/paraparesis, other brainstem signs (eg internuclear ophthalmoplegia) or evidence of sphincter dysfunction (eg suprapubic or transurethral catheter).

- If the patient has had a cerebellar stroke, then there may be other features of a lateral medullary syndrome (ipsilateral Horner's syndrome, ipsilateral facial and

contralateral limb spinothalamic loss, ipsilateral palatal weakness and contralateral hemiparesis). The ataxia in such cases is ipsilateral and the patient may have evidence of other cardiovascular risk factors, eg coronary artery bypass graft scar, atrial fibrillation or diabetes mellitus. A cerebellar haemorrhage can have catastrophic consequences and lead to rapid deterioration in the patient's level of consciousness due to brainstem compression: there may be a surgical scar over the occiput where decompression has been performed and this should be looked for at the end of the examination.

- Cerebellar tumours usually present slowly but can present in a stroke-like manner. The patient may be pale and thin. The commonest tumours to metastasise to the cerebellum are from the lung and breast, and in routine clinical practice these systems need to be examined.

- Patients with chronic alcohol abuse often develop a chronic cerebellar syndrome that characteristically affects the lower limbs and gait more than the eyes and upper limbs. In such patients there may be signs of chronic liver disease and portal hypertension.

- Rare genetic syndromes may prominently affect the cerebellum and other neurological systems may be involved, eg spastic paraparesis and peripheral polyneuropathy in Friedreich's ataxia.

Further discussion

There are many rare causes of a cerebellar syndrome, but common ones such as alcohol

and anticonvulsants must not be forgotten and should be mentioned before the rarer causes in giving a differential diagnosis. The examiners may ask you to discuss the molecular mechanism of the spinocerebellar and Friedreich's ataxias, which are part of a group of rare genetic disorders called the 'triplet repeat diseases' because they are associated with an expanded number of trinucleotide repeats in disease states. If you are led into this line of questioning, then it is a good sign: the examiners think you have done well!

1.2.6 Weak arm/hand

Instruction

This 60-year-old woman has pain in her right arm and hand. Please examine her arms.

General features

It is unlikely in the context of PACES, but is the patient cachectic or clubbed? Is there lymphadenopathy? Any of these features would suggest malignancy. Check carefully for breast masses and also for any abnormal chest signs, particularly at the lung apex where a Pancoast tumour might be found (indicated by wasting of the intrinsic hand muscles and Horner's syndrome).

Are both radial pulses equally palpable, and is the BP the same in both arms? A positive Adson's test (decrease in the radial pulse when the patient turns the head to the affected side and breathes in deeply) may indicate subclavian artery compression, eg by a cervical rib, but the test may also be positive in normal subjects. Is there a characteristic skin rash of herpes zoster?

Musculoskeletal

- Observe how the woman moves her neck and shoulder, eg when removing her clothing before being examined. If movement of the neck is painful, then this will be held rigid. If the shoulder is painful, then the normal scapulohumeral rhythm of movement, whereby the arm moves in the shoulder joint before the scapula moves, will be reversed.

- Feel for local tenderness of muscles of the back of the scalp, neck and shoulder, and also for tenderness of the shoulder joint itself.

Neurological examination

Root/radicular lesion

Look for signs of nerve root lesions as shown in Table 17, the most common roots affected being C5–C7. Look also for the following.

- An inverted brachioradialis jerk, which occurs when finger flexion is the only response to an attempt to elicit the normal biceps or supinator jerk. This may indicate a spinal cord lesion at C5–6, resulting in lower motor neuron signs at the level of the lesion (ie loss of C5–6 reflexes) and upper motor neuron signs below the lesion [ie brisk C7 (triceps) and C8 (finger flexion) reflexes, and pyramidal signs in the legs].

- If there is dissociated sensory loss (loss of pain and temperature with intact proprioception) in a cape-like distribution (ie suspended sensory level, see Fig. 11) and lower motor neuron weakness, it is likely that there is an intrinsic cord lesion such as a syrinx. Other signs may include Horner's syndrome (if the lesion extends to the T1 segment) and pyramidal weakness below the level of the lesion.

> If the T1 nerve root is affected, Horner's syndrome may be present because of damage to the adjacent sympathetic plexus.

Peripheral nerve lesions
See also Section 2.1.

Median nerve lesion Look for evidence of the following.

- Signs and symptoms of carpal tunnel syndrome (see Section 2.1).

- If only the anterior interosseous branch of the median nerve is damaged, the patient will be unable to perform the ring sign (pinch grip), resulting in the thumb and index fingers assuming an extended position. Also there is pronation weakness when the elbow is in a flexed position (the latter is due to weakness of pronator quadratus). The ring sign involves flexion of the distal phalanges of the thumb (flexor pollicis longus) and index finger (flexor digitorum profundus); there are no sensory changes (pure motor branch).

- In an elbow lesion (pronator teres syndrome), apart from weakness of thumb abduction there is weakness of flexion of the distal phalanges of the thumb and the adjacent two fingers (anterior interosseous branch function); sensory changes are as in carpal tunnel syndrome plus there is decreased sensation over the thenar region extending up to the wrist.

Ulnar nerve lesion Look for evidence of the following.

- Most commonly damaged at the elbow.

- Wasting of first dorsal interosseous appears first, but later there may be involvement of the other dorsal interossei and hypothenar eminence.

- Difficulty abducting and adducting outstretched fingers.

- Froment's sign: distal thumb flexion (adductor pollicis weakness) when a patient is asked to pinch a sheet of paper between the thumb and second metacarpal.

- Sensory loss over the little finger and the medial half of the ring finger.

TABLE 17 SIGNS IN AFFECTED CERVICAL NERVE ROOTS			
Nerve root	Weakness	Hyporeflexia	Sensory changes
C5	Deltoid, infraspinatus, supraspinatus	Biceps, brachioradialis	Shoulder tip, outer part of upper arm
C6	Biceps, brachioradialis, wrist flexors	Brachioradialis	Lateral aspect of forearm, thumb and index finger
C7	Triceps, wrist extensors	Triceps	Middle finger
C8	Intrinsic muscles of hand	Triceps, finger	Little and ring fingers
T1	Intrinsic muscles of hand	None	Medial aspect of forearm

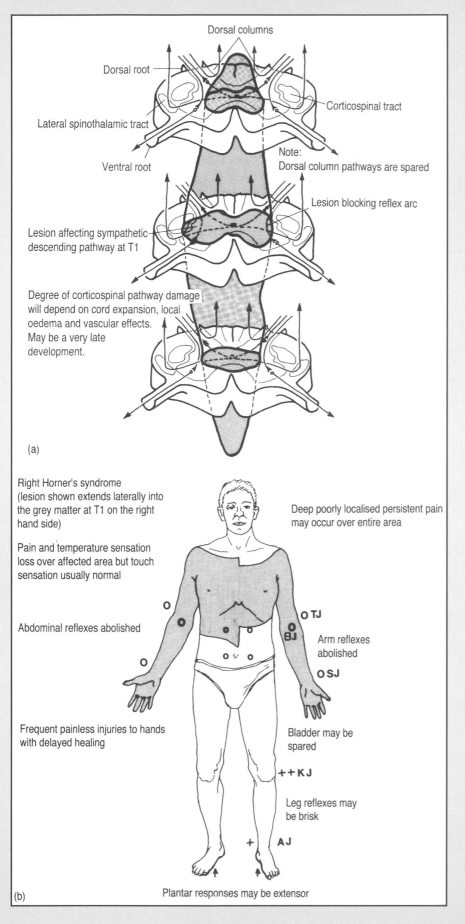

(a)

Dorsal columns

Dorsal root

Lateral spinothalamic tract

Ventral root

Corticospinal tract

Note:
Dorsal column pathways are spared

Lesion blocking reflex arc

Lesion affecting sympathetic descending pathway at T1

Degree of corticospinal pathway damage will depend on cord expansion, local oedema and vascular effects. May be a very late development.

Right Horner's syndrome (lesion shown extends laterally into the grey matter at T1 on the right hand side)

Pain and temperature sensation loss over affected area but touch sensation usually normal

Abdominal reflexes abolished

Frequent painless injuries to hands with delayed healing

Deep poorly localised persistent pain may occur over entire area

○ TJ
● BJ
Arm reflexes abolished

○ SJ

Bladder may be spared

++ KJ

Leg reflexes may be brisk

+ AJ

(b)

Plantar responses may be extensor

- If the deep palmar branch (purely motor) is compressed in Guyon's canal (which runs between the pisiform and hook of the hamate), there will be wasting and weakness of the interossei, especially the first dorsal and adductor pollicis; hypothenar muscles are usually spared.

Radial nerve lesion Look for evidence of the following.

- Most commonly damaged at the spiral groove of the humerus.

- Major feature is weakness of wrist and finger extensors (wrist drop).

- Weakness of forearm flexion with forearm midway between pronation and supination (due to brachioradialis involvement).

- Sparing of triceps occurs if the lesion is at or distal to spiral groove.

- Sensory loss over dorsum of hand between the lateral two digits.

- If only the posterior interosseous branch of the radial nerve is involved there is wrist extension, but with radial deviation because the extensor carpi radialis muscle is spared; brachioradialis and triceps normal; and there are no sensory changes (pure motor branch).

Axillary nerve lesion Look for evidence of the following.

- Wasting of deltoid.

- Weakness of shoulder flexion, abduction and extension.

- Sensory loss over lateral deltoid.

◄ **Fig. 11** Lesion in central cord at C5–T6 level. **(a)** Anatomical diagram. Note that the decussating spinothalamic pathways are blocked across the length of the central lesion. This may be slightly asymmetrical as shown, extending from C3 to T9 on the right and from C4 to T8 on the left. Spinothalamic sensation below this level would be unaffected. **(b)** The clinical picture.

🔑 Generalised axonal peripheral neuropathies will affect the legs before the arms and are generally symmetrical. Inflammatory or demyelinating neuropathies may damage individual nerve fibres and so could affect an arm first.

⚠ Myopathies that affect distal before proximal muscles are rare. However, one form of inflammatory muscle disorder should be considered: inclusion body myositis (see Section 2.2). In this there is typically disproportionate and marked weakness in the wrist and finger flexors relative to the corresponding extensors (so would cause difficulty carrying a briefcase), and disproportionate weakness of knee extensors compared with hip flexors.

Further discussion

What are the neurological causes of pain in the arm?

See Table 18.

Neuralgic amyotrophy (brachial neuritis)

This is characterised by acute onset of excruciating unilateral (although it may be bilateral) arm (usually shoulder) pain, followed by shoulder and parascapular muscle weakness several days later; the pain is so severe that it is often confused with the pain of a myocardial infarction. Presentation and nerve involvement can be variable. Sensory changes are minimal. There may be subsequent rapid wasting of arm muscles. Phrenic nerve involvement can result in significant breathlessness. Precipitating factors include recent trauma, severe exercise, surgery, infection or vaccination. It may rarely be hereditary. The prognosis is good, with a spontaneous recovery rate of over 90%.

1.2.7 Proximal muscle weakness

Instruction

This man has muscle weakness which has got progressively worse over the last 6 months. Please examine his limbs.

General features

Look for signs that may give diagnostic clues to the causes of proximal muscle weakness (Table 19), particularly the following.

- Skin, eg purpura of steroid treatment, and much less likely malar rash in systemic lupus erythematosus (SLE), Gottron's papules and heliotrope rash in dermatomyositis.

- Skeletal, eg joint swelling in SLE and rheumatoid arthritis.

- Endocrine, eg cushingoid apperance in glucocorticoid excess and tremor in hyperthyroidism.

Consider if this man could have myotonic dystrophy, which is very much commoner in PACES than in routine clinical practice: look for myopathic facies (drooping eyes/mouth and a sad/lifeless expression), ptosis, frontal balding and wasting of facial/neck/shoulder girdle muscles.

In routine clinical practice also check the following factors.

- Cardiovascular, eg cardiomyopathy in alcoholism, amyloidosis, glycogen storage diseases, inflammatory myopathies and muscular dystrophies.

- Gastrointestinal, eg hepatomegaly in metabolic storage diseases and amyloidosis.

Neurological examination

Look particularly for muscle wasting and also for the presence of pseudo-hypertrophy of the calf muscles, most typically seen in Duchenne's or Becker's muscular dystrophy.

It is very important to determine the distribution of the weakness, eg bilateral, proximal or distal, or more focal. If the patient has difficulty rising from a squatting position (hip muscles) or combing his hair (shoulder girdle), then the weakness is proximal; if the patient has difficulty standing on his toes (gastrocnemius/soleus) or doing fine movements with the hands (intrinsic hand muscles), then the muscle weakness is distal.

TABLE 18 NEUROLOGICAL CAUSES OF ARM PAIN

Site of lesion	Diagnoses
Cerebral	Thalamic lesion, extrapyramidal disorder
Spinal cord	Syringomyelia, tumour
Nerve root	Disc prolapse, vertebral collapse, trauma, post-herpetic
Brachial plexus	Pancoast's syndrome and brachial plexopathy, eg neuralgic amyotrophy, cervical rib, subclavian artery aneurysm, trauma
Peripheral nerve	Entrapment neuropathies, paraneoplastic, vasculitis, diabetes
Muscle	See Section 2.2

If myotonic dystrophy is a possibility, try to elicit myotonia by asking the patient to grip your fingers as hard as he can, relax, and then repeat the grip/relaxation cycle a few times (offer two fingers, but not more or you may get hurt if the patient is strong!).

⚠ Myopathy does not cause sensory signs. Do not diagnose a purely myopathic condition if sensory signs are present.

🔑 Do not forget to check whether there is also wasting and weakness in sternomastoid muscles (eg myotonic dystrophy) and facial muscles (some forms of muscular dystrophy or myotonic dystrophy).

⚠ Is the weakness fatiguable? Think of myasthenia gravis! Don't forget to check for extraocular muscle weakness by examining eye movements.

Further discussion

What are the causes of proximal muscle weakness?
See Table 19.

What are the causes of predominantly distal muscle weakness?
Myotonic dystrophy, inclusion body myositis and genetic distal myopathies (the latter are rare). See Section 2.2.

1.2.8 Muscle wasting

Instruction

This man has muscle wasting in his right arm and hand. Please examine his cranial nerves and his arms.

TABLE 19 CAUSES OF PROXIMAL MYOPATHY

Cause	Diagnoses
Drugs	Alcohol, corticosteroids, statins
Endocrine	Adrenal insufficiency, Cushing's disease, hyperthyroidism, hypothyroidism, acromegaly
Inflammatory	Dermatomyositis, polymyositis
Rheumatological	SLE, rheumatoid arthritis, polymyalgia rheumatica
Metabolic	Glycogen and lipid storage diseases, mitochondrial disease
Genetic	Limb girdle muscular dystrophies, fascioscapulohumeral dystrophy, Duchenne/Becker muscular dystrophy

SLE, systemic lupus erythematosus.

General features
Lesions that affect the ulnar nerve, T1 trunk or cord of the brachial plexus, T1 nerve roots, or the equivalent group of anterior horn cells can all cause wasting of the small hand muscles. However, you need to establish whether the muscle wasting is limited to the hand or involves other regions as well, eg muscles in the shoulders or thighs, as the latter would indicate a more diffuse disease process, eg motor neuron disease (MND) (see Section 2.1).

Neurological examination

Cranial nerve examination

- Are there any upper motor neuron signs indicating a pseudobulbar palsy, eg brisk jaw jerk, spastic tongue or emotional lability? This would indicate disease involvement of the corticobulbar pathways above the brainstem, eg in MND.

- Are there any lower motor neuron signs indicating a bulbar palsy, eg poor elevation of the soft palate or tongue weakness and atrophy? This would indicate involvement of the motor nuclei of cranial nerves IX–XII of the brainstem.

- If the T1 nerve root is involved (eg in a Pancoast tumour), Horner's syndrome may be present.

Limb examination

- Are there any upper motor neuron signs (spastic tone, brisk reflexes or extensor plantar responses)? These would be found in spinal cord lesions, eg cervical myelopathy above the level of C5, or diffuse disease processes (eg MND).

- Are there any lower motor neuron signs (wasting, fasciculations hypotonia or hyporeflexia)? These would be found in MND, chronic inflammatory demyelinating polyneuropathy (CIDP), multifocal motor neuropathy (MMN) or spinal cord compression at the levels of C5–T1 (indicating local anterior horn cell or radicular involvement).

- Sensory examination: in MND and MMN there is no sensory involvement. In cervical spondylosis, radicular findings often do not conform to textbook dermatomal descriptions. In CIDP there is often impairment of joint position and vibration sense, and less commonly of pain and temperature sensation.

MND and cervical myelopathy can sometimes be difficult to differentiate. The involvement of corticobulbar pathways, as suggested by the presence of a pseudobulbar palsy, would indicate the former as it places the disease process above the spinal cord.

It is crucial to differentiate MND from other potentially treatable conditions such as cervical spondylosis and MMN because of the better prognosis in the latter two conditions.

Further discussion

What are common mimics of MND?
See Table 20.

Wasting and weakness restricted to the small muscles of the hand (T1 lesion) should be considered the result of a Pancoast tumour until proven otherwise. Obtain a smoking history, look for nicotine staining and arrange a CXR immediately.

1.2.9 Hemiplegia

Instruction

This man has weakness in his left arm and leg. Please examine his arms and legs.

General features

The most likely diagnosis is stroke, so look for evidence of vascular risk factors/disease, eg xanthelasma, corneal arcus, nicotine stains, scars on the chest or legs indicating surgery for ischaemic heart disease, scars in the neck indicating previous carotid surgery, and the presence of a pacemaker.

When introducing yourself to the patient take particular note of how well he moves his limbs. Does he appear to have a visuospatial deficit, suggesting right parietal cortical involvement? You should also note the presence of speech and language problems. Aphasia is unlikely in a right-handed subject, but you do not yet know if he is right- or left-handed. It is important to know if it is his dominant or non-dominant hand that is affected.

Neurological examination

The neurological examination should be broken down into motor, sensory, visual and cognitive elements.

Motor signs

The key features to look for include the following.

- Wasting: this may be present on the affected side due to disuse over time.

- Tone: usually increased on the affected side (may be normal or even reduced in the acute setting).

- Power: typically power is reduced in a pyramidal distribution (upper limb extensors weaker than flexors and lower limb flexors weaker than extensors, hence the arm tends to be held in flexion with a hyperextended leg).

- Reflexes: these are increased on the affected side.

- Plantar response: extensor (upgoing) on the affected side.

Do not forget to examine the power of the facial muscles. If weakness is present on the opposite side to the limb weakness, this would suggest a brainstem stroke. If the weakness is on the same side, the damage is most likely in the middle cerebral artery territory.

Sensory signs

Sensory signs are likely to be in the same distribution as the motor signs. Sensory loss has a negative impact on functional recovery, so it is important to assess it. Do not forget to assess proprioception as impairment in this modality will cause specific difficulties with rehabilitation.

TABLE 20 MIMICS OF MND

Condition	Investigation(s)
Cervical/lumbar spondylotic myelopathy	MRI
Brainstem lesions, eg syrinx and stroke	MRI
MMN	Nerve conduction studies, anti-GM1 ganglioside antibody
Kennedy's disease (X-linked spinobulbar muscular atrophy)	Androgen receptor gene mutation
Myasthenia gravis	Single-fibre electromyography, anti-acetylcholine receptor antibody
CIDP	Nerve conduction studies, high protein in cerebrospinal fluid
Polymyositis or inclusion body myositis	Serum creatine kinase, electromyography, muscle biopsy
Thyrotoxicosis	Thyroid function tests
Paraproteinaemias	Serum protein electrophoresis

CIDP, chronic inflammatory demyelinating polyneuropathy; MMN, multifocal motor neuropathy; MND, motor neuron disease.

Visual signs

The presence of a homonymous hemianopia has value in localising the lesion site.

Cognitive signs

Determine whether the patient has any deficit in either of the following domains.

- Language function: briefly assess expressive and comprehension components (see Section 3.1).

- Visuospatial function: briefly look for visual and/or sensory inattention and/or extinction.

Once again, these features will have localising value to either the dominant (language) or non-dominant (visuospatial) hemisphere, and they suggest cortical involvement in the damage. Note that cortical signs can be present when only the white matter adjacent to the intact cortex is damaged, as this can effectively disconnect the cortical area from afferent and efferent connections. It is crucial to be aware of the presence of 'cognitive' signs when considering rehabilitation strategies.

Further discussion

In a patient with hemiplegic stroke the important questions are as follows.

- Where is the lesion?

- What is the pathology?

- What is the mechanism?

Where is the lesion?

Hemiplegia may be caused by a lesion affecting the cerebral cortex in the arterial territory of the anterior or middle cerebral artery, the deep white matter or the brainstem. The Oxfordshire Community Stroke Study (OCSS) classification is useful for determining the anatomical site of the lesion (Table 21).

What is the pathology?

Stroke is much the commonest cause of hemiparesis, but there are various stroke mimics that need to be considered, eg a space-occupying lesion (and in an acute setting, a seizure or hypoglycaemia). It is important to make the distinction between an ischaemic and a haemorrhagic stroke, but this cannot be reliably done by the bedside and neuroimaging is required to be certain.

What is the mechanism?

Stroke is broadly classified into ischaemic and haemorrhagic.

> ⚠️ It is not possible to distinguish an ischaemic from a haemorrhagic stroke on the basis of the history and examination alone. Neuroimaging (usually with CT in the first instance) is the only reliable method of doing so.

TABLE 21 THE OCSS SUBCLASSIFICATION SYSTEM

OCSS classification	Site of infarction	
Total anterior circulation syndrome (TACS)	Implies large cortical stroke in middle cerebral artery, or middle and anterior cerebral artery territories	New higher cerebral dysfunction (eg dysphasia, dyscalculia and visuospatial disorder) *and* Homonymous visual field defect *and* Motor and/or sensory deficit involving at least two of three areas of the face, arm or leg on the side opposite the lesion
Partial anterior circulation syndrome (PACS)	Implies smaller cortical stroke in the middle or anterior cerebral artery territories	Patients with two of the three components of TACS *or* New higher cerebral dysfunction alone *or* A motor/sensory deficit more restricted than those classified as LACS (eg isolated hand movement)
Lacunar syndrome (LACS)	Implies a subcortical stroke due to small-vessel disease	Pure motor stroke Pure sensory stroke Combined sensorimotor stroke Ataxic hemiparesis Dysarthria and clumsy hand Note that evidence of higher cortical involvement or disturbance of consciousness excludes a lacunar syndrome
Posterior circulation syndrome (POCS)		Ipsilateral cranial nerve palsy with contralateral motor/sensory deficit Bilateral motor and/or sensory deficit Disorder of conjugate eye movement Cerebellar dysfunction without ipsilateral pyramidal involvement (which if present is more likely to be ataxic hemiparesis; see LACS) Isolated homonymous visual field defect

Ischaemic stroke can be caused by thromboembolism from the heart or major vessels, or by occlusion of small penetrating cerebral vessels. The presence of atrial fibrillation or carotid bruits is helpful in indicating the likely source of embolus, which has implications for optimal secondary preventive strategies.

Almost all cases of intracerebral haemorrhage are caused by one of the following:

- hypertension;
- haemorrhagic infarction;
- ruptured saccular aneurysms or arteriovenous malformations;
- associated with bleeding disorders;
- amyloid angiopathy in the elderly.

Rarer causes include:

- tumours;
- trauma;
- cerebral vasculitis.

1.2.10 Tremor

Instruction

This woman has a 12-month history of tremor. Please examine her neurologically to determine the cause.

General features

The common causes of a tremor are listed and discussed in Section 1.1.6. The main differential diagnosis is between essential tremor (ET) and the tremor of idiopathic Parkinson's disease (PD).

Neurological examination

Is it Parkinson's disease?

Look specifically for these features, remembering that many of them may be asymmetrical.

- Hypomimia, ie paucity of facial expression, with 'mask-like' facies and a reduced blink rate.

- The tremor, when present, is classically pill-rolling and most marked at rest, although in severe cases it will often be seen with posture and action. Rest tremor of the hands is best seen with the hands resting, palms facing inwards, on the lap or over the edge of an armchair. The tremor may be intermittent and if not seen can be elicited by mental taxation (eg asking the patient to count backwards from 100 by subtracting three each time, while saying the numbers out loud as they do so – this is known as 'serial threes'), or it often comes on with walking.

- Bradykinesia, ie slowness and fatiguability of rapid movements. Ask the patient to open and close each hand as widely and as rapidly as possible, or to tap the thumb with each finger of the same hand in rapid succession with the widest amplitude possible. If not obviously slow, continue at least 10 times to demonstrate decrement in rate and amplitude. An extrapyramidal syndrome cannot be diagnosed without this feature.

- Extrapyramidal rigidity with 'cogwheeling', ie the combination of rigidity and tremor, is best demonstrated by slow and gentle rotation of the wrist.

 Tremor seen in the lower limbs is highly suggestive of PD.

- Ask the patient to write a phrase such as 'Mary had a little lamb' several times until micrographia develops or you are sure it is absent (eg after two lines of writing). Ask the patient to draw

a spiral, which may demonstrate tremor as well as micrographia.

- Note that the glabellar tap (which involves tapping the glabella and observing whether the patient blinks) is a non-specific test that is not clinically useful.

- Drug-induced parkinsonism may look identical to idiopathic PD, although it tends to be more symmetrical. Wilson's disease may present with parkinsonism and is associated with Kaiser–Fleisher rings (usually only visible with a slit lamp).

If time and the examiners allow, ask the patient to walk if the following are present.

- The posture is stooped, severe cases of which are referred to as 'simian'.

- The gait is typically short-stepped, shuffling and festinant, with reduced or absent arm swing. In early disease, a slight reduction in arm swing on one side may be the only abnormality. Freezing of gait occurs later in the disease.

Is it benign essential tremor?

This can look quite similar to the tremor of PD, but notice the absence of other signs of parkinsonism.

- Examination may be normal except for the tremor of outstretched arms, which may be worsened as the patient changes posture, eg holding the palms of the hands downwards under the nose or performing the finger–nose test.

- If possible, ask the patient to hold a cup and saucer, or a glass of water, which often exacerbates tremor.

- The key difference in distinguishing ET from the tremor of PD is that ET occurs mostly with posture and action and not at rest, whereas the tremor of PD is mostly at rest, although there is often a postural component.

- The tremor of ET interferes with activities, whereas some patients with PD do not notice the tremor initially or find it socially embarrassing because it is worst when they are not active.

Is it cerebellar disease?

The tremor of cerebellar disease is called an 'intention' tremor because it occurs with action, although when severe it can also occur at rest. The tremor is often severely functionally disabling and can render a patient virtually incapable of walking or using the arms. There will be other signs of cerebellar disease, as outlined in Section 1.1.6.

Further discussion

The examiners may ask how you would proceed to differentiate the tremor types by investigation and their management. If there is still doubt after clinical examination, then brain imaging can rule out other rarer diseases of the basal ganglia: fluoro-L-dopa or fluorodeoxyglucose positron emission tomography can sometimes be very helpful in demonstrating the characteristic asymmetrical reduction in signal in the basal ganglia seen in PD. Beta-blockers, anticholinergics and some anticonvulsants may help tremors, but often they only have a relatively modest effect. The use of anticholinergics in the elderly needs to be undertaken with caution because they can produce neuropsychiatric deterioration, eg hallucinations and confusion.

1.2.11 Visual field defect

Instruction

This man has been noted by his optometrist to have restricted visual fields. Please examine his eyes.

General features

Is the patient thin and pale with 'waxy' skin (suggesting panhypopituitarism) or does he have features of acromegaly? Does he have signs of a previous stroke (facial asymmetry, upper limb held flexed and internally rotated and a lower limb extended)? Are there any aids for those with visual impairment present (white stick, magnifying glass or Braille books beside the bed)?

Examination of vision

> In determining the site of the lesion, it is important to decide whether the visual field defect affects one or both eyes.

Monocular field defects

Visual field defects affecting one eye only are due to lesions in the visual pathway anterior to the optic chiasm, either within the eye or in the optic nerve (Fig. 12a).

- A central or paracentral scotoma (loss of the visual field within or adjacent to the central area of vision) usually indicates damage to the macular photoreceptors, eg macular degeneration, or macular nerve fibres at or within the optic nerve, eg optic neuritis. It is important to look for associated features such as reduced visual acuity, colour desaturation and a relative afferent pupillary defect. Is there papilloedema suggesting a local compressive lesion, such as optic nerve glioma?

- A dumb-bell shaped scotoma that covers both the central visual field and the blind spot is termed a cecocentral scotoma, which strongly implies optic nerve pathology.

- It is occasionally difficult to distinguish between an enlarged blind spot and a paracentral scotoma. Fundoscopy will reveal an abnormality of the optic disc, eg drusen or papilloedema, in the case of an enlarged blind spot.

- Horizontal/altitudinal field defects extend to the periphery but do not cross the horizontal midline. They most commonly occur in anterior ischaemic optic neuropathy due to vascular disease or giant-cell arteritis.

- A monocular segmental defect, for example a quadrantanopia in one eye only, may be due to retinal disease, such as ischemia from a retinal artery branch occlusion or retinal detachment. Careful fundoscopy of the dilated eye is usually diagnostic.

Binocular field defects

Field defects affecting both eyes may be due to bilateral ocular pathology, eg glaucoma or macular degeneration, or bilateral optic nerve pathology, eg due to toxins or multiple sclerosis. More frequently, however, binocular field loss is due to chiasmal or retrochiasmal lesions.

- Does the field defect respect the vertical midline? If so, the lesion is either chiasmal (bitemporal hemianopia) or retrochiasmal (homonymous hemianopia). Chiasmal lesions will eventually progress to involve the other visual field if left untreated.

- If the field defect crosses the vertical midline in each eye, the lesion must be anterior to the optic chiasm, indicating either ocular or optic nerve pathology.

- Bitemporal hemianopias (Fig. 12b) are seen in lesions affecting the optic chiasm.

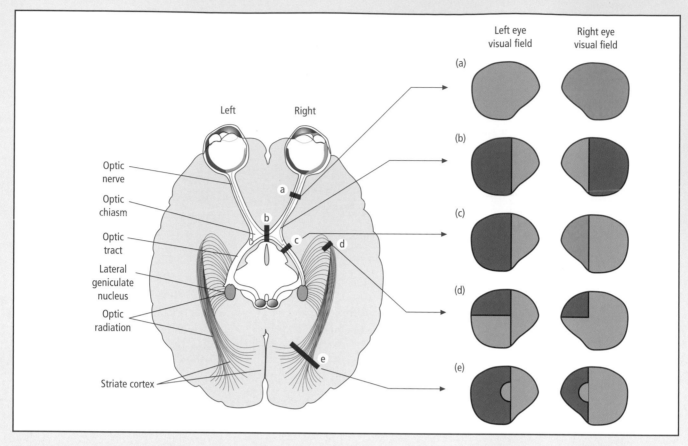

▲ **Fig. 12** Patterns of visual field loss depend on the site of the lesion.

Typically, pituitary lesions expand upwards into the optic chiasm resulting in a predominantly superior bitemporal hemianopia. Hypothalamic lesions expand downwards resulting in a bitemporal hemianopia that is most dense inferiorly.

- Lesions within the optic tract, optic radiation or striate (occipital) cortex cause homonymous visual field defects. These are typically hemianopic (Fig. 12c), although quadrantanopias (Fig. 12d) are seen in focal lesions within the temporal lobe (superior quadrants affected) or parietal lobe (inferior quadrants affected). The field defects tend to become more congruous, ie become more similar in each eye, the more posterior the lesion.

- Macular-sparing homonymous field defects implicate the striate cortex (Fig. 12e), which is commonly affected in a posterior circulation ischaemic event. The occipital pole, which is important in resolving the macular visual field, may additionally receive some blood supply from the middle cerebral artery.

Other examination

Once the characteristics of the visual field have been elucidated, it may be important to extend the clinical examination outside the visual system.

- If a pituitary lesion is suspected, look for features of acromegaly or panhypopituitarism.

- Other signs of multiple sclerosis should be sought in a young patient with signs of optic neuropathy: reduced visual acuity, a central scotoma, reduced colour appreciation and a relative afferent pupillary defect. Look for ataxia and spastic paraparesis, etc.

- Check the vascular status in a patient with a homonymous hemianopic visual field defect. Look for signs of coexistent hemiparesis or hemisensory loss. Are there any cortical parietal signs such as dyslexia, dyscalculia or dyspraxia?

In patients with monocular visual loss, check the carotid arteries for bruits, auscultate the heart for murmurs and feel the pulse for atrial fibrillation. Palpate the temporal arteries looking for tenderness, suggesting giant-cell arteritis. Check the inflammatory markers, particularly in any patient over the age of 50 years.

TABLE 22 CAUSES OF OPTIC NEUROPATHY

Type of lesion	Example
Hereditary	Leber's hereditary optic neuropathy, Friedreich's ataxia
Compressive	Optic nerve gliomas, sphenoidal wing meningiomas, dysthyroid eye disease
Vascular	Ischaemic: due to arterial or venous compromise
Inflammatory	Sarcoidosis[1]
Demyelinating	Multiple sclerosis[1]
Infections	Syphilis[1] or tuberculosis[1]
Toxic	Tobacco–alcohol ambylopia or heavy metals
Nutritional	Vitamin B_{12} and folate deficiency
Iatrogenic	Chloramphenicol, isoniazid or ethambutol
Other	Paraneoplastic

1. Also a cause of optic neuritis.

Further discussion

What are the possible causes of optic neuropathy?
See Table 22.

1.2.12 Unequal pupils

Instruction

This woman has an abnormality of her eyes. Please examine them.

Note that this case might also be found in Station 5: Eye examination.

General features
The causes of unequal pupils (anisocoria) are listed in Table 23. There is a clear clinical distinction to be made between patients who are noticed to have anisocoria but are asymptomatic, and those in whom the unequal pupils are part of a well-defined symptomatic disorder, eg brainstem stroke. Patients in PACES will virtually always fall into the former category. In a normal pupil miosis is caused by stimulation of the parasympathetic efferent fibres in the oculomotor nerve, whereas mydriasis is caused by activation of the sympathetic fibres from the superior cervical ganglion.

> Simple or physiological anisocoria (<0.6 mm) is seen in about 20% of normal people.

Eye examination
Which is the abnormal pupil? If the pupils respond to direct light, proceed to inspect them in bright and dim light.

- If anisocoria is greater in bright light than dim, then the iris sphincter on the side of the lesion is defective. This indicates that there is a local iris problem or a parasympathetic defect such as oculomotor palsy, ie the problem is on the side of the large pupil.

- If anisocoria is greater in dim light than bright, then the iris dilator muscle on the side of the smaller pupil is defective. This indicates simple anisocoria or Horner's syndrome, ie the problem is on the side of the small pupil.

Having decided which is the abnormal pupil, then look for those of the following specific features that are relevant.

- Ptosis.

- Irregularity of pupil.

- Inflammation of the iris.

- Light–near dissociation: the pupil does not react to light but does to accommodation. This is tested by asking the patient to look at something in the distance and then to focus on your finger held reasonably close to the patient's nose (Table 24).

- Afferent pupillary defect: the pupil will not react to light because of optic atrophy or severely diminished visual acuity from another cause. The swinging light test is used: on shining a light directly into the normal pupil, it will constrict and so will the affected pupil through the consensual response to light. On quickly moving the light to shine directly on the affected pupil, it

TABLE 23 COMMON CAUSES OF MIOSIS AND MYDRIASIS

Abnormality	Unilateral	Bilateral
Miosis	Horner's syndrome Iritis Pilocarpine	Argyll Robertson pupils Pontine bleed
Mydriasis	Holmes–Adie syndrome Oculomotor nerve palsy Midbrain lesion Atropine Unilateral afferent pupillary defect	Bilateral afferent pupillary defect, eg bilateral optic atrophy

TABLE 24 CAUSES OF LIGHT–NEAR DISSOCIATION

Pupil size	Diagnoses
Small pupils	Argyll Robertson pupils
	Long-standing Holmes–Adie pupils
	Diabetic neuropathy
Large pupils	Bilateral afferent pupillary defects
	Holmes–Adie pupils/tonic pupils
	Pretectal lesions

will dilate because it has an impaired direct response to light.

- Ophthalmoparesis.

- Optic atrophy.

When examining this woman, consider the conditions listed in Table 23, but particularly the following.

Horner's syndrome

Consists of miosis, ipsilateral partial ptosis and sometimes anhidrosis. Enophthalmos is not a useful sign. If anhidrosis affects an entire half of the body and face, then the lesion is in the central nervous system; if it affects only the face and neck, then the lesion is in the preganglionic fibres; and if sweating is unaffected, the lesion is above the carotid artery bifurcation (see Section 1.2.13 and Fig. 15). In the patient with Horner's syndrome, look for wasting of the muscles of one hand. This indicates a T1 lesion and flags the possibility of a Pancoast tumour.

Argyll Robertson pupils

This is almost always bilateral and consists of small irregular pupils that show light–near dissociation (poorly reactive to light, with better constriction to accommodation).

Holmes–Adie syndrome

There is usually unilateral pupillary dilatation with poor constriction to light and accommodation, occurring in association with depressed deep

tendon reflexes. This commonly affects young women. The pupil may become small over time.

Further discussion

Would you like to ask this woman some questions?

Your initial question would naturally be to ask the woman if she was aware of the problem with her pupil(s) or had any other problems with her eye(s) or brain. Regarding ocular/visual symptoms, check the following, the answers to which may be 'no'.

- Is there any pain or redness, which might indicate iritis or acute angle closure glaucoma?

- Does she have any diplopia, suggesting oculomotor palsy in this context?

- Does she suffer from headache? Both migraine and cluster headache can cause episodic Horner's syndrome, which may become permanent.

- Does she suffer from photophobia when moving from dark to light? This is caused by a fixed dilated pupil failing to protect the retina in bright light.

- Is there a history of poor night vision in a patient with small, poorly reactive pupils?

If she says that she has no ocular/visual symptoms, then it

would be appropriate to make brief enquiry about any general medical problems and follow any leads that this produces. Note new chest symptoms, particularly if she is a smoker (Pancoast tumour); also check vascular risk factors and take a drug history, which must include the use of eye drops.

What would be your approach to investigations and management?

This depends on the findings of history and examination. Remember the following.

- Any patient with bilateral tonic pupils, poorly reactive or irregular pupils, or pupils with light–near dissociation should have a VDRL (Venereal Disease Research Laboratory) test.

- Perform a CXR in cases of Horner's syndrome (especially if preganglionic) (Fig. 13).

- Imaging of the carotid artery in postganglionic Horner's syndrome.

- Imaging of the head is only required if other neurological features are present.

> ⚠ Think of Pancoast tumour! Look for unilateral wasting of small hand muscles. Obtain a CXR.

1.2.13 Ptosis

Instruction

This woman has an abnormality of her eyes. Please examine them.

Ptosis is abnormal lowering of the upper eyelid and is due to a problem with the levator palpebrae superioris muscle or its nerve supply (third cranial nerve) or involvement of the

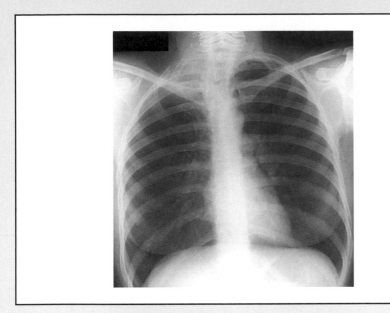

▲ **Fig. 13** Right Pancoast tumour.

sympathetic supply of the smooth muscle fibres of the superior tarsal muscle (Table 25). In assessing this patient, remember that many of the causes of ptosis would not be asymptomatic; those that might present without symptoms include congenital ptosis, disinsertion of levator, myasthenia gravis or Horner's syndrome.

General features
Look for the following.

- Are there any scars on the neck or chest wall that may be the result of previous surgery or trauma?

- Is there any evidence of malignancy?

- Is there any wasting of the small muscles of the hand? This indicates involvement of the C8/T1 nerve roots, which may be affected, along with the sympathetic supply to the eyelid, by lesions in the neck.

Eye examination
The upper eyelid normally covers 1–2 mm of the cornea, and the lower lid just reaches the level of the cornea. Are the pupils normal? Are ocular movements normal? Are the irises different colours (iris heterochromia) indicating either a congenital Horner's syndrome or Horner's syndrome occurring before the age of 2 years?

Look for the following patterns.

- Miosis, anhidrosis and enophthalmos with partial ptosis in Horner's syndrome. The pupillary asymmetry is more pronounced in low light conditions.

- Complete ptosis and abnormal eye position and movement in third nerve palsy, with a normal or dilated pupil.

- Partial ptosis with a sixth cranial nerve palsy and numbness in the distribution of the first or second division of the trigeminal nerve suggests a cavernous sinus or postorbital lesion.

- Fatiguability of the ptosis on looking up persistently, which would suggest myasthenia gravis; this may appear unilateral at onset.

- A loss of upper eyelid skin crease is suggestive of levator disinsertion.

Levator disinsertion

Disinsertion of the aponeurosis of levator palpebrae superioris from the tarsal plate is a common cause of unilateral ptosis in the elderly population, and is also associated with trauma. The important clinical sign is that the crease normally found on the upper eyelid is lost. There are no disorders of the pupil or external ocular movements. It is important to realise that these patients may complain of increasing ptosis at the end of the day, and may even report subjective (without objective) improvement after an edrophonium chloride (Tensilon) test. Therefore, differentiation from myasthenia gravis should be made on different grounds (other neurological signs or the presence of anti-acetylcholine receptor antibodies). Surgical reinsertion can be offered for symptomatic cases.

It may be important to proceed with examining the remaining cranial nerves and the limbs, particularly if Horner's syndrome is present. For example, a brainstem lesion may present with a central Horner's syndrome, hemisensory loss, dysarthria, dysphagia, ataxia, vertigo, and nystagmus. An assessment of limb fatiguability should also be made if myasthenia gravis is suspected.

Further discussion

What are the causes of ptosis?
See Table 25.

What are the causes of Horner's syndrome?
See Figs 14 and 15.

What is the localising significance of anhidrosis?
Depending on the level of the lesion, impaired flushing and sweating may be found ipsilaterally. Anhidrosis

TABLE 25 CAUSES OF PTOSIS

	Type of disorder	Example
Unilateral	Neuromuscular	Third nerve palsy Horner's syndrome Levator palpebrae muscle paralysis
	Local anatomical	Levator aponeurosis dehiscence/disinsertion Inflammation (eg chalazion) or infiltration (eg amyloidosis) of eyelids or conjunctiva Lost contact lens
	Congenital	
Bilateral	Neuromuscular	Myasthenia gravis Myotonic dystrophy Chronic progressive external ophthalmoplegia Ocular dystrophy Oculopharyngeal dystrophy Guillain–Barré syndrome
	Congenital	

affects the ipsilateral side of the body with central lesions. Lesions affecting second-order neurons, which exit the spinal cord at the level of T1, pass in close proximity to the pulmonary apex before synapsing in the superior cervical ganglion, and may cause anhidrosis of the ipsilateral face. With postganglionic lesions, anhidrosis is either absent or limited to an area above the ipsilateral brow.

⚠ **Think of Pancoast tumour** in any patient with Horner's syndrome and look for associated wasting of the intrinsic hand muscles, which is consistent with a T1 root lesion.

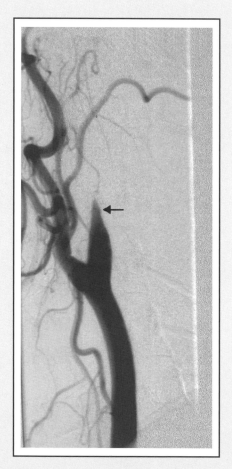

▲ **Fig. 14** Carotid artery dissection, a possible cause of Horner's syndrome.

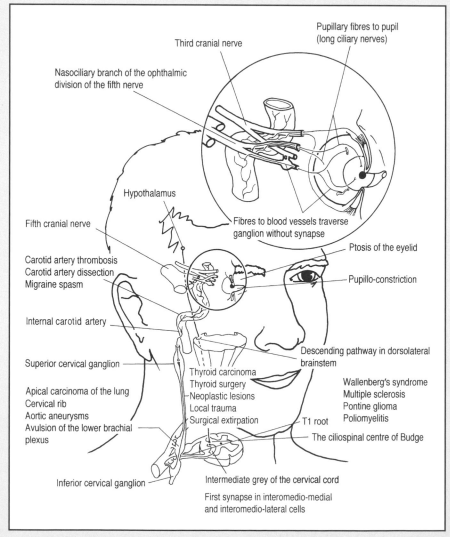

▲ **Fig. 15** Horner's syndrome.

TABLE 26 CAUSES OF DIPLOPIA

Eyes involved	Causes	Diagnoses
Binocular	Physiological	At extremes of vision

	Pathological	Neuromuscular: any cause of third, fourth or sixth nerve palsy, eg multiple sclerosis
		Myasthenia gravis
		Brainstem ischaemic event (not isolated diplopia)
		Miller Fisher variant of Guillain–Barré syndrome
		Cavernous sinus thrombosis
		Chronic progressive external ophthalmoplegia
		Mitochondrial diseases, eg Kearns–Sayre syndrome
		Local anatomical
		    Orbital infiltration, eg metastases
		    Dysthyroid eye disease

Monocular	Psychogenic	
	Pathological	Astigmatism Cataract Retinal pathology, ie detachment Foreign body in aqueous or vitreous media Poor optical equipment, eg defective contact lenses

1.2.14 Abnormal ocular movements

Instruction

This woman has worsening diplopia. Please examine her eyes.

Diplopia is caused by misalignment of the visual axes. You need to establish whether this is an isolated local problem or whether it is due to neurological disease (Table 26).

General features

- Is there a head tilt? The head tilts in the direction of action of the weak muscle. For example, in a left fourth cranial nerve palsy, the head tilts towards the right to compensate for the loss of intorsion of the left eye.

- Are there any signs of thyroid disease?

- Does the patient have a pacemaker? The presence of a pacemaker, in

conjunction with an external ophthalmoplegia, would suggest a diagnosis of the rare mitochondrial disorder Kearns–Sayre syndrome.

Eye examination

On inspection, look for the following.

- Proptosis: suggests an orbital lesion (unilateral) or thyroid eye disease (bilateral).

- Ptosis and a dilated pupil: indicates a third cranial nerve palsy (Fig. 16).

- Partial ptosis and a small pupil: indicates Horner's syndrome, which may be associated with ophthalmoplegia (see Section 1.2.13).

Does covering either eye relieve the diplopia? If not, the two images are coming from the same eye, which is relatively unusual. This can be due to refractive error (in which case asking the patient to look through a pinhole will relieve the symptoms) or a retinal problem (evident on fundoscopy).

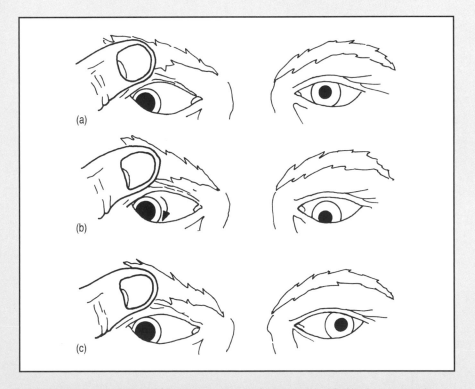

▲**Fig. 16** Right third-nerve palsy. (**a**) The patient is at rest when the eyelid is lifted by the examiner, the eye is looking down and out, and the pupil is fixed and dilated. (**b**) On attempted down-gaze the affected eyeball will be seen to rotate inwards, best demonstrated by watching a conjunctival vessel during the attempt. (**c**) Attempted gaze to the left. The right eye remains stationary while the left lateral achieves full abduction.

Analysis of diplopia

- In which direction is the diplopia worse? This occurs on looking in the direction in which the weak muscle has its purest action (Fig. 17).
- Are the images separated horizontally or vertically? Horizontal separation is likely to indicate sixth nerve palsy (Figs 18 and 19). The common cause of isolated vertical diplopia is superior oblique palsy, in which the patient may describe difficulty looking down, often notable when reading or walking down stairs.

The most important aspect is to check eye movements and at the point of maximum separation of an image, cover one eye. Loss of the lateral image indicates that the covered eye is the abnormal one; careful consideration of Figs 16–19 should then enable you to decide which muscle or nerve is causing the problem.

Always deliberately consider the question 'Is there internuclear ophthalmoplegia?' (nystagmus in abducting eye and failure of adduction of the affected side), which would suggest multiple sclerosis (Fig. 19).

A complete neurological examination is required to look for clues to differentiate the possible causes of diplopia given in Table 26, eg reduced visual acuity, optic

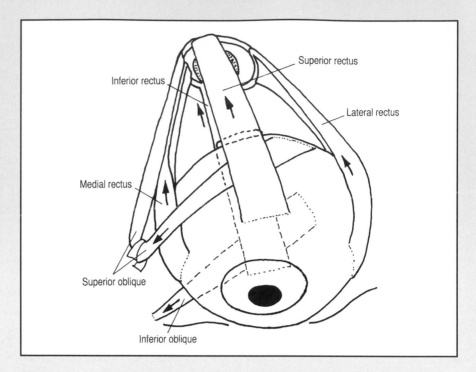

▲ **Fig. 17** The eyeball and eye movements. The left eyeball is shown from above, and the optic nerve is shown cut off so that the inferior rectus muscle can be seen. Note that due to the angulation of the orbit, the superior and inferior rectus muscles have their main elevating and depressing effect when the eyeball is looking laterally, whereas the oblique muscles (superior and inferior) that depress and elevate the eyeball (respectively) are maximally effective when the eye is looking medially. The medial and lateral recti simply pull the eyeball inwards and outwards.

▶ **Fig. 18** Eye movements in internuclear ophthalmoplegia and sixth nerve palsy.
(a) Normal on right gaze: both eyes move normally and single vision is retained with no nystagmus.
(b) Sixth nerve palsy (produced by a lesion at position B on Fig. 19) at rest: the left eye is slightly medially deviated giving a disconcerting diplopia best prevented by closing the eye or tilting the head round to the left, such that the normal right eye abducts to line up its ocular axis with the abnormal left eye. (c) Sixth nerve palsy on attempted left lateral gaze: the right eye achieves full adduction and the left eye remains static, producing widely separated images. (d) Internuclear ophthalmoplegia (produced by a lesion at position A on Fig. 19) prevents activation of the right medial rectus muscle on attempted left lateral gaze. On attempted lateral gaze the left eye abducts nearly completely but shows nystagmus. The right eye makes little or no movement medially, but due to minimal displacement no nystagmus occurs.

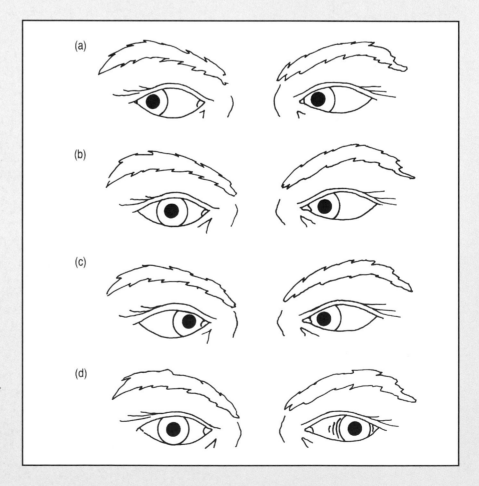

atrophy or cerebellar signs in multiple sclerosis, or fatiguability in myasthenia gravis.

Further discussion

What are the causes of a third cranial nerve palsy?

See Table 27 and Fig. 19.

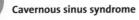

Cavernous sinus syndrome

This may result in ophthalmoplegia, pain, proptosis, Horner's syndrome (resulting in a mid-sized pupil caused by combination with a third nerve palsy, ie both sympathetic and parasympathetic paresis) and prominent scleral vessels. Intracavernous carotid artery aneurysm, mass lesions or thrombophlebitis may be causes; the latter is sometimes due to mucormycosis in the case of immunocompromised or diabetic patients.

What if the diplopia is worse in the evenings?

Consider myasthenia gravis.

1.2.15 Facial weakness

Instruction
This woman has a problem with her face. Please examine her cranial nerves.

The differential diagnosis depends on whether the facial weakness is due to a central or peripheral (upper motor neuron versus lower motor neuron) lesion. This is assessed by testing the muscles of the forehead, which are generally affected in a lower motor neuron lesion but not with a central lesion (Fig. 20). Note, however, that some lower motor neuron lesions may spare the forehead, eg focal lesions within the lower parotid gland.

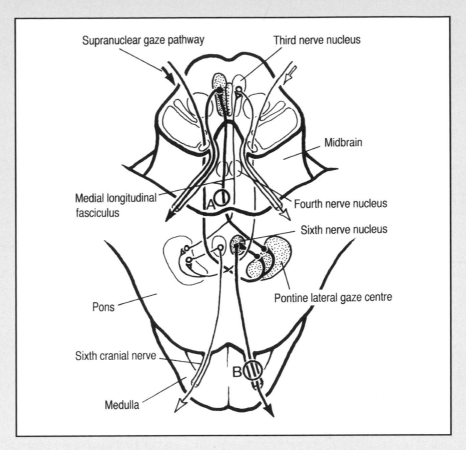

▲ **Fig. 19** Nerve pathways for lateral gaze. The pathways for achieving left lateral gaze are shown in thicker lines and stippled areas.

TABLE 27 CAUSES OF THIRD CRANIAL NERVE PALSY

Location	Diagnoses
Central (brainstem)	Infarction Haemorrhage Tumour Abscess
Subarachnoid space	Aneurysm Infectious meningitis: bacterial, fungal/parasitic, viral Carcinomatous/lymphomatous/leukaemic infiltration and granulomatous inflammation (sarcoidosis, lymphomatoid granulomatosis, Wegener's granulomatosis)
Cavernous sinus	Tumour: pituitary adenoma, meningioma, craniopharyngioma, metastatic carcinoma Giant intracavernous aneurysm Carotid artery–cavernous sinus fistula Cavernous sinus thrombosis Ischaemia from microvascular disease in vasa nervosa Inflammatory: Tolosa–Hunt syndrome (idiopathic or granulomatous inflammation)
Orbit	Inflammatory: orbital inflammatory pseudotumour, orbital myositis Endocrine (thyroid orbitopathy) Tumour (eg haemangioma, lymphangioma, meningioma)

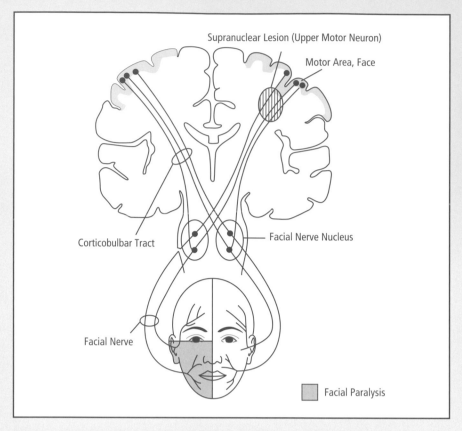

▲**Fig. 20** An upper motor neuron (supranuclear) facial nerve lesion causes weakness of only the lower half of the face (hatched area) because the upper part of the face receives bilateral upper motor neuron (supranuclear) input.

General features

- Does the patient have a stick, frame or other walking aid, suggesting the presence of limb weakness or ataxia?

- Does the patient wear a hearing aid, which clearly suggests the possibility of an eighth nerve lesion in this context?

- Is there a generalised rash, such as erythema nodosum, suggesting an inflammatory or infective cause? (This is unlikely in PACES.)

Neurological examination

If unilateral facial weakness is due to a lower motor neuron lesion, it is important to look for a number of other abnormalities to aid localisation.

- Is there involvement of the fifth, sixth and eighth cranial nerves, with ipsilateral ataxia suggesting a

lesion at the cerebellopontine angle? Large acoustic neuromas at this site may also expand to involve the ninth, tenth and eleventh cranial nerves, although this is uncommon.

- Is the sixth cranial nerve affected, either in isolation or with contralateral upper motor neuron limb signs suggesting a pontine lesion, such as a glioma?

- Are an extensive number of cranial nerves affected ipsilaterally? This may be seen in an infiltrative neoplastic process such as meningioma en plaque.

- Multiple cranial nerve palsies may also be due to a leptomeningeal process, eg sarcoidosis or malignant meningitis.

- Is there hyperacusis, implying a lesion proximal to the branch to

stapedius muscle? This is seen in approximately one-third of patients with Bell's palsy.

Facial nerve palsy

The head and neck must be carefully inspected for masses, eg parotid tumours, and scars, particularly just behind the ear (surgical removal of cerebellopontine angle tumours).

Further discussion

What is the course of the facial nerve?
See Fig. 21.

What are the causes of upper motor neuron facial weakness?
This may be due to any process above the level of the facial nerve nucleus in the pons. Remember that cerebral hemispheric lesions such as stroke, tumour or demyelination result in contralateral upper motor neuron signs affecting the face and limbs.

What are the causes of bilateral facial palsy?
The differential diagnosis for bilateral facial palsy includes the following.

- Myasthenia gravis: look for fatiguable weakness, complex ophthalmoplegia and lack of sensory signs.

- Myotonic dystrophy: check for grip and percussion myotonia; wasting and weakness of temporalis and masseter and sternocleidomastoid muscles.

- Facioscapulohumeral dystrophy: look for winging of the scapulae, bilateral foot drop and normal eye movements.

- In the acute setting, Guillain–Barré syndrome must also be considered.

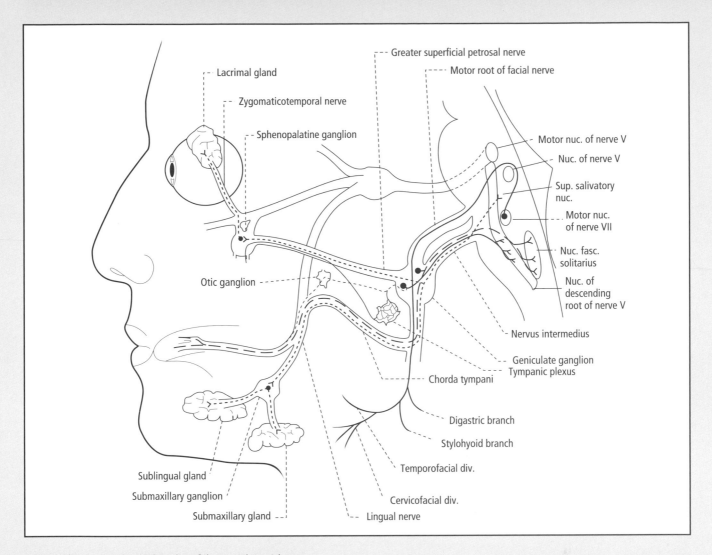

Greater superficial petrosal nerve
Motor root of facial nerve
Lacrimal gland
Zygomaticotemporal nerve
Motor nuc. of nerve V
Nuc. of nerve V
Sphenopalatine ganglion
Sup. salivatory nuc.
Motor nuc. of nerve VII
Nuc. fasc. solitarius
Nuc. of descending root of nerve V
Otic ganglion
Nervus intermedius
Geniculate ganglion
Tympanic plexus
Chorda tympani
Digastric branch
Stylohyoid branch
Temporofacial div.
Sublingual gland
Submaxillary ganglion
Cervicofacial div.
Submaxillary gland
Lingual nerve

▲**Fig. 21** The course and major branches of the seventh cranial nerve.

What is the prognosis and treatment of idiopathic Bell's palsy?

Bell's palsy is a common idiopathic facial palsy, possibly caused by viral infection (particularly herpes simplex virus 1) and oedema of the seventh nerve within the facial canal. There is an increased incidence during pregnancy and in cases of diabetes mellitus. Maximal deficit occurs within 48 hours. Postauricular pain is experienced by about 50% of patients, typically shortly before facial paralysis occurs. Treatment with steroids and antiviral agents will improve the outcome if given within 3 days of symptom onset. Complete recovery is seen within 60 days in 75% of patients.

What if the patient presenting with facial palsy has a rash on the ear?

In Ramsay–Hunt syndrome, herpes zoster vesicles may be seen in areas supplied by the sensory portion of the seventh nerve, ie tympanic membrane, external auditory canal, pinna, buccal mucosa and neck.

1.2.16 Lower cranial nerve assessment

Instruction

This woman has trouble swallowing fluids. Please examine her cranial nerves.

General features

The instruction suggests that any abnormality is most likely to be found in the lower cranial nerves, but check the following from the foot of the bed.

• Look at the patient's nutritional status: is she cachectic, suggesting difficulty with swallowing solids as well as fluids?

• Look for generalised loss of muscle bulk, perhaps due to motor neuron disease.

• Is there any evidence of previous trauma or surgery, eg any scars in the neck?

- Is there anything to suggest a stroke, eg hemiparesis or speech disturbance? This could mean carotid artery dissection in the neck causing lower cranial nerve palsies by direct compression or ischaemia of the nerves.

- Look for signs of conditions associated with dysphagia, eg myasthenia gravis, myotonic dystrophy and polymyositis.

- Is there any respiratory compromise, indicating a condition with respiratory muscle involvement, eg myasthenia gravis or motor neuron disease?

- Important in routine clinical practice, but less likely in PACES, is to check if there are any swellings in the neck. A swelling may indicate a tumour, which can compress or infiltrate lower cranial nerves, or cervical lymphadenopathy associated with a malignancy elsewhere.

Neurological examination

The lower cranial nerves comprise IX (glossopharyngeal), X (vagus), XI (spinal accessory) and XII (hypoglossal). Your examination should check the following.

- Voice (IX and X): note the quality and sound of the patient's voice. Is it weak, hoarse or nasal?

- Swallowing (IX and X): a drink should be available. Note any difficulty or regurgitation of fluid.

- Gag reflex (IX and X): observe the palate, which should rise symmetrically. If the cranial nerve is abnormal on one side, the palate will rise to the normal side. Also note elevation and symmetry of the uvula. Unilateral lesions usually result in deviation of the uvula away from the affected side.

- Trapezius and sternocleidomastoid (SCM) (XI): look for wasting,

weakness and asymmetry. Peripheral lesions of cranial nerve XI produce ipsilateral SCM weakness and ipsilateral trapezius weakness. Central lesions produce ipsilateral SCM weakness and contralateral trapezius weakness, because of differing sources of cerebral innervation. This is a common clinical misunderstanding.

- Tongue (XII): observe the tongue at rest in the mouth. Are there any fasciculations or wasting that may suggest motor neuron disease? Does the tongue deviate from the midline on protrusion? If there is a unilateral peripheral XII nerve lesion, the tongue will deviate towards the side of the lesion.

Although you have been asked to examine the cranial nerves, you should extend your examination as necessary.

- Is there bulbar weakness, eg depressed gag reflex or a weak cough, as well as a wasted and fasciculating tongue? A brisk jaw jerk, spastic tongue and emotional lability suggest psuedobulbar palsy (Fig. 22).

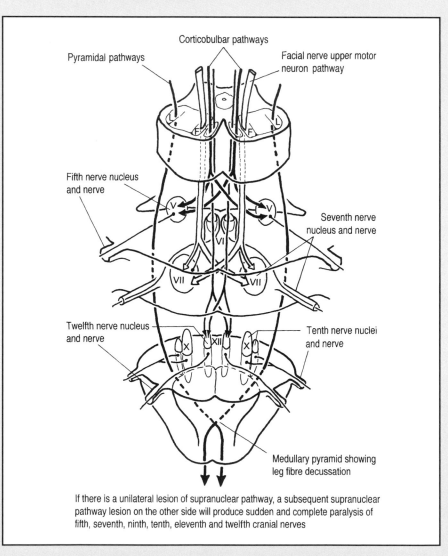

▲**Fig. 22** Anatomy of pseudobulbar palsy. The supranuclear pathways for the tenth nerve are not depicted, but are exactly like the fifth and twelfth nerves that are shown, with each supranuclear pathway contributing 50% to each right and each left nucleus. The facial nerve is different, with some 90% of fibres decussating; hence a lesion in the right supranuclear pathway will produce significant left facial weakness, whereas corresponding supranuclear lesions of the other motor cranial nerves will produce no abnormality (or at worst only transient abnormality).

TABLE 28 CAUSES OF MULTIPLE LOWER CRANIAL NERVE LESIONS

Site	Eponym	Cranial nerves involved	Usual cause
Extramedullary lower cranial nerve syndromes			
Cerebellopontine angle		V, VII, VIII, sometimes IX	Acoustic neuromas and meningiomas
Jugular foramen	Vernet	IX, X and XI	Tumours, aneurysms, trauma, Paget's disease
Posterior laterocondylar space	Collet–Sicard	IX, X, XI and XII	Tumours of parotid gland and carotid body
			Carotid artery dissection
			Tuberculous adenitis
Posterior retroparotid space	Villaret	IX, X, XI and XII	As above plus granulomatous lesions, eg sarcoid
Within the nerve		IX, X, XI and XII	Invasion of tumours, eg squamous cell cancer
			Granulomatous lesions
			Infectious, eg HIV, Lyme disease, herpes zoster
			Post infectious, eg Guillain–Barré syndrome
Intramedullary (brainstem) lower cranial nerve syndromes			
Tegmentum of medulla	Jackson	X and XII	Infarct or tumour
Lateral tegmentum of medulla	Wallenberg	Spinal V, IX, X and XI	Occlusion of vertebral or posterior inferior cerebellar artery

• In the limbs, upper motor neuron signs only (ie spasticity, hyperreflexia and extensor plantars) are seen in primary lateral sclerosis. Lower motor neuron signs only (ie flaccidity, atrophy, fasciculations and hyporeflexia) are seen in poliomyelitis and adult-onset spinal muscular atrophies. Both upper and lower motor neuron signs are seen in motor neuron disease. See Section 2.1 for further discussion.

Further discussion

It is rare to have isolated lower cranial nerve lesions. More often several lower cranial nerves will be involved together, especially cranial nerves IX, X and XI, which leave the skull together through the jugular foramen. Localisation of any lesion will usually require MRI of the head and neck.

The commonest causes of multiple lower cranial nerve lesions are shown in Table 28.

Swallowing is best assessed by asking the patient to take a small sip of water. If there is any difficulty with this, urgent speech and language therapy assessment is required. Having difficulty swallowing is a common occurrence after an acute stroke, but is of little localising value.

1.2.17 Speech disturbance

Instruction

This man is unable to communicate as well as he would like. Please examine his speech.

General features

The differential diagnosis of speech disturbance is determined by the type of disorder present: dysarthria, dysphasia or dysphonia.

• Dysarthria is a disorder of articulation in which the content of the speech is unaffected, the underlying diagnosis almost always being determined by eliciting other physical signs (Table 29).

• Dysphasia is a disorder of language caused by a cortical lesion of the dominant hemisphere (Table 30).

• In dysphonia, articulation and language content are normal but voice production is defective (Table 31).

The most important step in making the correct diagnosis of speech disturbance is to accurately characterise the abnormality: is it dysarthria, dysphasia or dysphonia?

General inspection should therefore look for clues that point to any of the cases indicated in Tables 29–31.

Look for evidence of neck surgery or swellings, indicating possible damage to the patient's vocal cords.

Is there anything to suggest a particular diagnosis associated with speech difficulties, eg myasthenia gravis, stroke or motor neuron disease?

Neurological examination

The type of speech defect is characterised by listening to the speech itself. Assessment of speech includes the following elements.

Phonation and articulation

When the patient talks, listen for dysphonia (a whispering, hoarse or otherwise abnormal voice) or disturbances of articulation that are characteristic of dysarthria. It may be possible to exaggerate dysarthria by asking the patient to repeat phrases such as 'biblical criticism' or 'West Register Street'. Repetition of particular letters can be used to assess individual parts of the articulatory process: lips ('pa'), tongue ('ta') and soft palate and posterior tongue ('ka'). Putting them all together rapidly ('pa-ta-ka') will uncover mildly dysarthric speech, but it is often difficult to characterise dysarthric speech purely on the basis of the way it sounds. It is frequently of mixed type, and the type(s) present can usually be deduced from the associated signs.

- Cerebellar speech is scanning or staccato, eg artillery pronounced 'art-til-ler-y', and associated with ataxic gait.

- Pseudobulbar or spastic dysarthria, caused by bilateral lesions in the upper motor neuron projections to the bulbar nuclei in the brainstem (see Section 1.2.16),

TABLE 29 CAUSES OF DYSARTHRIA

Cause	Diagnoses
Cerebellar dysarthria	Any cause of a cerebellar syndrome
Bulbar palsy	Myopathy or myositis Myasthenia gravis Motor neuron disease Bulbar poliomyelitis Guillain–Barré syndrome
Pseudobulbar palsy	Small-vessel cerebral ischaemic damage Motor neuron disease Multiple sclerosis
Hypokinetic dysarthria	Extrapyramidal disease, especially Parkinson's disease
Hyperkinetic dysarthria	Chorea or myoclonus
Isolated cranial nerve palsies	Cranial nerves V, VII, X and XII
Other	Hypothyroidism

TABLE 30 CAUSES OF DYSPHASIA

Cause	Diagnoses
Stroke	Dominant middle cerebral artery territory
Tumour	Dominant hemisphere
Trauma	
Cerebral abscess	
Herpes simplex encephalitis	
Degenerative CNS disease	Alzheimer's disease Frontotemporal dementia Progressive non-fluent aphasia

TABLE 31 CAUSES OF DYSPHONIA

Cause	Diagnoses
Paralysis of both vocal cords	Post thyroidectomy Neck malignancy Poliomyelitis Guillain–Barré syndrome Brainstem stroke Multiple sclerosis Syringobulbia
Paralysis of one vocal cord/recurrent laryngeal nerve palsy	Post thyroidectomy Carcinoma (bronchial, thyroid, lymphoma) Cervical node enlargement Aortic aneurysm Pulmonary tuberculosis
Neuromuscular respiratory failure	Guillain–Barré syndrome Myasthenia gravis Polymyositis
Spasmodic dysphonia	Associated with dystonia

is associated with dysphagia, small spastic tongue and a brisk jaw jerk. There may also be signs of small-vessel ischaemic damage such as *marche à petit pas*, brisk reflexes and extensor plantars.

- Bulbar dysarthria is due to a deficit in the bulbar cranial nerves (lower motor neuron type) or the bulbar muscles, hence there may be wasting and fasciculation of the tongue, proximal muscle weakness or fatiguability.

- Check carefully for isolated cranial nerve palsies.

Fluency

If phonation and articulation are normal, then consider whether the speech disturbance is a dysphasia. If the speech is not fluent (ie hesitant or 'telegraphic', missing out words such as 'and'), then this may indicate an expressive (anterior) dysphasia such as occurs with lesions in Broca's area. If the speech sounds fluent but patients substitute alternative words for those they may have forgotten (paraphrasias) or use nonsense words (neologisms), then this is compatible with a receptive dysphasia.

Comprehension

Early in the assessment it is wise to check that the patient understands what you are asking; indeed, it may be appropriate to do this right at the beginning if initial attempts at conversation with the patient are not rewarding. Comprehension is not an all-or-nothing skill, the level of comprehension being gauged by the complexity of the task that can be performed: one-, two- or three-step commands. You might approach testing as follows, starting with simple instructions and gradually increasing the complexity.

- 'I wonder if you are having some difficulty in understanding what I say?'

- 'I would like to test this . . .'

- 'Is that alright?'

- 'Can you open your mouth, please – open your mouth?' If the patient does not do this, then open your own mouth and see if he or she copies you.

- 'Can you show me your left hand?'

- 'Can you put your right hand on top of your head?'

- 'Can you touch your left ear with your right hand, and put your left hand on your nose?'

Naming

The patient may not be able to name objects (anomia), but may be able to describe them (circumlocution). This may indicate a lesion deep in the temporal lobe.

Repetition

Failure to repeat single words or phrases usually occurs as a result of a receptive dysphasia. However, there may be severe impairment of repetition with preserved comprehension. This dichotomy is said to be the essential feature of conduction aphasia in which the lesion is localised to the left sylvian fissure.

Reading

Test silently so as to test only visual comprehension, which is usually preserved in expressive dysphasia and impaired in receptive dysphasia.

Writing

Use verbal and written requests to get the patient to write something. Poor writing with errors similar to speech is a feature of expressive dysphasia.

Further discussion

Management of speech disturbance depends on the underlying cause and ranges from ENT referral for dysphonia to neurosurgery for some space occupying lesions causing dysphasia, so that patients with dysphonia may be referred to ENT and occasional patients with dysphasia may be referred to neurosurgery.

Types of dysphasia

Classification of language disorders has been based on various theoretical models, none of which show consistent correlation with anatomical lesions. Many consider it appropriate to think in terms of anterior or posterior dysphasia.

Anterior dysphasia This is characterised by the following.

- Non-fluent or hesitant speech, ie 'agrammatic' or 'telegraphic' speech, missing out words such as 'and'.

- Substitution of words or syllables.

- Poor writing, with errors similar to speech.

- Naming may be impaired.

- Comprehension, repetition (except for some word or syllabic substitution) and reading are preserved.

Posterior dysphasia This has the following characteristics.

- Fluent speech with normal rhythm. However, because of poor comprehension the patient is unable to monitor his or her speech and so it contains neologisms and paraphrasias as well as substitutions (ultimately ending up as incomprehensible jargon, so-called 'jargon aphasia'). The patient also talks incessantly.

- Poor comprehension, repetition and reading.

1.3 Communication skills and ethics

1.3.1 Genetic implications

Scenario

Role: you are a junior doctor in the neurology outpatient clinic.

Mr David Johnson, aged 54 years, is referred to the neurology clinic because of behavioural change and increasing cognitive difficulties. His son, who attends with him, has also noticed that his father has become increasingly 'fidgety'. Mr Johnson has no significant past medical history, but an extended family history, given by the son, reveals that Mr Johnson's mother (the son's grandmother) died in middle age with dementia, but this is something that 'the family don't talk about'. It is difficult to be sure how much Mr Johnson understands, but he tells you that you should 'talk about anything you want with my son'. He has also said the same thing to his GP, who arranged for the son to attend the clinic with his father. The view of the neurological team is that the most likely diagnosis is Huntington's chorea, which could be confirmed by genetic testing.

Your task: to discuss the implications of genetic testing for Huntington's disease with Mr Johnson's son.

Key issues to explore

- The son's knowledge of the disease and the diagnostic testing available.

- 'If you have Huntington's disease, would you like to know'?

- Why test when the disease is incurable?

Key points to establish

- The fact that any test results will have widespread implications for other family members, including the son himself.

- That testing may or may not clarify matters, but if the results are negative the problem will not be cured and so further investigations may be needed.

- That there is no treatment for Huntington's disease.

- Although it is difficult to produce 'black and white' rules in an area where much is grey, most physicians with experience of Huntington's disease feel that it is inadvisable to test in the following circumstances: children under 18 years; for insurance purposes; if the patient is reluctant; and if the result automatically reveals someone else (ie a parent) to have the disease without their consent.

- After any test, follow-up will be required whatever the result.

Genetic testing

Issues to consider if this is to be used include the following.

- Depression may follow a positive or negative result ('survivor guilt').
- Suicide after a positive result has occurred, but this is no more common than for any other disease or chronic disability.

Appropriate responses to likely questions

Son: I don't know about having the genetic test. Is there anybody else I can speak to about it?

Doctor: yes, I can make a referral to the regional specialist clinical genetics service, where you and your father would be able to receive further counselling regarding the test.

Son: can my father and I have the test done today?

Doctor: because of all the things that the test might mean, I feel it is important for you to have pretest counselling. This is provided by the regional specialist clinical genetics service. I will refer your father and you to them.

Son: what do you mean when you say 'all the things that the test might mean'?

Doctor: Huntington's is a genetic disease, which means that it runs in the family. If your father has Huntington's – and we don't know that at the moment – but if he does, then there is a 50% chance that he will have passed it on to each of his children. I'm afraid that means there's a one-in-two chance that you will have it, and also a one-in-two chance that any of your brothers and sisters will have it.

Son: if the test shows that someone's got Huntington's, can anything be done about it?

Doctor: I'm afraid that there is no specific treatment for Huntington's. There are things that can be done to help the symptoms, for instance drugs can sometimes help the distressing movements, but there isn't any treatment that will deal with the underlying disease.

Son: if I was tested and was positive, will I then know at which point the disease would start to cause me trouble?

Doctor: no, the timing can be variable and the onset of the disease could only be established by examining you neurologically.

Son: *so, do we have to have the test done?*

Doctor: no, you don't. As you can see it's a difficult issue, which is why I think that talking to someone in the clinical genetics service is necessary rather than just racing into the test. Some people decide that they want to know, and some people decide that they don't. There isn't a right and a wrong answer to the question.

1.3.2 Explanation of the diagnosis of Alzheimer's disease

Scenario

Role: you are the neurology junior doctor working in a general neurology outpatient clinic.

Mr Harry Wilson is a 69-year-old man who has come to clinic with his wife and one of his sons. He saw your colleague 2 months ago for investigation of memory difficulties. His symptoms have been coming on for several years and his wife initially took no notice of his memory lapses. Recently he has become disinterested in all activities, but his wife does not feel that he is depressed. His wife tells you that he is a shadow of his former self and can sit alone in a chair for hours without initiating conversation or activity. He recently had to be brought home by a friend after he was found wandering back and forward in front of his local shops. They have two sons in their forties.

The results of the blood tests, including thyroid function, erythrocyte sedimentation rate, syphilis serology and B_{12} were normal. His CT scan demonstrated some mild generalised atrophy, but there was no evidence of hydrocephalus, subdural haematoma, focal cortical atrophy or infarcts. His electroencephalogram demonstrated some diffuse slow waves but no overt epileptiform activity. The diagnosis is probable Alzheimer's disease.

His wife is finding it very frustrating as her husband does not appear to be aware of most of his problems. She would like to know what has caused his memory problems, and their son is anxious that it may affect him: 'Is it mad cow disease?' At the neurological meeting some of these issues have been discussed recently: the risk of inheriting late-onset Alzheimer's disease is not high, perhaps two to three times the risk of it occurring in a member of the general population with no family history.

Your task: to explain to the patient and his wife and son the diagnosis of probable Alzheimer's disease, its prognosis and treatment, as well as discussing the probability of inheriting late-onset dementia.

Key issues to explore

- A common problem with patients who have Alzheimer's disease is that they often have little insight into how they have been affected. This can cause significant problems, especially with frustration, within the family.

- The prognosis of the condition.

- The issue of symptomatic treatment with anticholinesterase inhibitors.

- Risk of family members developing the disease.

Key points to establish

- The diagnosis and prognosis of Alzheimer's disease.

- Possible treatment symptomatic options.

- Genetic risks in first-degree relatives.

- Future care involving the Alzheimer's Society, the patient's GP and social services in conjunction with regular outpatient follow-up.

Appropriate responses to likely questions

Wife: what is the diagnosis?

Doctor: the diagnosis is almost certainly a form of dementia called Alzheimer's disease, although doctors can never be 100% certain in life of the diagnosis. Other treatable causes of dementia have been excluded with the tests that have been done, and any other diagnoses would be degenerative brain conditions similar to Alzheimer's.

Wife: what do you mean by a degenerative brain condition?

Doctor: I'm afraid it means that the brain gradually deteriorates, and we don't have any treatments that will stop this happening.

Wife: how long has he got to live?

Doctor: I can't give you a definite answer, not because I'm hiding, but because I don't know. However, he is not imminently in danger of dying, but I'm afraid that his ability to do things for himself will slowly get worse and he is likely to need more and more care in the next few years.

Son: *what is the chance of me developing Alzheimer's disease?*

Doctor: your father has what we call late-onset Alzheimer's disease, so the risk of you developing Alzheimer's is higher than in the general population, perhaps two to three times more likely.

Son: *can I have any tests to find out whether I will get Alzheimer's?*

Doctor: no, there aren't any tests that will detect whether people are going to get late-onset Alzheimer's. It may be that such tests will become available in the future, but unless there's some sort of treatment that can be offered it will require very careful thought as to whether you, or anyone else, would want to be tested.

Wife: *is there any treatment or cure?*

Doctor: I'm afraid that there is currently no cure for Alzheimer's. But there is a group of drugs, called the anticholinesterase inhibitors, that are relatively new and may have a mild symptomatic benefit in some patients by increasing one of the chemicals in the brain that is low in those with Alzheimer's. However, it is not known if these drugs alter the long-term outlook. If your husband did want to try them, he would be monitored with memory tests every 3–6 months initially. If there was ongoing deterioration, then the drug would probably not be of benefit and would probably be stopped.

Wife: *are there any more tests that can be done?*

Doctor: no, there are no more specific tests that would be helpful. Neuropsychometry is a more formal and accurate way of assessing the degree and types of thinking problems your husband has, and it may be useful in monitoring progression of the disease and response to

treatment; but there aren't any other critical tests that need to be done.

Wife: *where can I get more information and help?*

Doctor: some patients and their carers find contact with the Alzheimer's Society helpful. I will write to your GP outlining our conversation and send you a copy of the letter. Your GP will be able to initiate contact with social services, nurses and other health professionals as and when they are needed.

1.3.3 Prognosis after stroke

Scenario

Role: you are the medical junior doctor working on a care of the elderly ward.

Mr John Smith, a 78-year-old man, was admitted to your ward yesterday following sudden onset of right-sided weakness and speech difficulties. He is also unable to swallow safely. There has been no change in his condition over the last 24 hours: he has no movement in his right arm or leg, he cannot speak and he does not respond to simple commands. A CT brain scan has shown a large left-sided middle cerebral artery infarct. His prognosis is very poor.

Your task: to explain to Mr Smith's wife that he has had a large stroke and may not survive; and also that if he does survive, there is a high chance of severe disability.

Key issues to explore

- What does the patient's wife know already about her husband's condition?

- What are her expectations? What does Mrs Smith already know and, in particular, what does she understand by the term 'stroke'?

Key points to establish

- That you would normally obtain permission from a patient to speak to the relatives, but this is not possible due to communication difficulties.

- That Mr Smith is very unwell having suffered a large stroke; that there is a large amount of damage seen on the brain scan, and that it is not possible to reverse this damage; that everything that can be done for Mr Smith is being done and that he is quite comfortable; that he could die from this illness and that the first few days are particularly unpredictable; and that even if Mr Smith does not die as a result of the stroke it is very possible that he will have some long-term disability as a result, but that the nature and extent of this cannot be determined at this early stage.

- That Mrs Smith is introduced to key members of the stroke team and encouraged to ask as many questions as she wishes.

Appropriate responses to likely questions

Wife: *why did this happen to him?*

Doctor: there are lots of reasons why people have a stroke, especially as they get older. Your husband's scan shows a type of stroke caused by a blood clot rather than a bleed, but we don't know exactly what caused this. At the moment we need to focus our attention on looking after him, but if he shows signs of recovery then he will have more tests to see if we can find the cause.

Wife: *does he need an operation?*

Doctor: no, that wouldn't help. We very rarely operate on patients who have had a stroke, unless the scan shows us that the brain is under a lot of pressure. We didn't see this on your husband's scan so an operation would not help him. In fact it would almost certainly make things worse.

Wife: can he be given a new 'clot-busting' drug?

Doctor: no, I'm afraid not. You are right that there are drugs available which can dissolve blood clots – they're often used for patients who have had heart attacks – but using them for people who have had strokes is not at all straightforward because they can cause severe bleeding in the brain that makes things worse. They are sometimes used, but only in people with some sorts of stroke and who have got to hospital very quickly. In your husband's case I'm afraid they wouldn't help – they wouldn't do any good and the risk of bleeding on his brain would be very high.

Wife: is he going to live?

Doctor: I'm not hiding anything when I say I don't know. As you know he's had a big stroke, but I don't know whether or not it's going to kill him. We have to take things hour by hour and day by day at the moment, but if there's any change in his condition then, assuming it's what you would like, we will let you know immediately.

Wife: if he does survive, then what sort of disability could he have?

Doctor: again, I'm afraid that I can't give you a definite answer as to what will happen but the stroke is on the left side of his brain, which controls the right side of his body and his speech. At the moment he is unable to move his arm and leg and he cannot speak. The extent to which these functions will recover is

unpredictable, but if he stabilises and shows progress over the next few days then our team of physiotherapists, speech and language therapists and occupational therapists will make some assessments. They will then devise treatment plans with the aim of recovering as much function as possible. If he does survive, the rehabilitation programme will last many months and he still may require help to look after himself. There is a high chance that he will need to use a wheelchair, at least in the early stages and perhaps in the long term, and he may also have persistent problems with understanding and speech.

Wife: should I tell my son to fly home from his holiday?

Doctor: your husband is in a stable condition for now, but he could become worse at any time. This can happen suddenly and he could deteriorate very quickly and even die. I would suggest that you should speak to your son and ensure that he understands this. He can then make a decision based on this information as to whether or not to return.

> Despite recent advances in the management of acute stroke, the prognosis remains poor, with up to 20% of patients dying within 30 days of the onset of the stroke. It is important when breaking the news of a large stroke to relatives that you are realistic about the chances of survival and full recovery.

1.3.4 Conversion disorder

Scenario

Role: you are the neurology junior doctor working on the neurology ward.

Miss Kate Beaumont was originally referred to the epilepsy clinic with a 2-year history of frequent episodes of apparent loss of consciousness. She is taking antiepileptic medication. These attacks were recently witnessed on the neurology ward while she was undergoing video-electroencephalogram (EEG) telemetry. The episodes do not have an epileptic basis on either clinical or EEG grounds. Other investigations have also been normal, and a diagnosis of non-epileptic attack disorder has been made. The neurology team have agreed that no further investigations are required. Miss Beaumont wishes to know what the cause of her attacks is and how you are going to treat them.

Your task: to explain to Miss Beaumont that the attacks are not due to epilepsy but have a psychological basis and are best managed with help from the neuropsychiatry team.

Key issues to explore

- What does the patient think is the cause of her attacks?

- What were the possible triggers more than 2 years ago that led to the attacks emerging?

- Is there any relevant past psychological history, eg depression, anxiety or self-harm?

Key points to establish

- Appropriate tests have given reassuring results and further tests are not indicated.

- The episodes will not improve with antiepileptic medication, which should be gradually withdrawn.

- The most appropriate therapy is psychological, and this is usually successful in reducing the attack frequency or stopping the attacks altogether.

> The patient is not considered to be 'putting it on' or 'faking illness'. The patient has little control over the nature of the episodes.

Appropriate responses to likely questions

Patient: so you think I am putting on the attacks?

Doctor: no, not at all. The attacks that you have are real, disabling and outside your conscious control: they could be thought of as involuntary episodes of 'switching off' or going into a 'trance'. For example, we have all had times when we do not hear our name being called when we are engrossed in a book or film, or remembering nothing of a familiar journey home. We can all therefore be unaware or have no memory of episodes that we have experienced.

Patient: why do I have the attacks?

Doctor: we don't fully understand what causes this disorder, but two-thirds of people with it have suffered some sort of traumatic experience in the past. This may be important for us to talk about further. We can't explain the link for certain, but it may be that when people are exposed to repeated frightening incidents they learn to switch off. Initially this is a helpful thing for them to do; it protects them emotionally at the time. But it may come back later in life as these

attacks, so it may be that your attacks are brought on by stress. However, sometimes people are initially unable to identify the triggers of their attacks; and when they are found they often turn out to be fleeting stressful or unpleasant thoughts that you may barely be aware of, and which have little to do with your circumstances at the time of the attack.

Patient: aren't there any more tests you can do?

Doctor: as you probably know, there are always more tests that doctors can do, but I don't think that any more tests would be helpful for you. You've had thorough tests done, including monitoring of the brain waves when you've been having an attack, and we've discussed the results with everyone in the neurology team. We think we should move on from doing tests to focus on how we can try and treat the problem.

Patient: how do you treat the attacks?

Doctor: in some patients clarification of the cause of the attacks and withdrawal of antiepileptic medication is enough for the episodes to stop or greatly improve. If your attacks do not improve, then it is likely that we will need to refer you to another part of our team, the neuropsychiatrists, with whom we work very closely. They will need to see you and talk more about the cause of your attacks. Usually they suggest some form of counselling or therapy involving changing your body's response to a certain trigger or experience.

Patient: will I come to any harm from having these attacks so frequently?

Doctor: there is no evidence that the attacks that you have cause you any

harm, other than minor injuries that you may already have experienced such as biting your tongue or friction burns from the carpet. It is theoretically possible to be hurt more seriously if an attack occurs at the roadside or on the stairs, but this is extremely unusual and it's very rare for patients with this sort of problem to come to serious harm because of them.

1.3.5 Explaining the diagnosis of multiple sclerosis

Scenario

Role: you are the neurology junior doctor in an outpatient clinic.

Miss Marlene Cox is a 34-year-old woman who is coming back to the neurology clinic for the results of her recent scans. She was initially referred by her GP with numbness and tingling in the legs, and she has a past history of episodes of blurred vision 6 months ago. An MRI scan of her brain and spinal cord has shown several high-signal white matter lesions in both cerebral hemispheres and a high-signal lesion at the level of C4 typical of demyelination. Visual evoked potentials and the results of a lumbar puncture are all consistent with this diagnosis. No further investigations are required. She needs referral to the specialist multiple sclerosis (MS) service for discussion of further management.

Your task: to explain to Miss Cox that the most likely diagnosis is MS.

Key issues to explore

- What does the patient know/fear about MS?

- The prognosis and treatment options.

Key points to establish

- That the most likely diagnosis is MS.

- That there is no definitive test to make a diagnosis of MS, but that the combination of typical symptoms and results from various tests help to make the diagnosis.

- That MS can manifest in many different ways and is not always disabling. Often patients with MS seen in the media are those with more severe disability. There are many thousands of patients with MS who live relatively normal lives, hold down jobs and raise families.

- That there are now several treatments available: these cannot cure the condition but can help to keep patients as healthy as possible for as long as possible.

- That the patient has the contact details of someone she can call when she leaves the clinic (the MS specialist nurse if possible).

Appropriate responses to likely questions

Patient: how can you be sure I've got MS?

Doctor: there isn't one single test that can ever prove the diagnosis of MS, but the problems that you've had – with the vision and now with the legs – coupled with the test results, the scans, the vision tests and the lumbar puncture all point to MS. I wouldn't be telling you the truth if I said anything different.

Patient: will I need to use a wheelchair?

Doctor: I'm not hiding anything when I say that I don't know whether or not you will need to use a wheelchair in the future, but hopefully you will stay as well as you are now for a long time. As you know some patients with MS do deteriorate, but very many don't. However, it tends to be the ones with severe disease that you see in the papers or on the television. We will make sure we see you regularly so that you will be able to report any changes in your condition to us.

Patient: do I need any treatment now?

Doctor: I'm afraid that there isn't any treatment that has a magical effect in MS, but there are some treatments that can possibly help in some cases. I'm not an expert on this, but I want to suggest that I will make an appointment for you to see someone from the MS specialist service so that they can discuss things with you.

Patient: what should I do if I develop new symptoms?

Doctor: you should still see your GP as the first port of call if you are worried about any new symptoms, because not everything you experience will necessarily be caused by MS. Also, you can always contact the MS specialist nurse to discuss new symptoms or problems with medication. You may also find it helpful to keep a diary of symptoms so that when you come to clinic you are able to report any changes.

Patient: have I passed this on to my children?

Doctor: that's very unlikely. We don't know exactly what causes MS. There is a lot of research being done that is trying to establish what factors can increase the risk of developing the condition, but it is not a genetic condition that is inherited from parents. So although there is a slightly higher risk that children with an affected parent will develop the condition, the risk is still very small indeed.

> ⚠ Beware of making a diagnosis of MS in patients who have had only one episode of central nervous system demyelination. This is referred to as a 'clinically isolated syndrome' and the patient may not ever have any further symptoms. Making a diagnosis of MS has many implications for the patient medically, socially and psychologically.

1.4 Acute scenarios

1.4.1 Acute weakness of legs

Scenario

A 27-year-old woman is referred urgently with a 3-day history of progressive weakness of her legs.

Introduction

What are the main priorities in this case?

It is critical that you think of acute spinal cord compression. In the acute stage it may be difficult to differentiate upper and lower motor neuron weakness since even in spinal cord lesions the legs may initially be flaccid. However, on the basis of the history and examination it should be possible to pick up enough clues to distinguish between an acute cord syndrome, acute neuropathy and muscle disease.

What are the causes of acute leg weakness?

See Table 32.

TABLE 32 CAUSES OF ACUTE LEG WEAKNESS

Site of lesion	Diagnoses
Brain	Stroke, tumour (especially parasagittal), multiple sclerosis (MS)
Spinal cord	Spinal cord infarction, tumour, disc protrusion, transverse myelitis, abscess, MS, poliomyelitis
Peripheral nerve	Guillain–Barré syndrome, porphyria, diphtheria
Neuromuscular junction	Myasthenia gravis, aminoglycosides, botulism
Muscle	Polymyositis, dermatomyositis, inclusion body myositis, periodic paralysis, metabolic myopathy (eg hypokalaemia)

History of the presenting problem

What would indicate that the patient had a spinal cord syndrome?

- Is there a problem with the bladder? Any involvement suggests spinal cord or cauda equina pathology in this context.

- Is there a sensory level, or even a band of tightness (suspended sensory level) around the torso? These features would suggest a cord lesion.

If a cord lesion is likely, then a sudden onset indicates a probable vascular cause (cord stroke or arteriovenous malformation). Compression or transverse myelitis would typically come on over hours to a few days.

> 🔑 A suspended sensory level is a band of impaired sensation below and above which sensation is normal. It may be unilateral or bilateral and is indicative of an intrinsic cord lesion.

What features would suggest Guillain–Barré syndrome?

- A history of preceding illness, particularly diarrhoea.

- Ascending symptoms.

Other rare acute neuropathies may need to be considered. Ask about any episodes of colicky abdominal pain or acute delirium/confusion (suggesting porphyria), which can also occasionally cause an acute neuropathy. Systemic features together with fever should alert you to the possibility of an infective myeloradiculitis, eg due to tuberculosis.

> 🔑 **Back pain and weak legs**
> - Back pain is often thought to indicate pathology in the vertebral bodies or discs, but it may equally be a feature of transverse myelitis or an epidural abscess.
> - Back and proximal muscle pain is commonly seen in early stages of Guillain–Barré syndrome.

What features would be suggestive of muscle or neuromuscular involvement?

- Muscle disease or neuromuscular junction disease is likely to be generalised if it is causing this particular clinical picture, so ask carefully about symptoms in the arms and cranial nerves (particularly diplopia and dysphagia) and whether fatiguability has been a recent feature (myasthenia gravis).

- Is there any shortness of breath suggesting respiratory muscle involvement? This could equally indicate progressive Guillain–Barré syndrome.

- Is there any muscle pain, eg in myositis?

- Is there a rash, eg in dermatomyositis?

Other relevant history

Drugs may cause a motor neuropathy (eg dapsone) or a myopathy (eg zidovudine), impair neuromuscular transmission (eg aminoglycosides) or precipitate an acute attack of porphyria (eg phenytoin).

Neurological examination

What features would be suggestive of a spinal cord syndrome?

- Brisk reflexes, extensor plantars and a clear sensory level make localisation easy, but not all of these may be present. Look very carefully for any of them. If you find an extensor plantar, go back and re-examine for tone, power and reflexes, looking more carefully for upper motor neuron features.

- It is crucial to examine carefully for a sensory level or a suspended sensory deficit, as either of these strongly suggests the spinal cord is the site of any lesion.

> 🔑 The presence of cranial nerve signs does not necessarily mean the lesion is in the brainstem. There may be multiple lesions, as in MS (acute cord syndromes are a common way for MS to present), and cranial nerve palsies are common in Guillain–Barré syndrome.

- Look at the patient's back for evidence of trauma, and also for superficial vascular markings/malformations that may indicate an underlying vascular malformation as a cause of cord stroke. Auscultate over the spine for bruits: these are very rare, but if you do not check you will never hear one.

⚠ Although a sensory level points to the spinal cord as the site of pathology, it is notoriously inaccurate at localising the level. You should therefore use all possible clinical signs to help you, eg a patient with a sensory level at the umbilicus (T10), and who also has brisk arm reflexes, is likely to have a lesion in the cervical cord above C5, rather than at T10. The significance of this is that it is the cervical cord that requires imaging, not the thoracic cord. It is generally much better to start imaging at the top (cervical) and work down, rather than the other way around.

What features would be suggestive of Guillain–Barré syndrome?

In the presence of a suggestive history, the finding of symmetrical weakness of the legs (this may be more proximal or more distal, as this is a demyelinating neuropathy), minimal sensory loss and areflexia is virtually diagnostic (see Section 2.1).

What features would be suggestive of muscle or neuromuscular disease?

- The presence of more extensive weakness, in particular of proximal arm muscles and neck flexors.

- Muscle tenderness suggesting myositis.

- A heliotrope rash over the eyelids or extensor surfaces

of joints suggesting dermatomyositis.

- Fatiguability of muscle power, ptosis or bulbar features, suggesting myasthenia gravis.

Investigation

An MRI scan should be performed to rule out a compressive lesion that is amenable to neurosurgical decompression. A scan reported as normal should exclude a compressive lesion but does not rule out the spinal cord as the site of the lesion: cord stroke and (sometimes) inflammatory lesions may be difficult to visualise.

Further comments

Treatment depends on the underlying disorder.

- Urgent intervention is needed in acute spinal cord compression and may include surgical decompression, high-dose steroids and radiotherapy depending on the type of lesion.

- Disc protrusions causing cord compression need surgical removal.

- In epidural metastasis, treatment is with high-dose steroids and radiotherapy, with the prognosis depending on the patient's condition at diagnosis and the radiosensitivity of the particular tumour.

- In epidural abscess, surgical decompression, drainage and intravenous antibiotics are needed in cases of spinal cord compromise.

- Neurosurgical intervention may be useful for some spinal tumours.

For management of other conditions see the relevant sections on individual diseases.

1.4.2 Acute ischaemic stroke

Scenario

You are called to the care of the elderly ward to see a 78-year-old woman who was admitted the previous day with palpitations. The ward staff found her slumped in bed, conscious but not communicating. You suspect she has had a stroke.

Introduction

How common is stroke?

Stroke is the second commonest cause of death in the UK and is the leading cause of long-term acquired adult disability in most countries. It is the most common life-threatening neurological condition and is responsible for around 5% of the expenditure of the entire NHS budget. Ischaemic infarction is responsible for about 80% of all strokes, with the remainder being caused by intracranial haemorrhage (15%) or rare causes (5%).

What is the prognosis?

The prognosis following a stroke is poor, with up to 20% of patients dying within the first 30 days after a first-in-a-lifetime stroke. The risk of dying following a stroke is highest immediately after the event and then falls over the next few weeks and months, although the risk of dying in the years following a stroke remains elevated compared with that in stroke-free individuals. The key to improving the outcome from stroke is to recognise it as a medical emergency and act quickly to make an early accurate diagnosis.

How can ischaemic and haemorrhagic strokes be differentiated?

It can be very difficult to distinguish a stroke caused by cerebral ischaemia from one due to primary intracerebral haemorrhage. Neuroimaging, particularly CT scanning, is the only way of making the distinction securely. It is crucial to make the distinction so that treatment and secondary prevention can be accurately targeted.

History of the presenting problem

Some features in the history help to make the diagnosis of stroke. The symptoms should be of sudden onset and maximal within minutes to hours. If the symptoms are more gradual in onset, then this should raise the suspicion of an alternative diagnosis such as a space-occupying lesion or cerebral infection. Symptoms should be predominantly negative, eg loss of power, loss of sensation and loss of speech rather than positive, eg involuntary movements or pins and needles.

Other relevant history

Who is at risk of having a stroke?

There are certain 'non-modifiable' vascular risk factors associated with an increased risk of any vascular occlusive event (eg ischaemic stroke, myocardial infarction and peripheral vascular disease). These comprise increasing age, male sex, history of a previous vascular event and a family history of vascular event(s). It is important to establish the presence of any modifiable vascular risk factors in order to reduce the future risk of stroke. These include hypertension, diabetes mellitus, smoking, hypercholesterolaemia, cardiac arrhythmias, physical inactivity and obesity.

Examination: general features

Is the patient in a stable condition?

Following an acute stroke patients are not usually critically unwell and are generally haemodynamically stable and fully conscious. However, if the stroke is large and causing mass effect or if there is significant brainstem involvement, then the patient may present in coma or deteriorate rapidly. Remember the following.

- Check airway, breathing and circulation. If the patient is not maintaining the airway, protect with an oropharyngeal tube and high-flow oxygen. Call for early anaesthetic support.

- Check score on the Glasgow Coma Scale (see Section 1.4.5).

- Check vital signs: temperature, pulse rate, BP and respiratory rate. Raised BP is common following a stroke (whatever the cause).

- Check for neck stiffness: this raises the possibility of intracranial infection (and haemorrhage).

- Look specifically for signs of atrial fibrillation, cardiac valve disease, cardiac failure and carotid bruits.

Neurological examination

A neurological examination will enable accurate identification of the site of the lesion, but in routine clinical practice this degree of accuracy has no value over and above a bedside system of classification such as the Oxfordshire Community Stroke Study (OCSS) classification (see Section 1.2.9). Therefore, perform a rapid neurological examination based on the OCSS classification, concentrating on motor, sensory, visual and cognitive domains.

Cranial nerves

- Check for facial asymmetry.

- Check for Horner's syndrome (may suggest carotid artery dissection).

- Check visual fields: is there hemianopia? This can be difficult to ascertain in a patient who is not communicating. Hold the patient's eyelids gently open and present a visual threat from the left and then from the right side: does the patient shut his or her eyes in response to one stimulus but not the other?

- Check for papilloedema: this suggests an alternative diagnosis such as a space-occupying lesion, although malignant hypertension complicated by stroke is another possibility.

- Look for deviation of the eyes and check eye movements if possible (ophthalmoplegia suggests brainstem involvement).

- Check palatal elevation and gag reflex: this is commonly affected following a stroke and can lead to aspiration pneumonia. If there is any suspicion that swallowing is affected, the patient must be made nil by mouth and a nasogastric tube inserted until an assessment can be made by a speech and language therapist.

Limbs

- Look at the posture of the patient. Slumping to one side suggests a weakness and/or inattention on that side.

- Tone: in the acute setting this may be normal or even low, only becoming increased on the affected side after hours or days.

- Power: this will be reduced in the affected limbs. There may be complete hemiplegia or a hemiparesis, in which case the weakness may be in a pyramidal distribution (arm flexors weaker than extensors and leg extensors weaker than flexors).

Quadraparesis suggests brainstem or spinal cord pathology.

- Reflexes: in the acute setting these may be normal, but they soon become increased on the affected side.

- Coordination: this may be impossible to assess if the patient is very weak. Any suggestion of ataxia should raise the possibility of a cerebellar or brainstem lesion.

- Sensation: it may be impossible to ascertain whether sensation is preserved in a patient who is obtunded/not communicating. Sensory disturbance in affected limbs may range from inattention, to a subjective impression of reduced light touch and pinprick sensation on the affected side, to a complete loss of all sensory modalities.

Speech (see Section 1.2.17)

- It is important to assess the patient's ability to communicate as this will help diagnostically and also have major bearing on recovery.

- Check for dysarthria (a disorder of articulation with normal speech content).

- Check for dysphasia (a disorder of language), indicating a lesion in the dominant (usually left) hemisphere: there may be receptive or expressive problems, or both.

- Dysphasia should be distinguished from acute confusion or cognitive impairment.

Investigation

The diagnosis of stroke is made on clinical grounds, but investigations help to localise the problem, distinguish the pathology and establish the cause. An urgent CT

brain scan should be the first test ordered and the necessary tests include the following.

- CT scan: this is primarily to exclude intracranial haemorrhage and should be done urgently in all patients presenting with stroke. Where it is necessary to prioritise patients in order to obtain a CT scan, it is imperative that those with a fluctuating level of consciousness and those on anticoagulants are scanned immediately.

- Blood tests: FBC, electrolytes, renal/liver/bone function tests, glucose, inflammatory markers and cholesterol should be taken in the first instance.

- CXR: check for signs of aspiration pneumonia, cardiac failure, left atrial enlargement or widened mediastinum.

- ECG: is the patient in atrial fibrillation or any other cardiac arrhythmia? Check for signs of a previous myocardial infarction.

- MRI brain scan with diffusion-weighted imaging (where available): this is a useful tool for detecting ischaemia within minutes of the onset of stroke (which is often not seen on an early CT scan).

Further investigation will depend on the individual case and may include the following.

- Echocardiogram if the clinical examination suggests a cardiac valve abnormality or cardiac failure.

- 24-hour ECG if the patient has a history of palpitations or for any reason it is suspected that there is a cardiac arrhythmia.

- Carotid Doppler ultrasound scan in all patients with an anterior circulation stroke who make a reasonable recovery.

- MRI axial T1-weighted scan from the skull base down to C4 if carotid dissection is a possibility (Fig. 23).

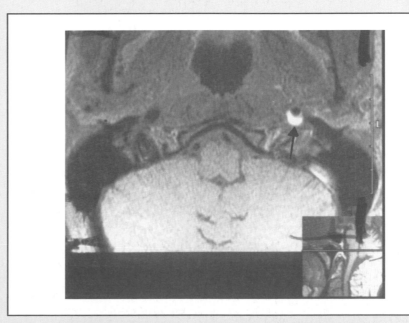

▲ **Fig. 23** Axial T1-weighted MRI through the neck. Arrow indicates crescentic shape of blood in the wall of the left internal carotid artery.

Management

The management of acute stroke has moved on significantly in the past decade with the widespread introduction of specialised stroke units. In addition, a few centres in the UK are treating eligible ischaemic stroke patients with intravenous thrombolysis. Management is as follows.

- Patients should be transferred to a specialised stroke unit as soon as possible.

- Early assessment of swallowing is crucial in improving outcome and a nasogastric tube should be inserted if swallowing is not safe.

- Hydration should be maintained either with intravenous fluids or via a nasogastric tube.

- Feeding should be started early unless there is any contraindication to doing so, eg vomiting or the possibility of surgery.

- Once intracranial haemorrhage has been ruled out, start treatment with aspirin 75 mg once a day.

- Hyperglycaemia may need to be managed with a sliding scale of insulin.

- Hypertension is common in the acute setting, but because of the disturbance of cerebral autoregulation much harm can be done by inappropriate treatment. Most authorities would recommend giving antihypertensive agents to a patient who has just had a stroke only if hypertension were extreme (>240/140 mmHg) or there were other pressing indications, eg aortic dissection.

- Turning regularly to prevent pressure sores is required for patients with severe hemiparesis.

- Thromboembolic stockings and prophylactic doses of low-molecular-weight heparin reduce the incidence of deep vein thrombosis and subsequent pulmonary embolism.

- Early assessment by physiotherapists and occupational therapists is vital to provide a personalised, integrated programme of therapy to aid recovery.

How do stroke units benefit patients?

A systematic review of randomised trials that compared the outcome for acute stroke patients cared for in a specialist stroke unit with those who were cared for in general medical wards showed that care on a stroke unit reduces mortality, physical dependency and the need for institutionalisation: the result is an overall odds reduction of 23% in patients treated on a stroke unit for the outcomes of death or living in an institution within 6–12 months of randomisation. This benefit probably arises because stroke units contain knowledgeable and enthusiastic multidisciplinary teams that implement well-coordinated care. Stroke units are potentially the most effective treatment available for acute stroke, principally because they can be applied to most stroke patients. The National Service Framework for Older People (a UK government document) states that all patients who have a stroke should have access to integrated stroke care services.

What are the benefits and risks of thrombolysis?

A systematic review of randomised trials comparing thrombolytic agents with placebo in patients with acute ischaemic stroke included 18 trials comprising 5,727 patients. Despite an increase in intracranial haemorrhage and death at 3–6 months, thrombolysis also reduced the proportion of patients with poor functional outcome at 3–6 months follow-up (odds ratio 0.84, 95% confidence interval 0.75–0.95). Subgroup analyses established that the most favourable risk–benefit ratio was obtained using tissue plasminogen activator within 3 hours of the onset of symptoms.

Why are we not using thrombolysis more often?

Thrombolysis is a complex treatment to administer, requiring a trained team, access to rapid neuroimaging and high-dependency monitoring facilities. In addition, the proportion of acute stroke patients eligible to receive thrombolysis is very small because intracranial haemorrhage must be excluded and the drug started within 3 hours of onset of symptoms. Therefore, despite the clear benefits seen in randomised trials, the realistic impact of thrombolysis on the burden of stroke is likely to be limited.

Further comments

Complications of acute stroke include the following.

- Cerebral oedema: this is the commonest cause of death and is usually associated with deterioration in the condition of the patient 4–5 days after the onset of stroke.

- Haemorrhagic transformation.

- Seizures: may complicate up to 10% of strokes (whatever the cause).

- Depression: this is particularly common following left anterior circulation lesions and may complicate up to 50% of all strokes.

- Syndrome of inappropriate antidiuretic hormone secretion (SIADH): this typically occurs at around 7–9 days after the onset and should be monitored by checking serum sodium frequently in the early stages after stroke.

- Pressure sores.

- Pulmonary embolism.

- Aspiration pneumonia.

> The Royal College of Physicians *National Clinical Guidelines for Stroke*, 2nd edn (2004) (http://www.rcplondon.ac.uk/pubs/books/stroke/) is a useful document for all aspects of stroke care. NHS trusts have a responsibility to ensure that local guidelines for the management of acute stroke are produced and followed.

1.4.3 Subarachnoid haemorrhage

Scenario

You are asked to see a 19-year-old man in the resuscitation area of the Emergency Department. His mother tells you that he had been out for the night and came home early complaining of severe headache and nausea. He went straight to bed and when she checked on him later he had vomited and was drowsy, so she called an ambulance. There was no history of headaches and no prodromal illness.

Introduction

Your first priority is to rule out subarachnoid haemorrhage (SAH).

What causes subarachnoid haemorrhage?

Most non-traumatic SAHs (around 80%) are caused by ruptured

saccular (berry) aneurysms, which are usually found at bifurcations and branchings of arteries of the circle of Willis. Other causes of SAH are much less common and include arteriovenous malformations, arterial dissection and hypertension. The commonest sites for aneurysms are:

- posterior communicating artery (30% of cases);

- anterior communicating artery (25% of cases);

- middle cerebral artery (25% of cases).

It is a common misconception that aneurysms are congenital; in fact they develop during the course of life.

What is the differential diagnosis?

Studies have shown that up to 30% of patients with SAH are misdiagnosed at presentation. It is important to rule out other causes of severe headache, nausea and neck stiffness such as meningitis, encephalitis and migraine. This should be possible with good history-taking and examination skills.

What is the prognosis?

The prognosis following SAH is poor, with mortality around 50%. Figures from neurosurgical units tend to be somewhat better than this, probably because they never see the most severely affected patients. A good clinical outcome is expected in 90% of patients admitted in a good clinical condition, ie with a Glasgow Coma Scale (GCS) score of 14 or 15. Although the clinical course of SAH is unpredictable and clinical signs do not reliably determine which patients will have a worse outcome, it is generally accepted that an impaired level of consciousness at presentation is a poor prognostic indicator.

History of the presenting problem

The key feature in diagnosing SAH is a history of severe sudden-onset headache ('like a blow to the head'). The headache usually begins when the patient is active, and sexual activity may precipitate an SAH (as well as other more benign headaches). There is little in the history that will distinguish aneurysmal versus non-aneurysmal bleeding, except perhaps a history of trauma. Other presenting symptoms include drowsiness, neck pain or stiffness, nausea and vomiting, back pain, seizures (10–20% of cases) and focal neurological symptoms such as limb weakness.

Other relevant history

Are there any identifiable risk factors for developing SAH, such as smoking or heavy drinking? A family history of SAH could be relevant: the risk in first-degree relatives of individuals who have suffered an SAH is increased three- to five-fold, and particular note should be taken of a family history of adult polycystic kidney disease.

Examination: general features

Is the patient stable?

Patients with SAH are often critically unwell and may be haemodynamically unstable with a depressed level of consciousness. To confirm their stability, assess the following.

- Start by checking the patient's airway, breathing and circulation. If they are not maintaining their airway, then the first priority must be for this to be protected with an oropharyngeal tube and high-flow oxygen. Call for early anaesthetic support.

- Check GCS (see Section 1.4.5).

- Check vital signs: temperature, pulse rate, BP and respiratory

MMC Core Curriculum

rate. The combination of hypertension and bradycardia should alert you to the possibility of raised intracranial pressure.

- Check for neck stiffness.

- Look specifically for head injury, hypertension, signs of alcohol excess or drug abuse, connective tissue diseases (unlikely) or abdominal masses (polycystic kidneys, although this is very unlikely).

Neurological examination

Cranial nerves

- Check the fundi, looking for papilloedema and retinal haemorrhages (thought to result from an acute increase in intracranial pressure that causes obstruction to the venous outflow from the eye).

- Check for visual field defects, which may be monocular (caused by anterior communicating artery aneurysms compressing the optic nerve after rupture) or hemianopic (caused by rupture of a posterior communicating artery aneurysm).

- Check pupil responses: small unreactive pupils may signify hydrocephalus as a consequence of raised intracranial pressure.

- Check eye movements: third nerve palsy is a well-recognised sign after rupture of a posterior communicating artery aneurysm. Ophthalmoplegia may suggest brainstem involvement. Bilateral sixth nerve palsies may occur due to increased intracranial pressure.

Limbs

- Examine the patient, looking for hemiparesis (occurs in 15% of patients with ruptured aneurysms).

- Check for cerebellar signs, which may suggest vertebral artery dissection as an aetiological factor.

Investigation

Investigation of the patient with suspected SAH is divided into tests needed to assess the patient's general medical condition, such as FBC, electrolytes, renal/liver/bone function tests, glucose, inflammatory markers, clotting studies, CXR (also to check for aspiration) and ECG, and those aimed at detecting the underlying cause with a view to treatment.

- CT scan: this is the immediate investigation of choice and should be done without contrast, taking very thin cuts through the base of the brain to optimise the chance of seeing a small collection of blood (Fig. 24). The sensitivity of modern scanners to detect SAH is very high: 98–100% if the scan is performed within 12 hours of onset of symptoms and 93% in the first 24 hours.

- A patient in whom SAH is strongly suspected but with a negative CT scan should have a lumbar puncture. Different laboratories use different cerebrospinal fluid (CSF) tests in cases of suspected SAH: some look for xanthochromia, whereas others look for elevated bilirubin in the context of normal serum bilirubin. Both these tests may be negative if the CSF is examined in the first 12 hours after onset. It is not always possible to distinguish true haemorrhage from a 'traumatic tap'; in particular, the three-tube method that looks for decreasing numbers of erythrocytes in successively collected specimens is not always reliable.

Further imaging studies may be appropriate in patients with confirmed SAH if intervention is

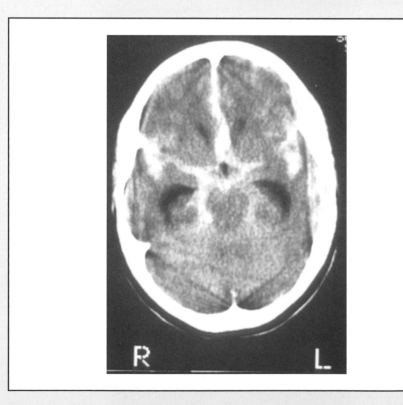

▲**Fig. 24** Non-contrast CT scan showing blood in the subarachnoid space and early ventricular dilatation.

contemplated. This can be done invasively (digital subtraction angiography) or non-invasively (usually with CT angiography) and helps to assess vascular anatomy, the site of bleeding (and possibly the location of the aneurysm that bled) and the presence of other aneurysms (about 20% of those with SAH have multiple aneurysms). Non-invasive imaging may be preferred in very unstable patients.

Management

The management of SAH involves general and specific measures aimed at stabilising the patient and intervening to control a haemorrhage or prevent complications.

General measures

- Transfer to a high-dependency or intensive-care bed as soon as possible.

- Strict bed-rest.

- Management of hypertension.

> **Hypertension in the acute phase of SAH can be left untreated, unless there are signs of end-organ damage. Existing antihypertensive drugs can be continued.**

Specific measures

Nimodipine (60 mg po every 4 hours or intravenous infusion at a rate of 0.5–2 mg/hour) should be given, provided the patient is not hypotensive. This helps to prevent or treat the ischaemic deficit that may occur due to vascular spasm.

Endovascular treatment of aneurysms is being used increasingly and is much less invasive than surgery. The aneurysm can be packed with coils, which ideally results in the lumen becoming

occluded by thrombus. Success of the procedure depends on having an experienced neuroradiologist and favourable characteristics of the aneurysm, such as having a narrow neck.

Surgery to clip the aneurysm, which may prevent rebleeding and which has been shown to improve outcome, may be required if the patient is not suitable for endovascular intervention. Although the timing of surgery has not been shown to be a critical factor in determining outcome, most neurosurgeons favour early intervention. Indications for surgery in patients with confirmed aneurysmal bleeding (and a technically accessible aneurysm) are:

- GCS ≥12;

- GCS <12 with space-occupying intracranial haemorrhage or hydrocephalus.

> ⚠ **If patients with large intracranial collections of blood become increasingly drowsy, they are candidates for immediate surgical evacuation of the haematoma.**

Long-term measures

After surgery or endovascular intervention it is important to address vascular risk factors. Patients must be advised to refrain from driving and contact the UK Driver and Vehicle Licensing Agency (DVLA); their licence is usually returned after 3 months if they have made a full recovery. They should be strongly advised to refrain from smoking and heavy alcohol consumption.

Further comments

Complications of SAH include the following.

- Delayed cerebral ischaemia secondary to vasospasm.

- Rebleeding: this occurs in around 50% of patients and is associated with a much worse prognosis.

- Hydrocephalus: this should be suspected in patients with a declining conscious level; early ventricular drainage may be required.

1.4.4 Status epilepticus

> ### Scenario
>
> A 33-year-old man with known epilepsy is brought into the Emergency Department by ambulance. He has had at least six convulsive seizures in quick succession over the last 45 minutes.

Introduction

What is the definition of status epilepticus?

Status epilepticus is defined as a condition in which epileptic activity persists for 30 minutes or more. This may take the form of either a prolonged seizure or recurrent attacks without recovery in between. From a pragmatic point of view, emergency treatment and investigations should be initiated for any convulsion lasting longer than 10 minutes.

What are the potential causes?

About 50% of patients with status epilepticus do not have pre-existing epilepsy. In this group, the commonest causes of status epilepticus are cerebral tumour and stroke (Table 33). Of patients with epilepsy, 5% will have at least one episode of status epilepticus at some point, commonly due to drug withdrawal, intercurrent illness or

TABLE 33 CAUSES OF STATUS EPILEPTICUS

Aetiology	No previous history of epilepsy (%)	Previous history of epilepsy (%)
Cerebrovascular disease	20	19
Cerebral tumour	16	10
Intracranial infection	15	6
Other acute event	14	3
Cerebral trauma	12	17
Acute metabolic disturbance	12	5
No cause identified	11	41

progression of the underlying disease.

What is the outcome of status epilepticus?

The 30-day mortality rate in status epilepticus is 10–20% and is determined by the aetiology and duration of the status. It is also increasingly recognised that, in addition to the morbidity resulting from the underlying cerebral pathological process and physiological derangement during status, persistent seizure activity may further damage the brain.

History of the presenting problem

It is clearly not possible to obtain any history from a patient in status epilepticus, but after rapid initial examination and instigation of treatment (see below) you should do the following.

- Talk with any available witnesses: family/friends who have accompanied the patient or ambulance/paramedical staff. Is the patient known to have epilepsy? Does the patient have any other medical conditions, eg diabetes? What were the circumstances surrounding the beginning of epileptic fitting, in particular has the patient been unwell recently (and in what way), suffered any injury to the head or been using alcohol or drugs?

- Read all records completed by ambulance staff or others.

Examination

- Check airway, breathing and circulation. Monitor oxygenation with pulse oximeter, but note that this may not read accurately while a patient is convulsing.

- Look for evidence of head injury.

- Note if there are any focal features to the status epilepticus: are both sides of the body convulsing and are the eyes (if they can be seen) deviated to one side?

- Look for clues that the patient may have epilepsy or diabetes, eg Medic-Alert bracelet, a bottle of antiepileptic drug (AED) or an appointment card for neurology outpatient clinic.

Investigation

Immediate

Check fingerprick blood glucose concentration: if it is <2.5 mmol/L, immediately give intravenous glucose/dextrose. It is unlikely that a blood glucose concentration >1.5 mmol/L will cause status epilepticus, but correct any hypoglycaemia as a therapeutic trial if there is even a remote possibility because neglected hypoglycaemia

can be fatal or cause permanent neurological damage.

Check FBC, clotting screen, glucose (laboratory), electrolytes (hyponatraemia), renal/liver/bone function tests (renal failure, hepatic failure and hypocalcaemia) and hypomagnesaemia. Take a venous blood sample for storage. Check arterial blood gases (consider poisoning if there is unexplained metabolic acidosis).

When fitting controlled

Perform a CT (or MRI) brain scan if cause of status epilepticus not clearly established. Also check the following.

- ECG: note that abnormalities mimicking cardiac ischaemia can be seen with some intracranial pathologies, eg subarachnoid haemorrhage.

- CXR: look for signs of aspiration.

- Other tests as dictated by clinical circumstances, eg thick film for malaria, blood cultures and lumbar puncture.

Management

Treatment should be started immediately (Tables 34 and 35; Fig. 25).

Early status epilepticus (0–30 minutes)

Supportive Ensure airway maintenance and high-flow oxygen with, if necessary, a nasopharyngeal airway if masseter trismus prevents placement of an oral airway.

⚠ Do not try to force an oropharyngeal airway into a patient who is fitting. Only two things will result: damage to the patient's teeth, tongue or mouth; and damage to your fingers.

TABLE 34 GENERAL MEASURES FOR THE PATIENT PRESENTING WITH STATUS EPILEPTICUS

Stage	Measures
First stage (0–10 minutes)	Assess cardiorespiratory function Secure airway (without causing damage; see text) and resuscitate Administer oxygen (high flow)
Second stage (0–30 minutes)	Institute regular monitoring (see text) Initiate emergency AED therapy (see text and Table 35) Set up intravenous lines Emergency investigations Administer glucose/dextrose (50 mL of 50% solution) and/or intravenous thiamine (250 mg) as high-potency Pabrinex where appropriate Treat acidosis if severe
Third stage (30–60/90 minutes)	Transfer to intensive care unit Escalate emergency AED therapy (see text and Table 35) Establish aetiology Identify and treat medical complications Pressor therapy when appropriate Establish intensive care and EEG monitoring (see text and Fig. 26) Initiate intracranial pressure monitoring where appropriate Initiate long-term maintenance AED therapy

Insert intravenous lines for fluid replacement and drug administration (preferably with 0.9% sodium chloride rather than 5% glucose solutions).

Drugs should not be mixed: if two AEDs are needed (eg phenytoin and diazepam), then two intravenous lines should be sited. The lines should be in large veins because many AEDs cause phlebitis and thrombosis at the site of infusion.

TABLE 35 EMERGENCY AED REGIMEN FOR STATUS IN NEWLY PRESENTING ADULT PATIENTS (SEE ALSO FIG. 25)

Duration of seizure	Treatment
Before admission	Diazepam 10–20 mg given rectally, repeated once 15 minutes later if status continues to threaten; or midazolam 10 mg given buccally *If seizures continue, treat as below*
Early status	Lorazepam 0.07 mg/kg iv (usually a 4-mg bolus, repeated once after 10–20 minutes; the rate is not critical) *If seizures continue 30 minutes after first injection, treat as below*
Established status	Phenytoin infusion at a dose of 15–18 mg/kg at a rate of 50 mg/min *or* Fosphenytoin infusion at a dose of 15–20 mg phenytoin equivalent/kg at a rate of 150 mg phenytoin equivalent/min *and/or* Phenobarbital bolus of 10 mg/kg at a rate of 100 mg/min (usually 700 mg over 7 minutes in an adult)
Refractory status	General anaesthesia, with propofol, midazolam or thiopental Anaesthetic continued for 12–24 hours after the last clinical or electrographic seizure, then dose tapered

Prevent injury to the patient by nursing with the cot sides up.

Monitoring Ensure there are regular neurological observations and recording of vital signs, eg ECG monitor. Metabolic abnormalities may cause status epilepticus or develop during its course, hence frequent repeated biochemical/haematological and arterial blood gas analysis is required in patients who are not improving.

Treatment Emergency anticonvulsant therapy should be started. Fast-acting benzodiazepines are indicated at this stage, with intravenous lorazepam (0.07 mg/kg to a maximum of 4 mg, repeated once if seizure activity does not stop) the drug of choice in most clinical settings. Other benzodiazepines such as diazepam, clonazepam and midazolam are alternatives, but lorazepam is preferred due to its more prolonged action.

If hypoglycaemia is suspected, 50 mL of a 50% dextrose solution should be given immediately by intravenous injection. If there is a history of alcoholism, or other compromised nutritional states, 250 mg of thiamine should also be given intravenously, with facilities for treating anaphylaxis. Routine glucose administration in non-hypoglycaemic patients should be avoided, as there is some evidence that this can aggravate neuronal damage.

Established status epilepticus (30–60/90 minutes)

Supportive The physiological changes of uncompensated status epilepticus may require specific therapy. Active treatment is most commonly required for hypoxia, hypotension, raised intracranial pressure, pulmonary oedema and hypertension, cardiac arrhythmias,

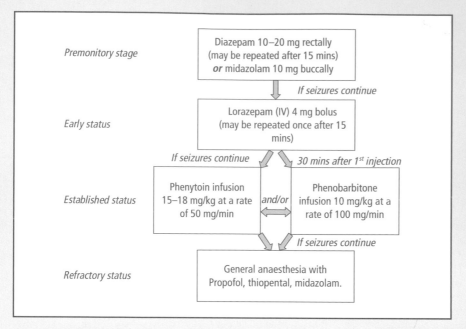

Premonitory stage	Diazepam 10–20 mg rectally (may be repeated after 15 mins) **or** midazolam 10 mg buccally
Early status	*If seizures continue* → Lorazepam (IV) 4 mg bolus (may be repeated once after 15 mins)
Established status	Phenytoin infusion 15–18 mg/kg at a rate of 50 mg/min *and/or* Phenobarbitone infusion 10 mg/kg at a rate of 100 mg/min
Refractory status	General anaesthesia with Propofol, thiopental, midazolam.

▲**Fig. 25** Flow diagram illustrating optimal treatment of status epilepticus.

cardiac failure, lactic acidosis, hyperpyrexia, hypoglycaemia, electrolyte disturbance, acute hepatic or renal failure, rhabdomyolysis or disseminated intravascular coagulation.

> It is frequently suggested that in the presence of acidosis the administration of bicarbonate may prevent shock and mitigate the effects of hypotension and reduced cerebral blood flow. However, in most cases this is unnecessary: adequate support of respiration and abolition of motor seizure activity is more effective.

Monitoring If seizures continue despite the measures taken above, the patient must be transferred to an intensive-care environment.

Treatment There are three alternative treatment options: fosphenytoin, phenytoin and phenobarbital (Table 35). All are given by intravenous loading followed by repeated oral or intravenous supplementation, eg phenytoin 5–6 mg/kg daily, titrated to serum levels.

There are numerous alternative treatment options. Although once popular, continuous benzodiazepine and clomethiazole (chlormethiazole) infusions are hazardous (on a general medical ward) and are not now recommended. There have been uncontrolled studies of intravenous sodium valproate at doses of at least 15 mg/kg followed by an infusion of 1 mg/kg per hour, but experience remains limited.

> **Establish the aetiology**
>
> The range of causes of status epilepticus depends primarily on the patient's age and the presence or absence of established epilepsy (Table 33). The investigations required depend on clinical circumstances, with CT/MRI scans and cerebrospinal fluid examination often required. The latter should be carried out only with facilities for resuscitation available as intracranial pressure is often elevated in status epilepticus. If the status epilepticus has been precipitated by drug withdrawal, immediate recommencement of the withdrawn drug will usually rapidly terminate the status epilepticus.

Refractory status epilepticus (after 60/90 minutes)

If seizures continue for 60–90 minutes after the initiation of therapy, the stage of refractory status epilepticus is reached and full anaesthesia is required.

Supportive Full intensive-care support should continue.

Monitoring In prolonged status epilepticus or in comatose ventilated patients, motor activity can be barely visible. In this situation, continuous electroencephalogram (EEG) monitoring using a full EEG or cerebral function monitor is necessary, and at the very least intermittent daily EEGs should be recorded, aiming for a particular EEG pattern termed 'burst suppression' (Fig. 26).

Continuous intracranial pressure monitoring is sometimes needed, especially in children experiencing persisting, severe or progressive elevated intracranial pressure.

Treatment Anaesthesia can be induced by barbiturate or non-barbiturate drugs, although few have been subjected to formal evaluation and all have drawbacks. Most commonly used are the intravenous barbiturate thiopental, the intravenous non-barbiturate propofol or continuous midazolam infusion.

Long-term maintenance anticonvulsant therapy must be given in tandem with emergency treatment. The choice of drug depends on previous therapy, the type of epilepsy and the clinical setting. If phenytoin or phenobarbital has been used in emergency treatment, maintenance doses can be continued orally (through a nasogastric tube), guided by serum level monitoring. Other maintenance AEDs can also be started with oral loading doses.

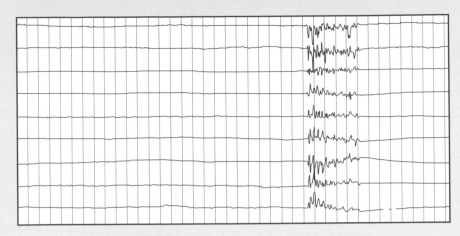

▲**Fig. 26** Electroencephalogram recording of burst suppression. Burst suppression provides an arbitrary physiological target for the titration of barbiturate or anaesthetic therapy. Drug dosing is commonly set at a level that will produce burst suppression, with inter-burst intervals of 2–30 seconds.

Care needs to be taken with nasogastric feeds, which can interfere with the absorption of some AEDs (especially phenytoin).

Anaesthesia should be slowly withdrawn once the patient has been free of seizures for 12–24 hours and provided that there are adequate plasma levels of concomitant antiepileptic medication.

⚠ Magnesium

Although effective in preventing eclampsia, there is no evidence that increasing magnesium serum concentrations to supranormal levels has any benefit in status epilepticus. Indeed, such a policy can result in motor paralysis, difficulty in detecting clinical seizure activity and hypotension. However, serum magnesium can be low in alcoholics and patients on medication for HIV, and in these patients intravenous loading with magnesium sulphate may help with seizure control and prevention of arrhythmias.

Further comments

Is it possible to avert status epilepticus at a very early stage?
In patients with established epilepsy, status epilepticus seldom develops without warning. Usually there is a prodromal phase (premonitory stage) during which seizures become increasingly frequent or severe. The earlier treatment is given the better, and urgent drug treatment will usually prevent the evolution into true status epilepticus. Diazepam has generally been the drug of choice. Alternatives include midazolam, which has the advantage over other benzodiazepines in that it can be administered by intranasal, buccal and intramuscular routes, with buccal midazolam (10 mg in 2 mL) seeming to be the most promising. The acute administration of either diazepam or midazolam will cause drowsiness or sleep, and occasionally cardiorespiratory collapse. Therefore, patients should be carefully supervised. If regular antiepileptic treatment has been reduced or stopped by the patient or doctor, then this should be reinstated.

Are there forms of status epilepticus other than convulsive?
The term 'typical absence status epilepticus' should be reserved for prolonged absence attacks with a continuous or discontinuous 3-Hz spike and wave occurring in patients with primary generalised epilepsy. There is no evidence that absence status induces neuronal damage and thus aggressive treatment is not warranted. Treatment can either be intravenous or oral, with intravenous benzodiazepines so effective that the response is diagnostic.

Complex partial status epilepticus
Complex partial status epilepticus has to be differentiated not only from other forms of non-convulsive status epilepticus but also from post-ictal states and other neurological and psychiatric conditions. It presents in a variety of ways, but typically with a confusional state with variable clinical symptoms. An EEG can be helpful, but often the scalp EEG changes are non-specific and the diagnosis is chiefly made on clinical grounds. Treatment with oral or rectal benzodiazepines is recommended; oral clobazam has proven to be an effective treatment. Treatment of the underlying cause (eg encephalitis or metabolic derangement) is paramount and can often lead to resolution of the status epilepticus.

⚠ Non-epileptic status (pseudo-status)

Due to the inherent morbidity and mortality of the management of status epilepticus, this is an extremely important diagnosis to make before escalation of AED treatment and admission to the intensive care unit. Often, however, the diagnosis is made only when EEG monitoring has been established.

1.4.5 Encephalopathy/coma

Scenario

A 70-year-old man is found collapsed in his home by a neighbour and is brought in by ambulance. He is unconscious with a Glasgow Coma Scale (GCS) score of 8. You are called to the Emergency Department to review him.

Introduction

What are the causes of encephalopathy/coma?

There is a wide differential diagnosis to encephalopathy, ie impairment of cerebral function associated with loss or disturbance of consciousness. A systematic approach to assessing the patient is required. A list of common causes of encephalopathy and coma is shown in Table 36.

History of the presenting problem

It is clearly not possible to obtain any history from a patient who is unconscious, but after rapid initial examination and instigation of immediate treatment (see below) you should do the following.

- Talk with any witnesses available: family/friends who have accompanied the patient or ambulance/paramedical staff. In this case, has the neighbour come to hospital with him and, if so, what were the circumstances in which he was found? Is the patient known to have epilepsy? Does he have any other medical conditions, eg diabetes? Has he been unwell recently (and in what way), suffered any injury to the head or been using alcohol or drugs?

- Read all records completed by ambulance staff or others.

Examination: general features

- Check airway, breathing and circulation. Monitor oxygenation with a pulse oximeter.

- Check vital signs: temperature, pulse, BP and respiratory rate.

- Look for evidence of head injury or neck stiffness: consider intracerebral bleeding or meningitis (much less likely).

- Look for clues that the patient may have diabetes, epilepsy or other medical condition, eg Medic-Alert bracelet, prescription/medications or an appointment card for an outpatient clinic.

Neurological examination

Check GCS (Table 37).

Are there any focal neurological features? Look in particular for facial asymmetry, ocular deviation and lateralising responses when assessing GCS. The presence of focal signs suggests a focal rather than metabolic cause. Place particular emphasis on those signs listed in Table 38.

If the patient can communicate, then an assessment of cognitive status should be made (see Section 1.2.17).

Investigation

Urgent in all patients

- Check fingerprick blood glucose concentration: if <2.5 mmol/L, immediately give intravenous glucose/dextrose (see Section 1.4.4).

- Conduct a CT brain scan if coma is worsening (GCS falling); this is also required (less urgently) if stable coma with focal neurological signs or diagnosis remains uncertain.

Routine in all patients

- Check FBC, clotting screen, glucose (laboratory), electrolytes

TABLE 36 CAUSES OF COMA AND ENCEPHALOPATHY

Causes	Diagnoses
Vascular	Ischaemic or haemorrhagic stroke; subarachnoid, subdural or extradural haemorrhage
Metabolic	Hypoglycaemia, uraemia, hepatic encephalopathy, carbon dioxide and carbon monoxide, hypoxia, acidosis (eg diabetic), hyponatraemia, hypernatraemia/calcaemia, hypothyroidism
Drugs	Alcohol, opioids, benzodiazepines and other central nervous system (CNS) depressants
Epilepsy	Post-ictal/status epilepticus
Infection	CNS sepsis, eg meningoencephalitis or an abscess
Hypothermia	
Trauma	Head injury

Note that any cause of severe hypotension can lead to encephalopathy/coma, in which case the primary aim must be to diagnose and correct the cause of hypotension, at which point the patient's conscious level can be reassessed. If it remains depressed, then the diagnoses listed here need to be considered.

TABLE 37 GLASGOW COMA SCALE

Domain	Finding	Score
Best eye opening response	Spontaneously	4
	To speech	3
	To pain	2
	None	1
Best verbal response	Orientated	5
	Confused conversation	4
	Words	3
	Sounds	2
	None	1
Best motor response (in any limb)	Obeys commands	6
	Localisation to painful stimuli	5
	Withdraws to pain	4
	Flexor (decorticate) response to pain	3
	Extensor (decerebrate) response to pain	2
	No response	1

1. Add scores in the three domains: minimum 3 and maximum 15, with coma defined as 8 or less.
2. Do not use methods of applying painful stimuli that cause bruising or bleeding: rubbing the sternum with your knuckles and applying pressure to the nail bed with a pencil or pen are recommended.

Contraindications to lumbar puncture

Do not perform lumbar puncture if there is:

1. clinical suspicion of raised intracranial pressure, such as drowsiness/coma, papilloedema or focal neurological signs, unless a CT scan shows no features of raised intracranial pressure; or
2. CT scan shows mass lesion or other evidence of raised intracranial pressure.

Risk is of transforaminal herniation or 'coning'.

Management

Management of coma

- Give 50 mL of 50% dextrose intravenously if fingerprick blood glucose <2.5 mmol/L.
- Give 0.4–1.2 mg naloxone intravenously if there is clinical suspicion of opioid overdose (small pupils and low respiratory rate).

and renal/liver/bone function tests.

- ECG: note that abnormalities mimicking cardiac ischaemia can be seen with some intracranial pathologies, eg subarachnoid haemorrhage.

- CXR: look for signs of aspiration.

Consider depending on clinical context

Lumbar puncture, if the diagnosis is not established and a CT scan shows no evidence of raised intracranial pressure. Also consider arterial blood gases; sepsis screen, including (when appropriate) thick film for malaria; MRI brain scan; and electroencephalogram.

General supportive care

- The most important priority is always to maintain the airway and ensure adequate ventilation.

TABLE 38 IMPORTANT NEUROLOGICAL SIGNS IN PATIENTS WITH COMA

Sign	Finding	Interpretation
Fundoscopy	Haemorrhages	Trauma or subarachnoid haemorrhage
	Hypertensive/diabetic retinopathy	Increased risk of cerebrovascular disease
	Papilloedema	Raised intracranial pressure
Pupillary reflexes	Dilated pupil/third nerve palsy	False localising sign
	Miotic pupil	Opioids or pontine lesion (Horner's syndrome)
Doll's head and caloric eye movements	Abnormal	Midbrain/pontine dysfunction
Corneal reflex	Absent	Pontine dysfunction
Gag reflex	Absent	Medulla dysfunction
Jaw jerk	Brisk	Suggests suprapontine lesion
Tone	Increased	Extrapyramidal/pyramidal disease (not acute)
Limb movements	Asymmetrical	Focal lesion in pyramidal tract
Reflexes	Asymmetry or hyperreflexia	Pyramidal tract lesions
Plantars	Extensor	Pyramidal tract lesions

TABLE 39 DIAGNOSIS OF BRAINSTEM DEATH

Conditions	Criteria
Preconditions	Diagnosis must confirm irreversible aetiology Patient must be in unresponsive coma (spinal reflexes do not exclude diagnosis)
Exclusions	Drugs, eg narcotics, hypnotics or muscle relaxants Metabolic or endocrine causes of coma Hypothermia (<35°C)
Clinical criteria	No pupillary response to light Absent corneal reflexes Absent vestibulo-ocular reflexes (no nystagmus with instillation of 20 mL of cold fluid into unblocked ears) No motor response within cranial nerve distribution to painful stimulation of face, trunk or limbs Absent gag reflex Absent cough reflex Absence of spontaneous respiration (after ventilating with oxygen to prevent hypoxia, disconnect from ventilator and allow $Paco_2$ to rise to more than 7 kPa)

The diagnosis of brainstem death must be confirmed by two competent medical practitioners who test the patient either separately or jointly on two occasions, usually 1–6 hours apart (other conditions also apply).

> ⚠️ Do not forget that *Listeria* meningitis is the second commonest cause of bacterial meningitis in the elderly and this responds to high-dose amoxicillin but not so well to third-generation cephalosporins.

Unless there is suspicion of an injury to the cervical spine, nurse the patient in the recovery position with high-flow oxygen delivered by face mask. In general, if the patient's GCS is <8, then an anaesthetist should be called immediately to monitor and protect the airway.

- Monitor the patient's pulse (continuous ECG), BP, respiratory rate, oxygenation (pulse oximeter) and temperature.

- Give intravenous fluids to maintain hydration and correct any electrolyte disturbance; also a urinary catheter to monitor urine output and protect the skin from soiling.

- Turn the patient over regularly to prevent pressure area damage.

- Give low-molecular-weight heparin to prevent thromboembolism (unless there is clear contraindication).

Specific care

As determined by cause of encephalopathy/coma.

- Anticonvulsants should be commenced for prolonged (>5 minutes) or recurrent seizures (see Section 1.4.4).

- Broad-spectrum antibiotics should be given if there is even a slight chance of bacterial meningitis.

- Consider herpes encephalitis when there is a preceding history of personality change, seizures or immunosuppression and give the patient empirical high-dose aciclovir. Other viral, bacterial and atypical organisms should be considered in the immunosuppressed patient, in which case close consultation with the local microbiologist is essential.

- If encephalopathy is prolonged (>24 hours), start nasogastric feeding.

Further comments

The prognosis of coma due to CNS suppressant drugs, metabolic/infective encephalopathies and seizures is often very good and patients may make a full recovery.

Patients in prolonged coma/encephalopathy with a persistent GCS of <8 have a particularly poor prognosis: 50% will die and only a small proportion will regain independent living.

Brainstem death is the legal definition of death in the UK (Table 39).

2.1 Peripheral neuropathies and diseases of the lower motor neuron

2.1.1 Peripheral neuropathies

Pathophysiology

Peripheral nerves contain bundles of nerve fibres, both large-diameter myelinated fibres and small-diameter non-myelinated fibres. The large myelinated fibres carry both efferent motor signals and afferent sensory signals (proprioception and vibration sense). The small non-myelinated fibres carry afferent pain and temperature as well as autonomic signals. The peripheral nerve can react to injury or insult in one of four ways: axonal degeneration, demyelination, Wallerian degeneration and neuronal cell body disease (neuronopathy).

Axonal degeneration

This is the commonest pathological process encountered in peripheral neuropathies, particularly those associated with systemic, toxic, nutritional and metabolic disorders. The commonest aetiology is diabetes mellitus (Table 40), the commonest cause of neuropathy in the UK (three-quarters of these cases being a distal symmetrical sensory or sensorimotor polyneuropathy). Large-diameter fibres are predominantly involved, and the longest fibres are affected first by this degenerative process.

Demyelination

Destruction of the myelin sheath, leaving the axon intact, leads to segmental demyelination, which is commonly secondary to an immune-mediated disorder (Table 41). Demyelination may occur distally or proximally and is patchy.

Wallerian degeneration

This is the name given to the degenerative process of the distal stump seen after nerve transection (or an equivalent insult). Regeneration from the proximal stump is slow and variable.

Neuronopathy

Neuronopathy describes a disease process that specifically attacks the neuronal cell bodies. In the case of motor nerves this occurs within the anterior horn of the spinal cord, and in the case of sensory nerves within the dorsal root ganglion. Examples of motor neuronopathies include motor neuron disease, spinal muscular atrophies and poliomyelitis. The sensory ganglion cell may be the primary site of injury in paraneoplastic neuropathies (see Section 2.11.1) or in Sjögren's syndrome.

Clinical presentation

The commonest type of neuropathy is the distal symmetrical sensorimotor axonal type. Patients will first complain of tingling, burning or band-like sensations in the toes or soles of the feet. As the symptoms progress the sensory disturbance will extend onto the dorsum of the foot and the ankle reflexes will be lost; there may also be weakness of dorsiflexion of the toes and ankle and possibly muscle wasting. Patients may complain of a feeling of walking on cotton wool or on stumps. Progression may lead to foot drop and a high-stepping gait; knee reflexes will be lost. Sensory symptoms in the fingertips do not develop until those in the leg have ascended to at least the knee. The patient's gait may become unsteady due to proprioceptive loss. Progression continues smoothly, moving centrally up the arms and legs in a symmetrical fashion, eventually affecting the anterior torso. In extreme cases involvement of the

TABLE 40 CLASSIFICATION OF DIABETIC NEUROPATHIES	
Type	Diagnoses
Symmetrical polyneuropathies	Distal sensory or sensorimotor polyneuropathy Large-fibre neuropathy ('diabetic pseudotabes')
Asymmetrical polyneuropathies	Cranial neuropathy (single or multiple) Limb mononeuropathy (single or multiple) Trunk mononeuropathy (single or multiple) Proximal diabetic neuropathy/diabetic amyotrophy

TABLE 41 CAUSES OF NEUROPATHIES

Type	Cause	Type	Cause
Sensorimotor polyneuropathy	Alcohol Diabetes mellitus Hypothyroidism GBS CIDP HMSN Vasculitis Paraneoplastic Paraproteinaemic	Painful	GBS Vasculitis Amyloidosis HIV Leprosy Malignant infiltration Diabetes mellitus Uraemia
Sensory polyneuropathy	Diabetes mellitus Hypothyroidism Drugs, eg isoniazid and vincristine Vitamin B_{12} deficiency Paraneoplastic Amyloidosis HIV Leprosy	Demyelinating	GBS/CIDP MMN Paraproteinaemic HIV Drugs (amiodarone) HMSN 1
Motor neuropathy	GBS/CIDP MMN Porphyria Lead Diphtheria	Axonal (small fibre)	Amyloid Leprosy HIV Diabetes mellitus (rare) HSAN Fabry's disease Tangier disease
Focal/multifocal neuropathies	Connective tissue disorders Vasculitis Granulomatous disorders, eg Wegener's granulomatosis and sarcoidosis Carcinomatous infiltration Nerve compression, eg common peroneal nerve palsy HIV Leprosy HNLPP Diabetes mellitus Fabry's disease	Axonal (large fibre)	Vasculitis Paraneoplastic Toxins Diabetes mellitus Porphyria Uraemia Vitamin B_{12} deficiency HMSN 2 Friedreich's ataxia
		Autonomic	GBS/CIDP[1] HIV Paraneoplastic[1] Porphyria[1] Diabetes mellitus Toxins[1] HSAN Amyloidosis

1. Predominantly acute.
CIDP, chronic inflammatory demyelinating polyneuropathy; GBS, Guillain–Barré syndrome; HMSN, hereditary motor and sensory neuropathy; HNLPP, hereditary neuropathy with liability to pressure palsies; HSAN, hereditary sensory and autonomic neuropathy; MMN, multifocal motor neuropathy with conduction block.

intercostal and diaphragmatic muscles leads to ventilatory disturbance.

Variations from this clinical picture are discussed below.

Axonal vs demyelinating neuropathies

Although the pathological process cannot be reliably distinguished clinically, the following may act as pointers.

- Concurrent proximal and distal involvement suggests a demyelinating process. Remember that axonal degeneration is a distal degenerative process, and demyelination can occur anywhere on the nerve.

- Loss of all reflexes early in the process, rather than sequential loss as described above, might suggest demyelination.

Asymmetry

Asymmetry of clinical findings suggests a multifocal process affecting individual nerve trunks or roots.

Large-fibre vs small-fibre neuropathies

In small-fibre neuropathies, the following are more likely.

- No significant weakness (motor fibres are large myelinated axons).

- Preserved reflexes (the fibres subserving the afferent limb of the muscle stretch reflex arc are large myelinated axons, as are the efferent motor fibres).

- Preserved balance (proprioceptive information is conducted in large myelinated axons).

- Reduced pinprick and temperature sensation.

- Sometimes autonomic disturbance.

Arms vs legs

It is unusual for the first symptoms of a peripheral neuropathy to be in the arms, and this should suggest the diagnoses below. Neuropathies that can present in the arms before the legs include:

- GBS/CIDP;

- porphyria;

- spinal muscular atrophy;

- HMSN;

- vitamin B_{12} deficiency (sensory symptoms).

Investigation

Peripheral neuropathies are often investigated with a blanket screening process. It is hoped that the preceding description of different types of neuropathy makes it clear that in some circumstances investigations can be targeted. Where this is not the case, blood screening is performed to consider the common or treatable causes of peripheral neuropathy.

Carpal tunnel syndrome

- Bilateral carpal tunnel syndrome may initially be mistaken for a peripheral neuropathy.

- Patients complain of nocturnal paraesthesia, numbness or burning sensations, often describing how they shake their hands or hang them over the side of the bed for relief.
- Symptoms may be confined to the thumb, index, middle and lateral half of the ring finger, but are often more diffuse, extending to the elbow and sometimes to the shoulder.
- Look for reduced sensation on the lateral part of the palm and splitting of the ring finger, and in more severe cases wasting of the thenar eminence and weakness of the abductor pollicis brevis.
- In mild cases the diagnosis is made on the history and confirmed electrophysiologically.

Other upper limb entrapment neuropathies

See Fig. 27 and Sections 1.2.2 and 1.2.6.

Lower trunk of brachial plexus

Mainly affected by cervical rib syndrome, altered anatomy, cervical outlet syndrome, brachial neuritis or Pancoast tumour of the lung apex.

Axillary nerve

Damaged by fracture of humeral neck, dislocation of shoulder and deep intramuscular injections (Fig. 27).

Radial nerve

May be damaged at the following sites.

- Axilla: damaged by weight-bearing on a crutch or resting the arm over back of chair while asleep or intoxicated.
- Spiral groove of humerus: vunerable to direct blow laterally (during anaesthesia or while drunk), medially or after mid-shaft humeral fracture (which may be either immediate or delayed as callus forms).
- Supinator muscle: the radial nerve (posterior interosseous nerve) passes through the supinator and may be damaged by occupational overuse or acute haemorrhage into muscle during trauma.

Ulnar nerve

May be damaged at the following sites.

- Elbow: often damaged by repeated minor trauma and prolonged bed-rest (patient resting on elbows), or delayed following fractures in childhood leading to minor anatomical abnormality (tardy ulnar palsy).
- Palm: deep branch damaged by trauma to the heel of the hand or idiopathically due to a ganglion. Confusing clinically as often there is no sensory loss and it is often mistaken for motor neuron disease (Fig. 28).

Median nerve

May be damaged at the following sites.

- Elbow: rarely damaged by direct trauma but may be involved in elbow fracture as deeply placed.
- Forearm: the anterior interosseous branch of the median nerve is a rarely damaged nerve that lies very deep; flexors of index finger and thumb are affected by it (ie pinch grip). Haemorrhage into the muscle during physical exertion is the most common cause of damage.
- Wrist: see carpal tunnel syndrome above (Fig. 28).

Blood tests

FBC, erythrocyte sedimentation rate, vitamin B_{12}/folate, urea and electrolytes, glucose, liver funtion tests, thyroid function tests and C-reactive protein. Special blood tests include antinuclear antibodies, extractable nuclear antigens, antineutrophil cytoplasmic antibodies, antineuronal antibodies, heavy metals, porphyrins and genetic testing.

Nerve conduction studies and electromyography

These tests should be able to determine whether the neuropathy is:

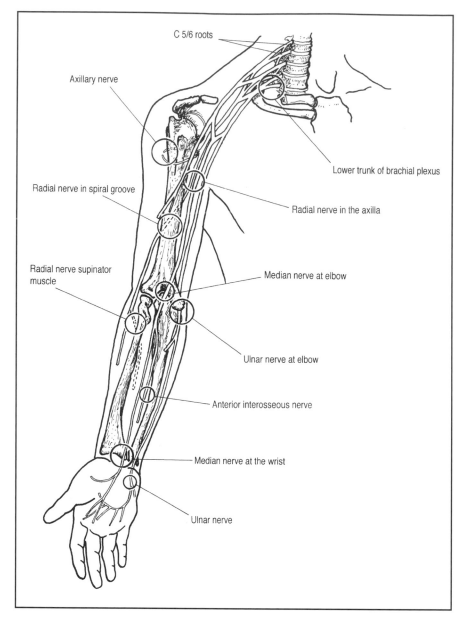

C 5/6 roots

Axillary nerve

Radial nerve in spiral groove

Radial nerve supinator muscle

Lower trunk of brachial plexus

Radial nerve in the axilla

Median nerve at elbow

Ulnar nerve at elbow

Anterior interosseous nerve

Median nerve at the wrist

Ulnar nerve

▲**Fig. 27** Neurological anatomy of the arm showing main locations of damage.

- generalised or multifocal;

- motor and/or sensory;

- axonal or demyelinating.

Standard nerve conduction studies (see Section 3.3) only detect abnormalities of large fibres. Hence a patient presenting with distal reduction in pain and temperature as well as preserved proprioception and reflexes may have normal nerve conduction studies. A more specialised test (detection of thermal thresholds) is required to detect an isolated small-fibre neuropathy.

If relevant, limited nerve conduction studies of affected family members should be performed.

Cerebrospinal fluid examination
This is not usually required for diagnosis, but may be helpful in inflammatory neuropathies with proximal involvement (elevated protein). Paraneoplastic neuropathies may also be associated with elevated protein. An elevated white cell count in a patient with suspected GBS should raise the possibility of HIV-associated inflammatory neuropathy.

Hunt for underlying malignancy
This is often unrewarding, but should be guided by other symptoms, eg chest, abdomen and blood film.

Nerve biopsy
Nerve biopsy is an invasive procedure and should only be carried out in a specialist centre. You need to consider whether management is being helped, as diagnostic yields are often low. It is usual to biopsy either the superficial radial or sural nerve, readily accessible pure sensory nerves. If the process is exclusively motor, another nerve must be used. As with other tissue sampling it is preferable that the chosen nerve is involved clinically but not severely affected, in which case only end-stage disease process may be seen with little or no diagnostic value. Biopsies may show diagnostic abnormalities in vasculitis or amyloidosis. In the case of hereditary neuropathies, the availability of genetic testing is making the role of nerve biopsies less important.

Management
Depends on the underlying cause. Remove any insult or correct any metabolic/endocrine abnormality as appropriate. While this may prevent further nerve damage, axonal recovery in particular is slow.

Inflammatory
Unlike GBS, CIDP may respond to steroids. Like GBS, both plasma exchange and intravenous immunoglobulin (IVIG) have equal efficacy. Some clinicians try a 6–8 week course of high-dose oral

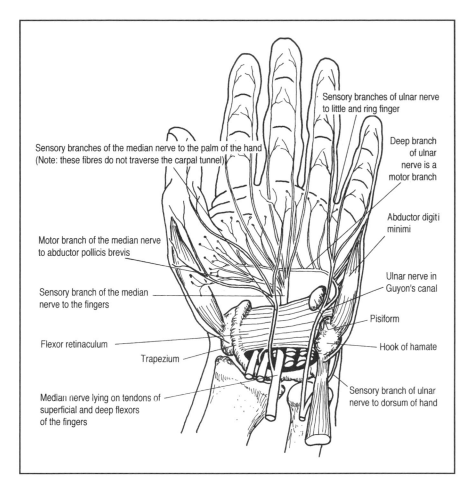

▲**Fig. 28** Anatomy of the median and ulnar nerves in the hand.

prednisolone and reserve IVIG for cases not responsive to steroids. Others use IVIG as a first-line treatment. Treatment courses may need to be repeated if the condition relapses and some patients become treatment dependent, requiring regular IVIG to maintain well-being.

Vasculitic neuropathy
Initial treatment is with high-dose oral prednisolone or, if severe, a short course of intravenous methylprednisolone followed by maintenance oral steroids. The use of IVIG is anecdotal but would appear sensible and is becoming more widely used. Systemic necrotising vasculitides may require cyclophosphamide.

Paraneoplastic neuropathy
See Section 2.11.1.

2.1.2 Guillain–Barré syndrome
This is an acute (postinfectious) inflammatory demyelinating polyneuropathy, affecting 2 per 100,000 per annum. It is usually monophasic, but relapses have been described.

Pathology
This is an inflammatory condition that leads to multifocal demyelination of spinal roots and peripheral nerves. Demyelination may occur anywhere along the lower motor nerve pathway, but the ventral (motor) roots, proximal spinal nerves and lower cranial nerves are most often affected, which accounts for the pattern of clinical features. Much evidence suggests that Guillain–Barré syndrome (GBS) is an organ-specific autoimmune disorder mediated by autoreactive T cells and humoral antibodies to peripheral nerve antigens. Preceding infections, particularly *Campylobacter jejuni*, may trigger this response through molecular mimicry.

Clinical presentation
Approximately 60–70% of sufferers report an illness in the preceding weeks (often 1–4 weeks prior to the onset). This is usually an upper respiratory tract illness or diarrhoea, and many pathogens have been implicated (Table 42).

The onset is subacute, usually over a few days, but can be rapid with complete paralysis in hours. However, the progression of symptoms may continue for up

TABLE 42 COMMON PATHOGENS IMPLICATED IN GBS	
Cause	**Diagnoses**
Viral	Cytomegalovirus
	Epstein–Barr virus
	HIV
	Hepatitis A
Bacterial	Mycoplasma
	Campylobacter jejuni
Immunisation	Tetanus toxoid
	Rabies
	Swine influenza

to 4 weeks (but no longer, by definition).

The main complaints are of ascending sensory symptoms (symptoms are more prominent than sensory signs) and ascending, or occasionally proximal, weakness. In most cases the legs are affected first and to a greater degree than the arms, but occasionally the arms can be worst affected. Muscle pain is common, frequently manifesting as deep intrascapular or lower back pain, or even initiating bilateral sciatica.

Physical signs

The main signs are of symmetrically reduced tone, areflexia, a varying degree of glove-and-stocking sensory disturbance (often mild), and lower motor neuron weakness. Facial involvement and ophthalmoplegia may be present.

Autonomic features occur in approximately half the patients (fluctuations in BP, heart rate, ileus and urinary retention).

> The clinician must be aware that fixed pupils can occur with autonomic involvement and this must not be confused with brainstem pathology.

Other clinical variants of GBS include:

- Miller Fisher syndrome (ataxia, areflexia and ophthalmoplegia).

- cranial nerve variant (polyneuritis cranialis);

- pure sensory variant;

- pharyngeal–cervical–brachial variant;

- acute autonomic variant;

- axonal variant (motor and sensory);

- acute motor axonal variant.

Investigations

If the condition is suspected clinically, your priorities are to monitor for potential complications, particularly respiratory and cardiac. Further investigations may confirm the diagnosis but are unlikely to be available immediately. Initial management therefore has to be based on clinical suspicion.

Measurement of respiratory function

Monitor forced vital capacity (not peak flow) at regular intervals, the frequency depending on the severity of the weakness or the rate of change.

Cardiac monitor

Doctors are aware of the respiratory complications of GBS but neglect the autonomic complications. Dysrhythmias can be fatal without intervention.

Cerebrospinal fluid

This may be normal in the first few days. Later protein rises as a consequence of inflammation in the proximal roots (within the subarachnoid space). If pleocytosis is present, consider other diagnoses (see Differential diagnosis below).

Nerve conduction studies

In GBS, peripheral nerve demyelination starts proximally at the nerve roots. Distal conduction velocities and distal motor latencies are therefore normal early in the illness, even in the face of profound weakness. The earliest electrophysiological abnormality is prolongation, impersistence or absence of the F wave. The electromyogram (EMG) will show denervation in later stages.

Antiganglioside antibodies

Gangliosides are sialylated glycosphingolipids found on nerves.

Anti-GQ1b antibodies appear to be present in all cases of GBS with associated ophthalmoplegia, particularly the Miller Fisher variant (triad of ataxia, areflexia and ophthalmoplegia).

Identification of the infective agent

- Results can often be negative, but may help with prognosis if positive.

- Stool culture for *Campylobacter jejuni*.

- Serology for atypical pneumonias.

- Cerebrospinal fluid (CSF) viral analysis.

Differential diagnosis

The differential diagnosis of acute/subacute weakness is broad but important. Given a good history together with examination features that are clear, then GBS is the commonest cause, but also consider the following.

- Other acute neuropathies including porphyria.

- Metabolic disturbances (severe hypophosphataemia, hypokalaemia and hypermagnesaemia) should be excluded.

- Myasthenia gravis may cause subacute onset weakness. Look for fatiguability.

- Occasionally central nervous system disease, such as acute brainstem stroke, spinal cord compression or transverse myelitis, may cause confusion, but a careful history and examination should prevent this mistake from being made.

- Poliomyelitis is now a less common differential. The presentation is usually strikingly asymmetrical, which helps differentiate it from the symmetrical picture of GBS.

- Typical features of GBS associated with CSF pleocytosis (cell count $>50 \times 10^6$/L) raise the possibility of meningoradiculitis caused by HIV, Lyme disease, tuberculosis or cytomegalovirus infection.

Treatment

The following points need to be considered.

- Patients who are deteriorating should be transferred to a unit able to deal with neuromuscular respiratory failure and autonomic dysfunction.

- Consider elective ventilation early if the patient is tiring.

- Cardiac arrhythmias should be treated as appropriate.

- Antihypertensive drugs must be used with extreme caution in the presence of autonomic dysfunction.

- Note that tracheal suction may trigger hypotension or bradycardia in the presence of autonomic dysfunction.

- Treat pain with NSAIDs or opiates.

- Feed patients via nasogastric tube or percutaneous endoscopic gastrostomy if necessary.

- Prophylactic subcutaneous heparin and thromboembolic stockings for immobile patients.

- Regular chest physiotherapy.

- Regular turning.

- Early physiotherapy.

- Psychological support for the patient and the family.

Specific treatment

A 5-day course of intravenous immunoglobulin (IVIG) (0.4 g/kg daily) is as efficacious as plasma exchange but with fewer side effects. Plasma exchange followed by IVIG does not confer a significant advantage. Patients with mild GBS do not require treatment.

> IVIG is easily administered. This should not dissuade the clinician from early transfer of the patient to a centre with a good intensive care unit. If a patient requires treatment, then transfer is necessary.

Prognosis

GBS begins with a period of deterioration, then a plateau phase, followed by a period of recovery. In series, up to 30% of patients require ventilation. Mortality remains about 4.5% despite treatment. On the whole this is a self-limiting disease. In very broad terms, one-third of patients make a full recovery (although remaining areflexic), one-third are left with mild disability and one-third have moderate to severe disability.

> Preceding illness with *Campylobacter jejuni* can result in a severe axonal variant with a poor prognosis.

FURTHER READING

Hughes RA and Cornblath DR. Guillain–Barré syndrome. *Lancet* 2005; 366: 1653–66.

2.1.3 Motor neuron disease

Aetiology

The causes of motor neuron disease (MND) are unknown, but many hypotheses have been suggested.

Mutations in the cytosolic Cu/Zn superoxide dismutase gene on chromosome 21 accounts for 20% of cases of familial amyotrophic lateral sclerosis (ALS) and 2% of the total cases of ALS. Glutamate is a major excitatory neurotransmitter, and overstimulation of glutamate receptors is associated with neurotoxicity in MND. Oxidative stress with free radical damage is also implicated in the pathogenesis of MND. Dysregulation of the vascular endothelial growth factor (VEGF), protein aggregation in the motor neuron, mitochondrial dysfunction and neuroinflammation modulated by non-neuronal cells may also play a part.

Epidemiology

The incidence of MND is 1–3 per 100,000, with the mean age of onset being 55 years. The male to female ratio is 3:2, and 10% of cases are familial, usually of an autosomal dominant inheritance. Most cases of MND are of the ALS type that has both upper motor neuron (UMN) and lower motor neuron (LMN) involvement. The other clinical variants, progressive muscular atrophy (PMA) with its purely LMN involvement and primary lateral sclerosis (PLS) with its purely UMN involvement, may just represent ends of the spectrum of ALS.

Clinical presentation

Muscle weakness is the most common presenting complaint, with onset in the arms more common than in the legs. Occasionally, one limb may become involved on its own. Some patients notice muscle twitching or fasciculations, muscle cramps and easy fatiguability.

> ⚠ Fasciculations are virtually never the sole presenting feature of MND.

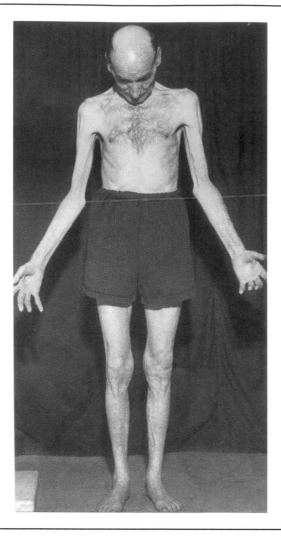

▲**Fig. 29** Wasted muscles in MND.

In 20% of patients, bulbar symptoms are the initial problem, eg dysarthria, dysphagia, difficulty chewing or coughing, and eventually sialorrhoea. Weight loss may occur. Rarely, respiratory muscle weakness causing breathlessness is the first symptom.

Physical signs

Cranial nerve examination may reveal lower cranial nerve involvement, eg facial weakness (VII), depressed gag reflex (IX/X), poor palatal movement (X) and a wasted fasciculating tongue (XII and bulbar palsy). A brisk jaw jerk (V), increased gag reflex or a spastic tongue indicates pseudobulbar palsy.

In the limbs, UMN involvement produces spasticity, weakness, hyperreflexia and Babinski sign, whereas LMN involvement produces atrophy (Fig. 29), fasciculations, flaccidity, weakness and hyporeflexia.

- In MND there is no extraocular or sphincter disturbance, and sensory examination is normal.
- You should never examine for fasciculations when the tongue is protruded, as you will often see 'abnormalities' that are not really present.

Investigation

See Sections 1.1.11 and 1.2.8.

Further points on investigation are as follows.

- Anti-GM1 ganglioside antibodies and electromyography are important in ruling out multifocal motor neuropathy (MMN).

- An MRI scan excludes cervical spine and foramen magnum lesions, eg syringomyelia, syringobulbia and cervical spondylosis.

Differential diagnosis

Misdiagnosis of MND is a common clinical problem with serious implications. Certain differentials should always be considered:

- Spondylotic cervical myelopathy: although this is a potentially treatable condition, there is increasing doubt as to whether it can actually mimic MND as it almost always causes only spastic paraparesis.

- It is important to diagnose MMN because it is potentially treatable with intravenous immunoglobulin or cyclophosphamide. It is associated with LMN signs only and anti-GM1 ganglioside antibodies (although these are not specific).

- X-linked bulbospinal neuronopathy (Kennedy's disease): this is associated with perioral fasciculation, LMN signs only, gynaecomastia, testicular atrophy, diabetes mellitus and a CAG expansion in the androgen receptor locus.

- Benign fasciculations, hexosaminidase A deficiency (Tay–Sachs disease), lymphoproliferative disorders and thyrotoxicosis may all mimic MND and should be excluded in atypical cases.

Treatment

Symptomatic treatment and supportive care are the mainstays of management in MND. The patient's right to self-determination should be respected at all times.

Riluzole, a sodium channel blocker that inhibits glutamate release, has only modest effects on disease progression and is expensive. A patient's FBC and liver function needs to be monitored when it is used.

Prognosis

Death usually ensues in 3–5 years as a result of aspiration pneumonia and respiratory failure.

Poor prognosis factors

- Older patients.
- Shorter duration between onset and diagnosis.
- ALS (rather than PLS or PMA).
- Low-amplitude muscle action potentials.

FURTHER READING

Shaw PJ. Molecular and cellular pathways of neurodegeneration in motor neuron disease. *J. Neurol. Neurosurg. Psychiatry* 2005; 76: 1046–57.

2.2 Diseases of muscle

A wide range of sporadic and hereditary insults can affect muscle, including:

- systemic disorders of metabolism;
- local and systemic inflammatory conditions;
- hereditary disorders of a muscle itself;

Cause	Diagnoses
Metabolic	Disorders of carbohydrate metabolism Disorders of lipid metabolism Mitochondrial myopathies
Inflammatory	Polymyositis Dermatomyositis Inclusion body myositis
Inherited myopathies	Disorders of dystrophin Limb girdle muscular dystrophies Facioscapulohumeral dystrophy Emery–Dreifuss muscular dystrophy Myotonic dystrophy Others
Channelopathies	Periodic paralysis Myotonia

TABLE 43 CLASSIFICATION OF MUSCLE DISEASE

- abnormalities of membrane ion channels.

Presentation may be with weakness, cramps, pain or a combination of these. The age of onset, presence or otherwise of a positive family history, nature of presentation and distribution of muscle involvement are all instructive pointers to the aetiology. A classification of muscle disorders is given in Table 43.

2.2.1 Metabolic muscle disease

Disorders of carbohydrate metabolism (glycogen storage diseases)

Pathophysiology

Figure 30 describes the biochemical pathway by which glycogen metabolism and glycolysis occurs within muscle cells. Deficiencies of the enzymes shown have all been associated with metabolic muscle disease. Clinically, enzyme deficiencies can be divided into those associated with exercise intolerance and those causing progressive muscle weakness.

The most important disease of each group is described below.

McArdle's disease

Also called myophosphorylase deficiency or type V glycogenosis. The same clinical picture is seen with phosphorylase b kinase deficiency (Fig. 30). First described by Dr Brian McArdle in 1952.

Genetics Myophosphorylase gene encoded on 11q13. Usually autosomal recessive but autosomal dominant inheritance has been described.

Clinical presentation Carbohydrate stores within muscle are necessary in the early stages of exercise prior to added energy supply being provided by lipid metabolism. Disorders of carbohydrate metabolism therefore present with exercise intolerance after minimal exercise. A 'second wind' phenomenon may be described if the patient exercises gently through the initial barrier, enabling diversion of blood flow to muscle and the onset of fatty acid metabolism.

Symptoms Often presents in the second and third decade, although

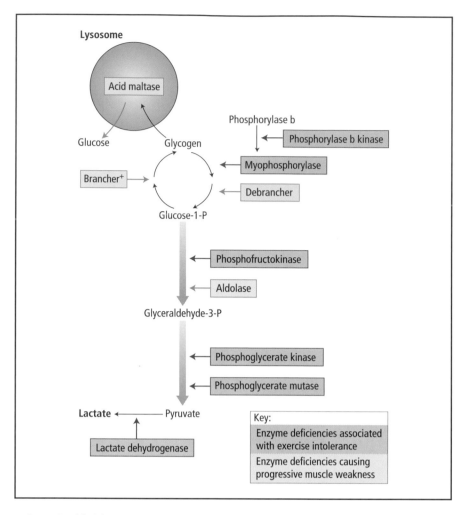

▲**Fig. 30** Simplified diagram of glycogen metabolism and glycolysis.

in retrospect there may have been poor exercise tolerance as a child. Symptoms include:

- muscle pain after minutes of exercise;

- painful muscle contractures;

- episodes of dark urine (myoglobinuria secondary to rhabdomyolysis).

Physical signs Usually no abnormal signs when resting. Patients may develop a mild myopathy late in the disease.

Investigation Consider the following.

- Provocative exercise tests to demonstrate increased creatine

kinase (CK) or a failure to increase lactate (ischaemic lactate test) may precipitate muscle necrosis and are potentially harmful.

- Electromyography (EMG): this may be normal. Painful contractures are electrically silent.

- Muscle biopsy: routine histology may be normal or may show some necrosis. This may show increased glycogen. Specific muscle biochemistry confirms enzyme deficiency.

Acid maltase deficiency
Also called Pompe's disease or type II glycogenosis. First described by Dr J.C. Pompe in 1932.

Clinical presentation There are four types: infantile, late infantile, juvenile and adult, the severity decreasing the later the age of onset. Cardiac involvement is almost invariable in the severe infantile type but is less frequent in the adult form.

Symptoms Progressive weakness. There may be respiratory involvement, often as the prominent feature.

Physical signs Muscle weakness with or without signs of cardiac or respiratory involvement.

Investigation The following will confirm the diagnosis.

- CK may be normal or moderately raised.

- EMG is usually myopathic with neurogenic changes and complex repetitive discharges late in the disease.

- Muscle biopsy demonstrates evidence of increased glycogen storage.

- Enzyme analysis: from muscle, leucocyte or fibroblast culture.

Treatment Supportive only.

Disorders of lipid metabolism: carnitine palmitoyltransferase deficiency

Pathophysiology Lipid metabolism, in particular the oxidation of fatty acids, takes over from carbohydrate metabolism on sustained exercise. The enzyme carnitine palmitoyltransferase (CPT) catalyses the coupling of carnitine to long-chain fatty acids, a reaction that must occur for the transfer of fatty acids across the mitochondrial membrane.

Clinical presentation Presents in young adults.

Symptoms Suspect this diagnosis if the following are features:

- bouts of weakness after prolonged exercise;

- myoglobinuria (more severe than in the glycogenoses);

- respiratory involvement may be associated with severe attacks.

The patient may subconsciously adapt to circumstances, preferring sprinting to long-distance running and snacking on sweet food to improve stamina.

Physical signs Examination may be normal.

Investigations Note the following.

- CK is normal unless soon after an attack.

- Muscle biopsy shows increased lipid storage.

- Biochemical analysis of muscle will show the enzyme defect.

Treatment Avoid precipitating factors.

Mitochondrial disorders

The respiratory chain of mitochondria is responsible for oxidative metabolism within cells. Diseases of mitochondrial function tip the cell towards anaerobic mechanisms and lactic acidosis. Mitochondrial myopathies are one group in a range of diseases of mitochondrial dysfunction, the mitochondrial cytopathies.

Mitochondria and their disorders are inherited through the maternal line. However, some aspects of their function are under nuclear control, and therefore some mitochondrial disorders may have a defect of nuclear, rather than mitochondrial, DNA.

2.2.2 Inflammatory muscle disease

Polymyositis and dermatomyositis have been covered elsewhere (see *Rheumatology and Clinical Immunology*, Section 2.3.5) and details are not repeated here.

Inclusion body myositis

Inclusion body myositis (IBM) can be sporadic or hereditary.

Sporadic IBM

Clinical presentation Look for the following.

- IBM affects men more than women. It is more common in those over the age of 50.

- Painless weakness and wasting, with selective involvement of long finger flexors and anterior thigh muscles (quadriceps). May be asymmetrical.

- Relentless progression.

Investigation Look for the following.

- Creatine kinase mildly elevated.

- Imaging: MRI can show the pattern of wasting and therefore distinguish sporadic from hereditary IBM (see below).

- Electromyography as in polymyositis, with spontaneous activity and myopathic features.

- Muscle biopsy shows myopathic changes with endomysial CD8$^+$ T-cell infiltrate. Rimmed vacuoles and characteristic tubulofilamentous inclusions are present. Interestingly, there is abnormal accumulation of proteins within the diseased muscle fibres including β-amyloid, amyloid precursor protein and prion protein.

Treatment IBM does not respond to steroids, despite the inflammatory changes. This may suggest that the

inflammation is a secondary phenomenon.

Hereditary IBM

This is far less common than the sporadic type, and can be differentiated as follows:

- usually autosomal recessive and linked to chromosome 9;

- dramatic sparing of quadriceps;

- no inflammation on biopsy.

FURTHER READING

Mastaglia FL, Garlepp MJ, Phillips BA and Zilko PJ. Inflammatory myopathies: clinical, diagnostic and therapeutic aspects. *Muscle Nerve* 2003; 27: 407–25.

2.2.3 Inherited dystrophies (myopathies)

These are a diverse group of hereditary muscle disorders.

Disorders of dystrophin

Pathophysiology

The key to understanding why a defect in dystrophin, or certain other proteins (see autosomal recessive limb girdle muscular dystrophy, or LGMD, below), can have such a devastating effect on muscle is the dystrophin–glycoprotein complex (DGC) shown in Fig. 31. This is a protein complex found within the sarcolemma that couples the contractile apparatus of the cell to the extracellular matrix through laminin 2. Each member of the DGC is an integral component, with deficiency of any one leading to disease.

Duchenne's muscular dystrophy

Clinical presentation Look for the following.

- X-linked.

- Presents in early childhood, often in second year, with clumsiness.

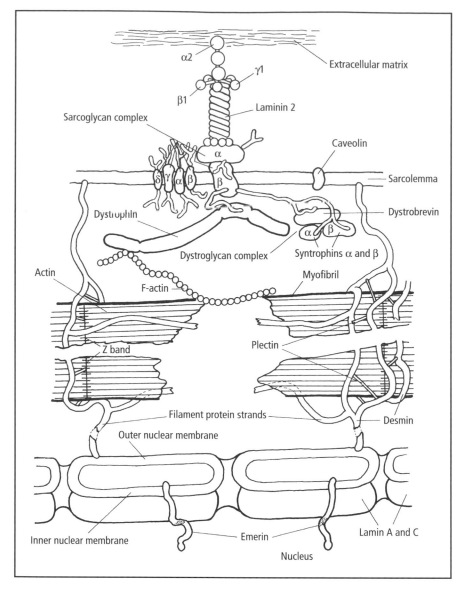

▲**Fig. 31** The dystrophin-associated glycoprotein complex is found in the muscle fibre membrane and is connected to the supporting and contractile apparatus of the muscle fibre.

- Proximal weakness and falls develop over the next few years.

- Pseudo-hypertrophy of the calf muscles is noticed.

- Wheelchair bound by the early teens, with the loss of mobility contributing to contractures and scoliosis.

- Cardiac involvement usually occurs and is characterised by cardiomyopathy.

- Death is from respiratory or cardiac involvement.

> 🔑 Gower's manoeuvre: the use of the upper limbs to push up on the knees to assist with rising from the floor.

Investigations Use the following tests.

- Creatine kinase (CK): often >10,000 mU/mL.

- Electromyography (EMG): myopathic.

- Muscle biopsy: severe dystrophic changes with characteristic hyaline fibres; absence of dystrophin on immunocytochemistry.

- DNA analysis: Xp21, molecular diagnosis available.

Treatment The use of corticosteroids is controversial, but some feel they are beneficial. Other than this, treatment is primarily supportive, although gene therapy may offer better outcomes in the future.

Becker's muscular dystrophy
Features include the following.

- X-linked.

- A milder form of Duchenne's muscular dystrophy caused by deficiency or defect in, rather than absence of, dystrophin.

- Presents late in the first decade of life.

- Patients may not be wheelchair bound until their third decade.

- Cardiomyopathy may be severe.

- Female carriers of an abnormal dystrophin gene may have a raised CK and cardiomyopathy.

Limb girdle muscular dystrophy
Various LGMDs have historically been lumped together to distinguish them from the X-linked muscular dystrophies (above) and facioscapulohumeral dystrophy (below). Recent developments have enabled molecular classification of these disorders. Only the briefest of synopses will be given here.

Autosomal dominant limb girdle muscular dystrophy (LGMD1)

- Less severe than autosomal recessive LGMD, often with adult onset.

- Most cases have been identified in a few large families.

- Numerous different genetic loci have been identified.

Autosomal recessive limb girdle muscular dystrophy (LGMD2)

- Often presents in childhood and can be clinically similar to the dystrophinopathies.

- Many subtypes have been identified, including those with deficiencies of the proteins calpain and dysferlin, and the arcoglycans (see Fig. 31).

Facioscapulohumeral dystrophy

Clinical presentation

An autosomal dominant condition with incomplete penetrance and sporadic cases. Clinically, it varies from mild facial weakness to severe generalised weakness involving particularly the face, scapular fixators, triceps, biceps, hip flexors and anterior thigh/calf muscles. The deltoid is often well preserved. Typically it commences around the early teens with only slow progression, but this is extremely variable.

Genetics

Tandem repeat deletion is identified at 4q35. The longer the deletion, the more severe the illness with earlier onset and more rapid progression. Anticipation is seen in families, suggesting an increasing deletion size with each generation. Penetrance varies, being 95% in males and 65% in females. The deletion appears to be located close by (possibly within regulatory DNA), but not within an actual gene.

Emery–Dreifuss muscular dystrophy

This rare disease is characterised by the following.

- Xq28, deficiency of emerin.

- Similar phenotype also recognised with normal emerin and autosomal dominant inheritance.

- Early contractures and cardiac complications.

- Female carriers may develop cardiac problems.

Myotonic dystrophy

Clinical features

Myotonia is best demonstrated by getting the patient to open and close the fist rapidly, or by percussing the thenar eminence with a tendon hammer, which causes the thumb to flex across the palm. It is difficult to demonstrate in the tongue as the mouth is warm, and myotonia is best demonstrated in the cold.

A mild progressive myopathy starting distally. Facial involvement with ptosis.

Look for the following associated features:

- cardiac conduction abnormalities;

- frontal balding;

- cataracts;

- gonadal atrophy;

- glucose intolerance;

- mental retardation.

Investigations

Genetics Autosomal dominant gene at 19q13.1 in which there is an abnormal large expansion of CTG trinucleotide repeats. The disorder shows anticipation (ie worse in successive generations) and may have been undiagnosed in older generations in whom signs may have been restricted to cataracts and mild ptosis.

Other investigations DNA analysis should be first line and it is no longer necessary to subject patients

to EMG. However, an EMG will demonstrate characteristic myotonic discharges (likened to a dive-bomber or motorcycle revving up).

Treatment
Mainly supportive.

> **FURTHER READING**
> Emery AE. The muscular dystrophies. *Lancet* 2002; 359: 687–95.

2.2.4 Channelopathies
A group of disorders characterised by episodic paralysis or myotonia due to mutations of either the calcium or sodium channel gene.

> **FURTHER READING**
> Graves TD and Hanna MG. Neurological channelopathies. *Postgrad. Med. J.* 2005; 81: 20–32.

2.2.5 Myasthenia gravis

Aetiology/pathophysiology

Myasthenia gravis (MG) is caused by an antibody-mediated autoimmune attack against acetylcholine receptors at neuromuscular junctions. This leads to degradation of acetylcholine receptors and reduced neurotransmission to skeletal muscle. Anti-acetylcholine receptor antibody titres tend to be higher in more severe disease, but 20% of patients (50% in ocular myasthenia) are seronegative; 75% of patients have thymic abnormalities (usually hyperplasia), but thymomas are only seen in 10% of cases. The thymus, with its antigen-presenting cells (T cells and B cells) is therefore thought to play a key role in the pathophysiology of MG.

Epidemiology

The prevalence of MG is estimated at approximately 10 per 100,000 population. It has a bimodal age distribution: the second and third decades in women and the seventh and eighth decades in men. The female to male ratio is 2:1. MG is often associated with other autoimmune diseases, eg Graves' disease.

Clinical presentation

Patients most commonly present with ptosis and diplopia (70%), not with fatigue. Oropharyngeal weakness (difficulty chewing, swallowing and talking) is the initial symptom in 15% of patients, and limb weakness in 10%. The severity of symptoms fluctuates during the day, being less severe in the morning and more severe as the day goes on. Exacerbation of symptoms may occur in intercurrent infections, pregnancy, menses and with certain drugs, eg aminoglycosides, beta-blockers, calcium antagonists, procainamide, quinidine and neuromuscular blocking agents. Penicillamine may induce MG.

> **!** Since many drugs have been observed to worsen weakness, all patients with MG should be monitored when a new drug is started.

MG remains purely ocular in 10% of patients, and the rest develop generalised weakness, usually within 2 years. After 10–15 years the weakness becomes fixed with little fluctuation.

Physical signs

In MG the weakness shows fatiguability. Repetitive testing is therefore needed to fully appreciate this feature. The pattern of weakness does not conform to the distribution of any particular nerves. In the eyes there is ptosis and extraocular muscle weakness, particularly of the medial rectus with sparing of the pupillary reflexes. There may be facial weakness that characteristically gives a 'myasthenic snarl' on attempted smiling, dysarthria, hoarseness, nasal speech, dysphagia and difficulty chewing.

> 🔑 **Weakness of neck flexors** is often a good indicator of weakness. However, any limb or trunk muscles may be weak. Deep tendon reflexes are normal. Patients are occasionally diagnosed as hysterical because of the odd distribution of weakness and the fatiguability.

Investigation

The following may be useful.

- The edrophonium chloride (Tensilon) test is positive in about 90% of those with MG. It is performed as follows: first identify what you want to measure, the best results being obtained with diplopia, ptosis and dysarthria. The patient is pretreated with atropine 400 μg iv, then edrophonium in doses of 2, 3 and 5 mg with at least 1–2 minutes between each injection. Observe for a transient response.

- Serum anti-acetylcholine receptor antibodies are present in 80% of patients with generalised MG and 50% with ocular MG. Anti-striated muscle antibodies are associated with thymoma.

- Plasma from patients with generalised MG who do not have detectable anti-acetylcholine receptor antibodies contains various other immune factors, and about 50% have an IgG antibody against the muscle-specific kinase (MuSK). The majority of patients with anti-MuSK antibodies have prevalent involvement of facial and bulbar muscles.

- An autoantibody screen and thyroid function tests should be done because of the association of MG with other autoimmune diseases.

- Single-fibre electromyography shows increased jitter in those with MG, but this also occurs in other neuromuscular transmission disorders.

- Electromyography shows a decremental response to repetitive nerve stimulation in muscles.

- A CXR (Fig. 32) and CT thorax should be done to look for a thymoma.

> 🔑 **Single-fibre electromyography** is performed by simultaneously recording the evoked responses from two muscle fibres of the same motor unit. In a normal muscle, action potentials recorded from two such muscle fibres are not synchronous. This variation in interpotential interval is defined as 'jitter'. Because of the variable neuromuscular transmission, this jitter is increased in disorders of the neuromuscular junction.

Differential diagnosis

Genetic forms of myasthenia are not immune mediated, but are caused by mutations of the acetylcholine receptor. These need to be excluded. Lambert–Eaton myasthenic syndrome usually occurs in association with malignancy, mostly small-cell lung cancers. Autoantibodies against voltage-gated calcium channels are thought to result in insufficient release of acetylcholine on depolarisation of the presynaptic membrane. Unlike in MG, muscle strength increases after exercise (postexercise facilitation), deep tendon reflexes are depressed (but

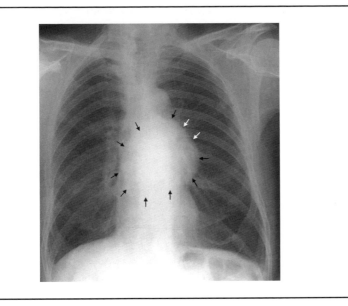

▲ **Fig. 32** Thymoma. (Reproduced with permission from Ray KK, Ryder RE and Wellings RM. *An Aid to Radiology for the MRCP*. Oxford: Blackwell Science, 2000.)

Respiratory failure may be due to the disease it self and/or inadequate doses of anticholinesterases (myasthenic crisis) or overdose of anticholinesterases (cholinergic crisis). It ought to be simple to distinguish the two, but in practice it can be difficult. Therefore the safest option is to discontinue all anticholinesterases temporarily and ventilate the patient if necessary.

FURTHER READING

Keesey JC. Clinical evaluation and management of myasthenia gravis. *Muscle Nerve* 2004; 29: 484–505.

increase with exercise), extraocular muscles are spared, autonomic dysfunction may be prominent and there is incremental response to repetitive nerve stimulation (see also Sections 1.1.11 and 1.2.14).

Treatment

Drugs

Anticholinesterases produce temporary improvement. Immunosuppressives are effective but take weeks or months to work. Steroids should be started at low doses to prevent exacerbation of weakness after initiation. Plasma exchange or intravenous immunoglobulin is used for temporary but rapid benefit in those with sudden worsening of MG.

Patients with anti-MuSK antibodies tend to respond less well to anticholinesterases, but the majority do relatively well with immunosuppressive agents.

Thymectomy

Thymectomy should be considered for most patients, but remember the following.

- The maximum response is seen 2–5 years after surgery.

- The best response is seen in young patients, although benefit can occur in late disease and older patients should certainly be considered.

- Is not generally recommended for patients with purely ocular disease, but occasionally dramatic benefit is also seen in this patient group.

- Occasionally thymic tissue is left behind, so repeat surgery should be considered for chronic or relapsing disease if this is felt to be the case.

Complications

The most serious consequence of MG is neuromuscular respiratory failure.

2.3 Extrapyramidal disorders

2.3.1 Parkinson's disease

Pathophysiology

Idiopathic Parkinson's disease (IPD) is a neurodegenerative disease and is characterised by death of the dopaminergic cells in the substantia nigra that project to the striatum. Recently, α-synuclein has been found to be the major constituent of Lewy bodies, which are proteinaceous inclusions within the degenerating dopaminergic cells. Other groups of neurons also eventually die and this is possibly responsible for the lack of response of some of the symptoms of IPD to dopamine replacement.

Aetiology

The precise cause of sporadic IPD is unknown. A small proportion of cases are familial and associated with genetic mutations, eg α-synuclein and parkin. Unknown environmental influences are almost certainly important. Mitochondrial and proteosomal function as well as cell trafficking and signalling are impaired, but the exact mechanisms and triggers that cause neurodegeneration remain elusive.

Epidemiology

- Prevalence increases with age: ~1% in over-sixties (~0.1% in the general population).

- No geographical differences exist, and it is equally as common in males as females.

- Previous epidemiological studies indicated a lower incidence in smokers, but it is unclear whether smoking is actually protective.

Clinical presentation
See also Section 1.3.

Common presenting features

- Gait disturbance: festinant, stooped and flexed with poor turning.

- Asymmetrical slowness (bradykinesia)/decreased dexterity.

- Asymmetrical stiffness ('lead pipe' or 'cogwheel' rigidity) in limbs.

- Deterioration in handwriting: fatiguing and smaller or 'micrographic'.

- Asymmetrical resting tremor.

Non-motor features

- Depression.

- Anosmia.

- Erectile and urinary dysfunction.

- Constipation.

Later problems
These features would not normally be part of the presenting or early clinical picture.

- Loss of balance/falls.

- Dementia/visual hallucinations.

- Swallowing difficulties, drooling and severe speech impairment.

Treatment complications These may become the dominant clinical features later in the disease.

- 'Motor fluctuations': this encompasses a range of clinical problems and usually starts with 'wearing off' of medication at the end of doses of levodopa.

- Later in the disease, there are sudden changes between 'on' periods (medication working with symptom relief) and 'off' periods (medication ineffective).

- 'Peak dose' and 'end of dose/ beginning of dose' dyskinesias: usually choreoathetoid movements of all limbs and the neck and face. Dystonia during 'off' periods, especially of the feet, may also become problematic. These usually develop after 5–10 years of levodopa treatment.

- Gait 'freezing', even when otherwise 'on'.

- Hallucinations (usually visual) and psychosis, which may be drug related or due to an underlying Parkinson's disease (PD)-associated dementia.

> IPD is a clinical diagnosis, and in the context of a typical history and examination no investigations are required.

Investigations
If the diagnosis or response to dopaminergic therapy is unclear, a formal levodopa or apomorphine challenge can help; if it is markedly positive it strongly suggests IPD, although a small proportion of patients with other syndromes may respond partially. Where the diagnosis is still unclear, the passage

of time can make the diagnosis clearer.

Functional imaging of the basal ganglia (using single-photon emission CT or positron emmision tomography) can be very helpful by showing greatly reduced and asymmetrical striatonigral dopaminergic activity. In some cases the correct diagnosis may not be made until *post mortem*.

In younger patients, serum and urinary copper studies should be performed to exclude Wilson's disease, and the Westphal variant of Huntington's disease (with genetic counselling and testing) should also be considered (see Section 1.5).

Differential diagnosis
The commoner causes of parkinsonism are listed in Table 44.

> In the elderly, cerebrovascular disease is only very rarely a cause of true parkinsonism when an infarct damages the nigrostriatal pathway. Diffuse small-vessel cerebrovascular disease causes 'vascular parkinsonism' which can be misdiagnosed as IPD (see Section 1.2.4) and which can coexist with IPD.

Drug-induced parkinsonism is an important cause not to miss as it is usually treatable. The other neurodegenerative conditions causing parkinsonism (MSA and PSP) are rarer than IPD, but certain clinical features should alert the clinician to the possibility of an alternative diagnosis to IPD.

Clinical features that are atypical in the diagnosis of IPD include:

- early instability or falls;

- poor response to levodopa;

- absent levodopa-induced dyskinesias;

TABLE 44 COMMON CAUSES OF PARKINSONISM	
Diagnosis	**Characteristics**
Idiopathic Parkinson's disease (IPD)	Asymmetrical resting tremor, rigidity, bradykinesia
Drug-induced parkinsonism	History of dopamine antagonists, no tremor, symmetrical
Steele–Richardson–Olszewski disease [progressive supranuclear palsy (PSP)]	Frontal disease prominent with falls, symmetrical parkinsonism, characteristic supranuclear gaze palsy, staring face
Multiple system atrophy (MSA)	Symmetrical parkinsonism with cerebellar, pyramidal and autonomic features
Benign essential tremor	Tremor mainly affects actions and posture in the upper limbs
Vascular parkinsonism	Frontal apraxic gait with pyramidal signs and dementia

- rapid progression;

- pyramidal or cerebellar signs;

- dementia early in the disease;

- down-gaze supranuclear palsy (up-gaze palsy is non-specific and occurs in the elderly);

- severe dysphonia, dysarthria and dysphagia;

- respiratory stridor;

- myoclonus.

Treatment

See Section 2.12 for background to neuropharmacology.

Levodopa

Levodopa remains the gold-standard treatment for PD, and is the most effective and best tolerated of the antiparkinsonian drugs.

To understand the rationale for the various different treatment strategies in PD, it is necessary to consider levodopa metabolism (Fig. 33). Of peripheral levodopa, 70% is converted to dopamine via the dopa decarboxylase (DDC) pathway. This causes stimulation of peripheral dopamine receptors, which results in nausea and vomiting and reduces the bioavailability of the drug to the brain. Levodopa preparations therefore contain a DDC inhibitor (eg Sinemet contains levodopa and carbidopa; Madopar contains levodopa and benserazide). This increases central nervous system bioavailability from 1% to 10%. Inhibition of DDC shifts peripheral metabolism of levodopa to other pathways, such as via catechol *O*-methyltransferase (COMT).

There are several preparations of levopdopa that have certain clinical uses. A dispersible form of Madopar can be useful for patients first thing in the morning when they may be extremely rigid and slow. It may act quicker than tablet preparations, and a liquid may be easier to swallow than a tablet. Each dose of standard levodopa 100 mg takes approximately 30–60 minutes to take effect and lasts for up to 4 hours. A controlled-release preparation lengthens this period of action slightly and may be useful to take last thing at night to help patients sleep and to enable them to mobilise in the night to go to the bathroom.

Despite giving a DDC inhibitor in the levodopa preparation, peripheral dopaminergic side effects, such as nausea and postural hypotension (usually only a problem when starting treatment), can be controlled by co-administration with the peripheral dopaminergic antagonist domperidone (the only safe antiemetic to give to parkinsonian patients).

Central effects such as hallucinations, confusion and dyskinesias can become a problem in the later stages of the disease and may be dose-limiting. Some experts advocate delaying levodopa therapy to try to delay the onset of long-term complications, but this is still controversial.

Dopamine agonists

These act directly on postsynaptic dopamine receptors and mimic the effect of endogenous dopamine. They can be effective 'levodopa-sparing' agents and have longer half-lives than levodopa. Dopamine agonists can be useful in the later stages of disease, when motor fluctuations and dyskinesias become a problem. There is also growing evidence that the early use of

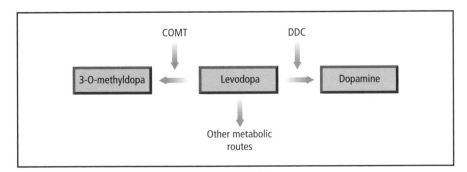

▲**Fig. 33** Pathway of levodopa metabolism in the periphery.

dopamine agonists, rather than levodopa, delays the onset of dyskinesias. However, the question as to whether early agonist monotherapy has long-term benefits remains controversial, although several studies show a reduction in long-term dyskinesias.

Bromocriptine, pergolide, ropinirole, pramipexole and cabergoline are the dopamine agonists generally used, although bromocriptine and pergolide are being used less frequently because they are ergot-based and can produce fibrotic reactions in the lung and heart over time.

The side-effect profile of agonists is similar to that of levodopa, although they tend to be less well tolerated, especially by the elderly who may develop psychosis, confusion and hallucinations. There have been some reports of sudden onset of sleep at the wheel, which is relevant when prescribing for patients who are still driving.

Apomorphine is a very potent dopamine agonist and is usually given subcutaneously because a very high rate of first-pass metabolism excludes the oral route. It may be given by intermittent injections or, in cases of severe disease, by continuous infusion or an 'apomorphine pump'. It is extremely effective in improving severe motor fluctuations and dyskinesias in late-stage disease. Domperidone is usually given at the start of treatment to avoid nausea and postural hypotension, but most patients can stop it after a few weeks. Autoimmune haemolytic anaemia is a rare but serious complication, and thus 3-monthly FBC and Coombs' tests should be performed on all patients on apomorphine.

Amantadine

This is an *N*-methyl-D-aspartate receptor antagonist, but its exact mechanism of action in IPD is unclear. Amantadine was previously used in early disease but fell out of favour. However, following new evidence that demonstrated an anti-dyskinetic effect, it is receiving renewed interest. Side effects include confusion, hallucinations and leg oedema.

Selegiline (Deprenyl/Eldepryl)

This is an irreversible monoamine oxidase B inhibitor. Two interesting issues have arisen surrounding this drug.

Experimental data in animals suggests that it is 'neuroprotective', ie slows disease progression, but this has not been substantiated in humans. The DATATOP study suggested it resulted in a delay in the need to commence levodopa, but interpretation of this trial has been questioned and long-term follow-up showed no lasting benefit.

Does selegiline increase mortality? The 1995 report by the UK Parkinson's Disease Research Group concluded that increased mortality was seen in patients taking a combination of selegiline and levodopa compared with levodopa alone. However, further studies suggest that any true increase in mortality is likely to be less than the 60% reported in this study, and no excess was seen in the long-term DATATOP follow-up.

COMT inhibitors

COMT inhibitors are used to optimise the effects of each dose of levodopa and are therefore useful clinically when the patient complains of end-of-dose 'wearing off'.

Side effects include the following.

- Potentiation of levodopa side effects.
- Gastrointestinal disturbance.
- A reduction in levodopa dose may be necessary.
- The first available COMT inhibitor, tolcapone, was withdrawn due to possible hepatic toxicity. It is now being relaunched and has the advantage of being more potent than entacapone. Entacapone does not appear to affect the liver but needs to be given with each dose of levodopa.

Anticholinergics (trihexyphenidyl/benzhexol)

Anticholinergics probably have a modest effect on tremor. They tend to be used in young patients with troublesome tremors and are avoided in the elderly because of neuropsychiatric side effects.

Side effects include:

- confusion (particularly in elderly patients);
- dry mouth;
- constipation;
- may worsen dyskinesias.

Surgery

Stereotactic surgery, either lesioning a specific target or by implanting a high-frequency stimulator, is increasingly used. Lesioning is irreversible, can only be performed unilaterally and may be more hazardous. In contrast, stimulation is reversible and can be performed bilaterally, but is much more expensive.

The targets are:

- thalamus for tremor;
- subthalamus and globus pallidus for dyskinesias and motor fluctuations.

General measures

The treatment of PD requires a multidisciplinary approach with the specialist nurse, speech therapist, occupational therapist and physiotherapist, all of whom are often able to contribute just as much as the doctor to improve a patient's quality of life.

Prognosis

Most patients with IPD have a near-normal life expectancy. Disease progression is extremely variable and it is important to reassure patients that it can run quite a benign course. Some patients may become disabled after many years, especially if hallucinations/psychosis and dementia limit treatment, whereas others will lead a fairly normal life, ultimately succumbing to other medical problems.

FURTHER READING

Colzi A, Turner K and Lees AJ. Continuous subcutaneous waking day apomorphine in the long term treatment of levodopa induced interdose dyskinesias in Parkinson's disease. *J. Neurol. Neurosurg. Psychiatry* 1998; 64: 573–6.

Developments in the treatment of Parkinson's disease. *Drug Ther. Bull.* 1999; 37: 36–40.

Lees AJ. Comparison of therapeutic effects and mortality data of levodopa and levodopa combined with selegiline in patients with early, mild Parkinson's disease. Parkinson's Disease Research Group of the United Kingdom. *BMJ* 1995; 311: 1602–7.

Pallanck L and Greenamyre JT. Neurodegenerative disease: pink, parkin and the brain. *Nature* 2006; 441: 1058.

Parkinson Study Group. Effect of deprenyl on the progression of disability in early Parkinson's disease. *N. Engl. J. Med.* 1989; 321: 1364–71.

Tolosa E, Wenning G and Poewe W. The diagnosis of Parkinson's disease. *Lancet Neurol.* 2006; 5: 75–86.

2.4 Dementia

2.4.1 Alzheimer's disease

Aetiology/pathology

Familial autosomal-dominant early-onset (usually between early forties and mid-fifties) Alzheimer's disease (AD) is caused in the majority of cases by mutations in one of three genes:

- presenilin 1 on chromosome 14;
- presenilin 2 on chromosome 1;
- amyloid precursor protein (APP) on chromosome 21.

In those over the age of 65 years, carrying the E4 allele of apolipoprotein E (encoded by a gene on chromosome 19) increases the risk of developing AD.

The neuropathological changes of AD are cerebral atrophy (especially of the medial temporal lobes), senile amyloid plaques with a central core of β-amyloid, neurofibrillary tangles of tau (Fig. 34) and β-amyloid in blood vessels or 'amyloid angiopathy'. An important step in the pathogenesis of AD is the cleavage of β-amyloid from the larger precursor protein APP, which results in the accumulation of β-amyloid. The mechanism of toxicity of β-amyloid and the association of β-amyloid with neurofibrillary tangles remain unclear.

Epidemiology

AD is the commonest form of dementia. Familial AD accounts for less than 5% of cases. Increasing age is the most important risk factor, but patients with Down's syndrome (trisomy 21) are also susceptible to developing AD which may be due to a gene dosage effect as the APP gene lies on chromosome 21.

Clinical presentation

Guidelines for the diagnosis of probable, possible and definite AD have been developed.

The earliest feature of AD is usually forgetfulness for recent events and

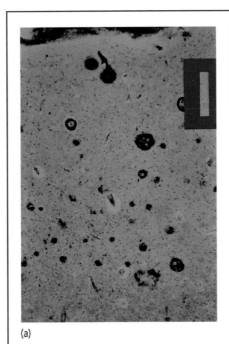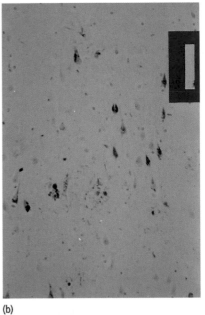

(a) (b)

▲ **Fig. 34** (a) β-Amyloid and (b) neurofibrillary tangles in AD.

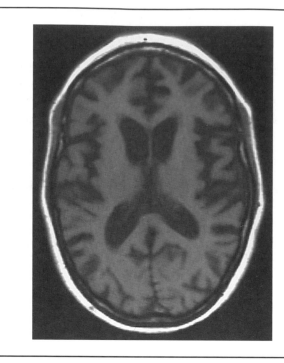

▲ **Fig. 35** Cerebral atrophy in AD.

repeating conversations. As the disease progresses, the patient develops:

- disorientation (initially to time);
- impairment of verbal fluency;
- loss of computational ability;
- inattentiveness and agitation;
- personality change;
- depression;
- difficulty with activities of daily living.

Late features include:

- severe memory impairment;
- loss of social awareness;
- complete disorientation;
- psychosis;
- delusions and hallucinations.

Patients may develop extrapyramidal signs (eg rigidity), pyramidal signs (eg hyperreflexia), seizures, myoclonus, mutism and incontinence. Progression of the disease is slow and gradual over several years, although more rapid forms have been described.

Investigation
An MRI scan of the brain may show cerebral atrophy, especially of the medial temporal lobes (Fig. 35). See also Section 1.1.7.

Differential diagnosis

Reversible or treatable causes of dementia must be ruled out at onset of presentation, eg hypothyroidism, vitamin B$_{12}$ deficiency, neurosyphilis and space-occupying lesions (such as hydrocephalus and subdural haematoma). See also Table 5.

Vascular dementia
Classicaly, multi-infarct dementia has been described as stepwise deterioration due to large-vessel sequential infarcts/haemorrhages. More commonly recognised is subcortical ischaemic leucoencephalopathy due to diffuse subcortical white matter ischaemia, often in association with hypertension, diabetes and smoking. Other features include:

- impaired executive function, eg planning actions;
- frontal gait apraxia;
- emotional lability;
- pseudobulbar palsy;
- urinary dysfunction;
- preservation of personality.

An MRI scan can often demonstrate diffuse white matter disease, lacunar infarcts and large-vessel strokes in the same patient.

Vascular dementia often coexists with AD.

Frontotemporal dementia
The main features are:

- loss of social awareness and appropriateness;
- loss of initiation, planning and motivation, termed 'abulia' (shallow affect);
- disinhibition;
- apathy;
- hyperorality;
- perseverative behaviour;
- decreased speech output.

An MRI scan may confirm focal frontotemporal atrophy.

Dementia with Lewy bodies
The main features are:

- progressive early cognitive deterioration;
- fluctuating symptoms;
- visual hallucinations;

- extrapyramidal signs (rigidity and bradykinesia more common than tremor);
- sleep pattern reversal;
- recurrent falls;
- syncope;
- hypersensitivity to neuroleptics (dopamine antagonists).

Other irreversible causes

- idiopathic Parkinson's disease with dementia;
- progressive supranuclear palsy;
- corticobasal degeneration;
- Huntington's disease (see also Sections 1.1.8 and 1.3.1);
- Creutzfeldt–Jakob disease (see Section 2.10).

Treatment

AD is not a curable disease, but quality of life can be maintained with the appropriate input. Supportive care is an integral part of management. A familiar environment reduces confusion and disorientation in patients with AD. Education and support of their caregivers is important. The Alzheimer's Society has excellent resources. Depression commonly coexists with AD and it is important that it is recognised and treated. Other behavioural disturbances may also require treatment, eg neuroleptics for agitation, aggression and hallucinations, and selective serotonin reuptake inhibitors or small doses of benzodiazepines for anxiety.

> ⚠ Tricyclic drugs have anticholinergic side effects that may worsen cognitive deficits. Selective serotonin reuptake inhibitors are a better choice.

Cholinesterase inhibitors, eg donepezil, galantamine and rivastigmine, modestly improve cognitive function by the equivalent of delaying symptoms of disease for approximately 6 months. Recent studies suggest that they may also improve non-cognitive functions, eg activities of daily living and behaviour. However, most of these trials are short (between 3 and 6 months) and the long-term benefits are uncertain. Memantine is a partial glutamate receptor antagonist and is licensed as treatment for moderate to severe AD. Memantine has also been found to be effective in mild to moderate AD. In practice, it is often used when cholinesterase inhibitors are ineffective or have intolerable side effects.

Selegiline, vitamin E and gingko biloba (a plant derivative) have been reported to benefit some patients with AD. Ginkgo biloba had a small but significant effect on cognition in a recent meta-analysis.

There is growing evidence that cholinesterase inhibitors have a beneficial effect in other dementias such as dementia with Lewy bodies (DLB), vascular dementia and dementia in Parkinson's disease. They may be especially helpful in patients with DLB for treating the neuropsychiatric manifestations such as visual hallucinations.

Prognosis

Mean survival is about 8 years after the onset of disease but many younger patients can now survive with a good quality of life for many years if they receive the appropirate management. Bronchopneumonia is the usual cause of death following a period of immobility.

FURTHER READING

Birks J and Harvey RJ. Donepezil for dementia due to Alzheimer's disease. *Cochrane Database Syst. Rev.* 2006; (1): CD001190.

Lleo A, Greenberg SM and Growdon JH. Current pharmacotherapy for Alzheimer's disease. *Annu. Rev. Med.* 2006; 57: 513–33.

Loy C and Schneider L. Galantamine for Alzheimer's disease and mild cognitive impairment. *Cochrane Database Syst. Rev.* 2006; (1): CD001747.

Overshott R and Burns A. Treatment of dementia. *J. Neurol. Neurosurg. Psychiatry* 2005; 76 (Suppl. 5): v53–9.

2.5 Multiple sclerosis

Aetiology/pathophysiology/pathology

The aetiology of multiple sclerosis (MS) is unknown. Several infectious agents have been suggested as a cause but none have been convincingly proven. There is also some evidence that MS is an autoimmune disease. Molecular mimicry of several viral and bacterial peptides with proteins of myelin may trigger an immune response. Myelin basic protein has been implicated as a target of attack.

> 🔑 Demyelination with preservation of axons has long been considered the pathological hallmark of MS. However, there is increasing evidence that axonal loss and remyelination also occurs, with the axonal loss contributing to the progressive neurological impairments. The loss of myelin makes it difficult to depolarise axons and interrupts conduction of an action potential.

Epidemiology

The prevalence of MS increases with increasing distance from the equator. People who migrate from a high-risk to a low-risk area at or after the age of 15 retain the risk of their birthplace; below the age of 15 they do not. The mean age of onset is 30, being slightly earlier in women than in men and in relapsing–remitting MS than progressive MS. The female to male ratio is 3:2. Polygenic inheritance is suspected in MS.

Clinical presentation

Common symptoms are weakness, sensory disturbances (numbness or tingling), blurred vision or loss of vision (optic neuritis), unsteadiness, incoordination, dysarthria, sphincter or sexual dysfunction and fatigue. Lhermitte's sign (an electric shock-like sensation down the spine on neck flexion) and Uhthoff's phenomenon (a worsening of symptoms when there is an increase in body temperature, such as when getting into a hot bath) may occur. Later in the disease course cognitive impairment can be a feature.

The risk of developing MS after an acute episode of optic neuritis or transverse myelitis may be as high as 75% and 90%, respectively, if MRI appearances are compatible with MS.

Four disease courses are recognised: relapsing/remitting, primary progressive, secondary progressive (relapsing/remitting followed by continuous progression) and progressive/relapsing (progressive disease from the start with distinct episodes of acute relapses) (Fig. 36).

Physical signs

Cranial nerves

Pale optic discs (indicating optic atrophy), scotoma, relative afferent pupillary defect in optic neuritis, internuclear ophthalmoplegia and objective facial numbness or weakness.

Motor and sensory

Upper motor neuron signs (eg spasticity, pyramidal weakness, hyperreflexia and extensor plantar responses), and impaired pain, temperature, vibration and joint position sense.

Cerebellar

Nystagmus, upper limb intention tremor, scanning dysarthria, dysdiadochokinesis and gait ataxia.

Investigation

MRI

An MRI scan is the investigation of choice, with good sensitivity but poor specificity. Demyelinating lesions are typically located in the periventricular white matter (Fig. 37), corpus callosum, pons, and mesencephalon and cerebellar hemispheres. In chronic MS, there are confluent plaques, cortical atrophy and ventricular enlargement. Enhancement with contrast is a sign of an acute lesion and indicates disruption of the blood–brain barrier.

Unfortunately, a lesion on MRI correlates poorly with disability scores. This is probably due to the fact that some lesions may be silent and some may be in strategic areas. This is likely to be more clinically relevant than the overall amount of inflammation at any given time.

Cerebrospinal fluid

The white cell count and total protein are usually normal, although a mild lymphocytosis (up to 30 cells) or slightly elevated protein are sometimes seen. Oligoclonal bands (bands in the IgG region) are found in cerebrospinal fluid (CSF) but not serum (indicating intrathecal synthesis) in 90% of cases of clinically definite MS. However, oligoclonal bands may also be detected in many inflammatory conditions affecting the central nervous system (CNS) or after CNS infection. If the oligoclonal bands in the CSF are matched by those in the serum, this is indicative of systemic inflammation and can occur in a wide range of conditions such as systemic lupus erythematosus, paraneoplastic disease and infections such as HIV.

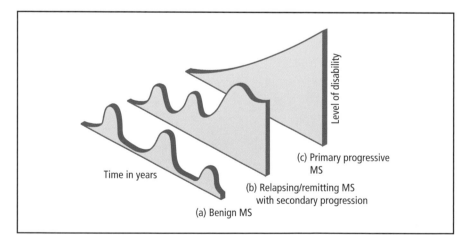

▲ **Fig. 36** Diagrammatic representation of the different clinical courses seen in MS. (**a**) Benign MS: there is no accumulation of disability between relapses for more than 10 years. (**b**) Relapsing/remitting MS becoming secondary progressive. At first, complete recovery is made between relapses. Then, a failure to recover fully from relapses leads to gradual accumulation of residual disability. Finally, the disability accumulates without clear relapses. (**c**) Primary progressive MS: gradual accumulation of disability without relapses.

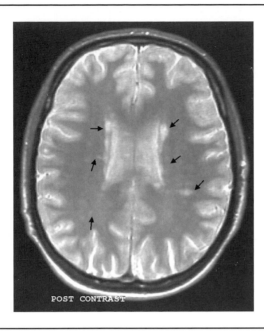

▲ **Fig. 37** Periventricular white matter lesions (arrows) in MS. (Reproduced with permission from Ray KK, Ryder RE and Wellings RM. *An Aid to Radiology for the MRCP*. Oxford: Blackwell Science, 2000.)

Visual, somatosensory and brainstem auditory evoked potentials

Visual-evoked potentials are a non-invasive test which may lend further support to the diagnosis of MS, particularly in patients who have had visual symptoms or those who do not wish to undergo lumbar puncture for CSF examination. These physiological studies may be abnormal in 50–80% of patients, but somatosensory- and brainstem-evoked potentials are usually only employed in difficult cases.

Differential diagnosis

The diagnosis of MS in the context of a young adult with two or more episodes of CNS dysfunction is straightforward. However, apparent monophasic illnesses may be caused by many pathologies including stroke, infections of the nervous system, inflammatory disease of the nervous system and tumours.

Progressive MS may be more difficult to diagnose clinically, but the most important diseases to exclude are potentially treatable causes of the symptoms, such as compressive spinal cord lesions, vitamin B_{12} deficiency, arteriovenous malformations and Arnold–Chiari malformation. The differential diagnosis in this category is broad and includes inflammatory and granulomatous CNS disease, CNS infections and hereditary disorders (such as adrenoleukodystrophy and metachromatic leukodystrophy).

Treatment

Relief or modification of symptoms

Modification of troublesome symptoms is currently the most effective way of helping improve the patient's quality of life.

Spasticity This impairs mobility and may cause painful spasms. The treatment options are as follows:

- baclofen (γ-aminobutyric acid agonist), oral or intrathecal;

- tizanidine (α₂ agonist);

- benzodiazepines;

- botulinum toxin;

- intrathecal phenol injection (last resort).

Although baclofen and tizanidine can be effective initially, the patient may require increasing doses if there is progression of disease. This often means the treatment becomes limited by side effects, particularly drowsiness.

Bladder disturbance This is a common problem, occurring in 50–80% of patients. Assessment is as follows.

- Establish whether the bladder empties using pre- and post-micturition ultrasound (the patient will not reliably be able to tell whether the bladder empties or not).

- If the residual volume is less than 100 mL, then use oxybutynin 2.5 mg two to three times daily (anticholinergic side effects are less likely to be a problem at this dose). Consider also antidepressants with anticholinergic action. Desmopressin nasal spray used at night may be helpful for nocturnal symptoms.

- If the residual volume is greater than 100 mL, it is not advisable to use these drugs until outflow obstruction has been overcome. Intermittent self-catheterisation is the best and simplest way to achieve this, but special training is needed.

Sexual dysfunction This is common but often not discussed with patients. You need to ask specifically about this, as patients are unlikely to volunteer the information. Sildenafil (Viagra) may be helpful for both men and women.

Fatigue This is a very common symptom, occurring in 70–80% of patients and is often out of proportion to the degree of physical disability, which may be relatively mild. Fatigue interferes with the patient's ability to perform the activities of daily living. Amantadine is often used without much success. An alternative is modafinil (100 mg once or twice a day), which seems to be more effective. However, some patients experience sleep disturbance when taking it, which may limit its use. It is important to look for correctable causes of fatigue, so check the patient's haemoglobin level and thyroid function tests.

Depression This occurs in 50–60% of patients at some stage during their illness, so it is important to identify and treat it.

Tremor This may be severe enough to impair the activities of daily living. Various drugs have been tried (antiepileptics, clonazepam and isoniazid) with only limited success. Thalamotomy may help in refractory disease.

Paroxysmal symptoms These include trigeminal neuralgia, pain, paraesthesiae, ataxia, dystonia and weakness, and they are thought to be due to ephaptic transmission of nerve impulses at sites of previous disease activity. Drugs used to treat neuropathic pain can be of some benefit (eg amitriptyline, gabapentin and pregabalin).

Treatment of acute attacks

Relapses are self-limiting but the following options are available to help speed recovery.

- High-dose intravenous methylprednisolone (1 g daily) with or without a follow-up short course of low-dose oral prednisolone or

methylprednisolone. Steroids may shorten an acute attack, but have no effect on disease progression.

- Rest may be just as effective.

- Physiotherapy at the time of the relapse is often of benefit.

Disease-modifying treatment

Disease-modifying drugs are a group of compounds that alter the progression of MS. They have been shown to reduce the frequency and severity of relapses, as well as slowing the development of disability in some people. There are currently two types of disease-modifying drugs used in the treatment of MS:

- beta interferons, which come in two forms, interferon beta-1a and interferon beta-1b;

- glatiramer acetate.

Beta interferons are licensed for use in relapsing/remitting MS, and immunosuppressive agents have also been used, but the results are not dramatic. There are numerous ongoing trials looking at the safety and efficacy of other agents designed to modify the disease course in MS.

- In relapsing/remitting MS, interferons beta-1a and beta-1b both reduce the frequency of relapses and the number of new lesions appearing on MRI, although the effect on clinical disability is less convincing. There is emerging evidence that interferons may also be effective in progressive forms of MS.
- Glatiramer acetate (a synthetic polymer) has been shown to reduce relapses and benefit disability in relapsing/remitting MS.
- Immunosuppressives that have been tried include azathioprine, methotrexate, cyclophosphamide, ciclosporin, mitoxantrone and total lymphoid irradiation.

The side effects of immunosuppression are a major drawback.

Prognosis

The following factors may be associated with a better prognosis:

- diplopia, optic neuritis or sensory symptoms at onset;

- female, rather than male, sex;

- earlier age of onset;

- long first remission.

FURTHER READING

Thompson AJ. Symptomatic treatment in multiple sclerosis. *Curr. Opin. Neurol.* 1998; 11: 305–9.

- - - - - - - - - - - - - - -

Triulzi F and Scotti G. Differential diagnosis of multiple sclerosis: contribution of magnetic resonance techniques. *J. Neurol. Neurosurg. Psychiatry* 1998; 64 (Suppl. 1): S6–S14.

- - - - - - - - - - - - - - -

Tselis AC and Lisak RP. Multiple sclerosis: therapeutic update. *Arch. Neurol.* 1999; 56: 277–80.

2.6 Headache

2.6.1 Migraine

Pathophysiology

The cardinal features of migraine are headache in the distribution of the trigeminal nerve and upper cervical roots, in association with transient neurological symptoms.

The pain is mediated through the trigeminal nerve fibres that innervate the large intracranial extracerebral vessels, transmitted via 5-hydroxytryptamine $(5HT)_{1B}$ serotonin receptors. These fibres project into the trigeminal nucleus

(5HT$_{1D}$ serotonin receptors) where they may receive projections from high cervical nerve fibres. This interaction accounts for the characteristic distribution of pain: the pain is likely to be related to episodic dysfunction of brainstem or diencephalic systems that modulate the trigemino-vascular system.

Epidemiology

- Lifetime prevalence is 5–10% for men and 15–25% for women.

- The first attack is experienced in the first decade by 25% of patients, and is less common after 50 years of age.

Clinical presentation

Common features

- Migraine headache is episodic, with complete resolution between attacks and each attack lasting from a few hours up to 3 days.

- Pain is often temporal and may be unilateral or bilateral. It is typically descibed as throbbing but may be constant.

- Patients with migraine will often describe how they take to their beds with the curtains closed. Although this is in marked contrast to the patient with cluster headache (see Section 2.6.3), aggravation by light, noise and movement experienced by those with migrane is common to many other types of headaches. Stress (and relaxation from stress), exercise, missing meals, menstruation, alcohol and various foodstuffs are often considered by patients to precipitate their attacks.

- Headache may be accompanied by nausea (90%) and vomiting (75%).

- The aura occurs prior to, but occasionally with or after, the headache and is most often visual.

By definition the aura should last between 5 and 60 minutes. Transient hemianopic disturbance, fortification spectra and spreading scintillating scotomata (but not blurring or non-specific spots) are symptoms of a migrainous aura. In addition, patients may describe unilateral paraesthesia, or even mild weakness, of their face and hand, and also occasionally aphasia.

Migraine variants

- Hemiplegic migraine: in true hemiplegic migraine the weakness is more marked than that ocasionally encountered in the common aura, and it may long outlast the headache, possibly lasting up to several days. For this diagnosis to be made, there needs to be a clear family history or a good history of preceding migraine with aura. It may be sporadic or familial, with some families carrying a dominant gene on chromosome 19. Traditionally, hemiplegic migraine responds well to flunarizine, a calcium channel antagonist, suggesting that the disorder is a channelopathy.

- Basilar migraine: this is accompanied by an aura in which there is frequently visual disturbance that is characteristically bilateral and associated with vertigo, ataxia, dysarthria, bilateral sensorimotor features and occasional drowsiness.

- Ophthalmoplegic migraine: the headache is associated with extraocular muscle palsies, particularly the third and rarely the sixth, which develop as the headache subsides.

- Retinal migraine: associated with monocular blindness, disc oedema and peripapillary haemorrhages. Vision may not recover for weeks or even months.

- Acephalgic migraine: this causes diagnostic problems, in that the presence of a typical migrainous aura without headache can be mistaken for transient cerebral ischaemia. A previous history of migraine with aura makes the diagnosis easier, but migraine equivalents can occur *de novo* in older patients. Characteristically, the symptoms evolve over a few minutes or longer, compared with transient ischaemic attacks (TIAs; see Section 2.8).

Investigations

Investigations do not contribute to the diagnosis of migraine, but if a secondary cause of headache needs to be excluded then an investigation may be appropriate (as discussed in Section 1.1.1).

Differential diagnosis

The main differentials are:

- episodic tension-type headache;

- cluster headache;

- chronic migraine (often in association with analgesia overuse) and other forms of chronic daily headache (see later in this section) can be very difficult to distinguish.

The aura, if it involves prominent sensorimotor features, may be confused with stroke or TIA. Migraine auras typically spread over many minutes or longer, whereas TIA symptoms do not spread. Furthermore, migraine auras are more likely to be positive phenomena (flashing lights, coloured spots and tingling) than TIAs. Occipital lobe simple partial seizures cause hemianopic visual disturbances, although these are typically multicoloured migratory blobs rather than monochromatic scintillations or angulated lines.

Treatment

Objectives and principles

- To minimise impact on the patient's lifestyle, as the tendency to headaches cannot be cured.

- To explain and reassure.

- To identify and avoid predisposing factors (stress, depression and anxiety) and triggers (alcohol, missed meals and change in sleeping habits) within reason. However, some of these may be unavoidable and so the patient should be encouraged to have regular habits.

Acute treatment

Step 1 Simple analgesia (aspirin 900 mg or paracetamol 1000 mg) or NSAIDs, with or without an antiemetic such as metoclopramide 10 mg or domperidone 20 mg. Consider suppositories (especially diclofenac plus domperidone) if nausea and vomiting is a persistent problem.

> ⚠️ It is extremely important to ask patients how much simple analgesia they take, particularly any compounds containing codeine or paracetamol. Medication-overuse headache may occur if simple analgesia is taken on more than 8–10 days in every month. However, NSAIDs appear to be less implicated and are an option, eg naproxen 500 mg bd for 2 weeks to help patients wean off other analgesia. A similar problem is seen with triptan overuse. Medication-overuse headache is important to diagnose as migraine preventives are ineffective unless simple analgesia is withdrawn to acceptable limits.

Step 2 Consider using the following.

- Specific antimigraine drugs (triptans, $5HT_{1B/1D}$ agonists). Different drugs may suit different patients, so it may be worth trying each one.

- At 2 hours the response rates (headache improving from severe/moderate to mild/absent) are approximately 50–65%, and the proportion of patients who are headache free is approximately 20–35%.

- Recurrence of symptoms occurs within 24 hours in 20–40% of patients for all triptans.

- Oral preparations are available, together with subcutaneous, nasal spray (sumatriptan) and a rapidly dispersible wafer that is placed on the tongue (rizatriptan). Subcutaneous or wafer preparations can be used if vomiting affects oral administration.

- Naratriptan is of slower onset, but there may be a lower recurrence rate with this drug.

Step 3 Before proceeding to step 3, review the diagnosis and then compliance. As a one-off treatment, intramuscular chlorpromazine 25–50 mg may improve headache that is not otherwise responding.

Prophylactic treatment

Patients are the best judge of when to commence a prophylactic agent, although generally agents tend to be considered for patients with two to three severe attacks per month. Continue with a prophylactic agent for 2–3 months, as long as it is tolerated, before deciding whether it has worked or not. Because migraine is cyclical, prophylactic agents that are effective should be continued for no more than 6 months.

The following agents may be tried.

- Atenolol 25–100 mg bd or propranolol LA 80–160 mg bd.

- Sodium valproate 600–2000 mg daily.

- Pizotifen 0.5–1.5 mg nocte.

- Amitriptyline 10–100 mg nocte.

- Topiramate 50–100 mg daily.

- Gabapentin 1800–3600 mg daily.

- Methysergide 1–2 mg tds. Often not considered because of associations with retroperitoneal fibrosis (1 in 2,000 risk), but if it is used in short courses, eg 6 months of treatment followed by a 1 month drug-free period, then this side effect can be avoided.

- For menstrual migraine, ie those attacks in which the onset of migraine can be predicted in relation to onset of menstruation, a 100-µg oestrogen patch starting 3 days before until 4 days after menstruation may be helpful in preventing attacks.

In pregnancy

Paracetamol is the safest option for acute headache and prochlorperazine is the safest option for nausea. Most migraines improve, but should a prophylactic agent be required then propranolol has the safest record.

Migraine and hormone-replacement therapy

Hormone-replacement therapy (HRT) is not contraindicated in the migraineur. Menopause may exacerbate migraine, so HRT may help the symptoms. Worsening migraine on commencement of HRT occasionally happens, but may be helped by changing the dose or formulation of the HRT.

> ⚠️ There is a small increased risk of stroke in women with migraine with aura who are taking the combined oral contraceptive pill, particularly in the presence of other vascular risk factors.

Prognosis

If migraine starts in childhood:

- 50% of males and 30% of females are migraine free at 30 years of age;

- over 50% of sufferers still get migraines at 50 years of age;

- in half of these cases the migraine is less severe.

If migraine starts in adulthood, 70% lose migraine or experience significant improvement over 15 years.

FURTHER READING

Goadsby PJ. Recent advances in the diagnosis and management of migraine. *BMJ* 2006; 332: 25–9.

2.6.2 Trigeminal neuralgia

Trigeminal neuralgia (TN) occurs predominantly in patients over the age of 40 years. It is attributed to compression of the sensory root of the trigeminal nerve, either by an aberrant blood vessel (Fig. 38) or occasionally by tumours in the cerebellopontine angle. In addition, TN may be seen in multiple sclerosis

(MS), with demyelination in the trigeminal sensory root.

Clinical presentation

- Patients characteristically describe a severe paroxysmal pain in the distribution of the trigeminal nerve (usually mandibular or maxillary, the ophthalmic branch being affected only rarely).

- The pain is described as lancinating or electric shock-like, and lasts only for seconds.

- Occasionally, the paroxysms are so frequent that they blur into one, giving the impression of lasting longer. There may also be a residual ache between bouts.

- Attacks may occur in clusters, but are clearly differentiated from cluster headache by the quality of the pain.

- Triggers are common, with almost any stimulus setting off an attack. Consequently, many patients are unable to wash, shave, chew or even talk during an attack.

- Pain is unilateral in over 95% of cases, and bilateral TN should raise the possibility of MS.

Physical signs

There are usually no physical signs. However, note that:

- the presence of a reduced corneal response, reduced sensation in the affected distribution or ipsilateral hearing loss should raise the possibility of a structural lesion;

- a larger compressive lesion may lead to weakness of the muscles of mastication, ipsilateral ataxia or other cranial nerve palsies.

> ⚠ If TN occurs in a patient under the age of 40 years this should raise the possibility of MS or a structural lesion.

Investigation

In the event of a structural lesion being suspected, MRI should be performed as this will detect demyelination as well as extra-axial mass lesions.

Differential diagnosis

When the patient describes the classical history of TN, the diagnosis is easy to make. If there is a chronic element to the pain, then the differential broadens (see Section 1.1.2).

Treatment

Medical

- Carbamazepine is the drug of choice, with a response rate of 75%. Start with 100 mg daily and increase at weekly or 2-weekly intervals, up to a dose of 1600 mg in divided doses. Lower doses usually suffice.

- If carbamazepine does not work, consider gabapentin, pregabalin, baclofen, phenytoin or clonazepam, but the chances of success are much lower with these drugs.

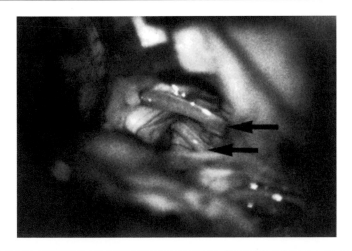

▲ **Fig. 38** Perioperative view of the trigeminal nerve root entry zone in contact with two divisions of the superior cerebellar artery (arrows) in a patient with trigeminal neuralgia. The arteries can be seen to indent the nerve. (From Hamlyn PJ. *Neurovascular Compression of the Lower Cranial Nerves.* Amsterdam: Elsevier Science, 1999 with kind permission of P.J. Hamlyn and Elsevier Science.)

The chances of medical treatment succeeding if carbamazepine fails are relatively small, so consider surgical options early.

Surgical

For patients with medically intractable TN, neurosurgical intervention should be considered. The options are as follows.

- Peripheral nerve block with alcohol or phenol injections may be used, but the effect is temporary (lasting 18–24 months). The injections may cause facial numbness.

- Percutaneous denervation, either by glycerol injection or radiofrequency thermocoagulation of the trigeminal ganglion. This may cause facial and corneal numbness. Anaesthesia dolorosa, a severe dysaesthesia that is generally unresponsive to therapy, occurs as a complication in 5–10% of cases.

- Microvascular decompression via a posterior fossa approach. The surgeon separates the trigeminal sensory root from the compressing aberrant blood vessel using a non-absorbable sponge. This approach is more likely to cause death, stroke, facial weakness or hearing loss, but is less likely to be associated with recurrence, dysaesthesias or anaesthesia dolorosa.

FURTHER READING

Brisman R. Surgical treatment of trigeminal neuralgia. *Semin. Neurol.* 1997; 17: 367–72.

– – – – – – – – – – – – – – –

Hamlyn PJ. *Neurovascular Compression of the Lower Cranial Nerves.* Amsterdam: Elsevier Science, 1999.

2.6.3 Cluster headache

Pathophysiology

- The mechanism of pain is similar to migraine, in that the trigemino-vascular system is involved.

- The central disorder is likely to involve the pacemaker regions of the posterior hypothalamus.

Epidemiolgy

Migraine is 20 times more common. Cluster headache occurs predominantly in males (male to female ratio 6:1) over the age of 20 years.

Clinical presentation

Characteristic features

- Severe unilateral orbital, supraorbital and/or temporal headache described as an intense, constant and boring pain.

- Typically each attack lasts for 15–180 minutes, occurring one to three times daily for 4–8 weeks, with each cluster occurring once or twice a year. There is, however, considerable variation.

- 80–90% of patients will have recurrent attacks at the same time each day, particularly in the early hours of the morning ('alarm clock' headache).

- There are several important associated features (see below).

- During a bout, alcohol seems to be a potent trigger.

- A chronic form of cluster headache may develop from episodic cluster or may occur *de novo*, in which the patient experiences recurrent attacks for more than a year with few or no remissions.

Associated features

Patients should have one or more of these features in order to be diagnosed as having cluster headache:

- conjunctival injection;
- lacrimation;
- nasal congestion;
- rhinorrhoea;
- ptosis;
- miosis;
- eyelid oedema.

Physical signs

In chronic cluster headaches a permanent Horner's syndrome may develop, but examination is usually normal between attacks.

Differential diagnosis

- Episodic cluster headache is simple to diagnose, but the chronic form may be more difficult (see Section 1.1.2).

- Attacks with the features of cluster headache, but with a shorter duration (3–45 minutes) and occurring more frequently (20–40 times per day), have been termed 'chronic paroxysmal hemicrania', and are almost invariably responsive to indometacin.

In a patient with unilateral facial pain and a Horner's syndrome, any contralateral focal neurological signs should make you consider a carotid artery dissection (see Section 1.1.2).

Treatment

Acute

Try the following.

- 100% oxygen via a close-fitting mask at a rate of 15 L/min relieves approximately 80% of attacks within 15 minutes.

- Sumatriptan 50–100 mg orally or 6 mg subcutaneously are as effective as oxygen.

- Ergotamine tablets or suppositories may be used the night before in anticipation of 'alarm clock' headaches.

- Verapamil 80 mg qds is effective in stopping a bout.

- Corticosteroids are also effective in stopping a bout, but recurrence is a problem.

Prophylaxis
The following agents may be helpful.

- Verapamil 240–600 mg daily has been used in the prevention of both episodic and chronic cluster headache, and is the drug of choice as a prophylactic agent. High doses need to be used.

- Lithium carbonate is efficacious in the suppression of chronic, but less so of episodic, cluster headache in doses of 300–600 mg daily (maintaining serum levels at less than 1.2 mEq/L).

- Sodium valproate, topiramate and methysergide have also been used with some benefit.

FURTHER READING

Goadsby PJ and Lipton RB. A review of paroxysmal hemicranias, SUNCT syndrome and other short-lasting headaches with autonomic features, including new cases. *Brain* 1997; 120: 193–209.

Goadsby PJ. Mechanisms and management of headache. *J. R. Coll. Physicians Lond.* 1999; 33: 228–34.

2.6.4 Tension-type headache
Tension-type headache (TTH) is described as a constant tight or band-like sensation (non-pulsatile) around the head, which is usually bilateral (80–90%) and not aggravated by physical activity. It may be episodic (occurring on less than 15 days each month) or chronic (more than 15 days each month).

The term 'chronic daily headache' is often used for this type of headache, but is a descriptive, not diagnostic, term. Varieties of primary chronic daily or near-daily headache include:

- chronic tension-type headache;

- transformed or chronic migraine (analgesic overuse);

- chronic cluster headache;

- chronic paroxysmal hemicrania;

- new persistent daily headache.

Secondary causes are discussed in the Differential diagnosis section.

Pathophysiology
The pain of TTH is probably generated by the activation and sensitisation of second-order trigeminal neurons. The current phenotypic classification is likely to be reorganised once the underlying biological and genetic processes are better understood.

Epidemiology
Daily headache is common, with a lifetime prevalence of approximately 5% of the population.

Clinical presentation
Characteristic features include the following.

- The quality of the headache, as described above, may be of band-like bifrontotemporal pressure, or like a weight pressing down on top of the head.

- Occasional unilateral stabbing sensations may occur.

- Mild nausea (but not vomiting) and photophobia are common.

- Chronic forms are worsened by anxiety and stress, but pain is not limited to these occasions.

- Alcohol may relieve TTH, unlike migraine.

- There are no abnormal features on examination.

Investigation
Many patients are anxious to have a brain scan, but if there are no abnormal physical signs and the headache has the characteristic features described above then a scan is not indicated, and reassurance is appropriate.

Differential diagnosis
If the headache is of more recent subacute onset, then the following can present with generalised non-specific headaches, and so must always be considered in the appropriate age group.

- Expanding intracranial lesion: any age, but will produce symptoms more quickly in a young brain rather than atrophic one.

- Progressive hydrocephalus: any age, but as for intracranial lesion.

- Temporal arteritis: in those over 55 years old.

- Idiopathic intracranial hypertension: in young females.

- Primary angle-closure glaucoma: headache and eye pain associated with coloured haloes around lights, but may cause bilateral pain. Rare before middle age.

Overdiagnosed causes of chronic headache

Headache should not be attributed to:

- sinus disease, unless there are other symptoms supporting this;
- disease of the ears, teeth or temporomandibular joint, unless there are other symptoms supporting this;
- errors of refraction, as this only occasionally causes a very mild frontal headache not present on waking.

Treatment

Principles

Reassurance is a key component of treatment. It is essential to identify contributory factors such as:

- functional or structural cervical or cranial musculoskeletal abnormalities;
- depression;
- analgesic overuse (see Section 2.6.1).

Non-pharmacological

These approaches are also useful.

- Encourage regular exercise in the sedentary.
- Suggest stress management if stress is prominent in the history.
- Physiotherapy may help to correct posture and to improve symptoms secondary to trauma such as whiplash, but it may be less successful in degenerative disease of the neck.

Pharmacological

Simple analgesia Regular simple analgesia is inappropriate as it may be implicated in the genesis of the headache, although a single course of naproxen 500 mg bd for 3 weeks occasionally breaks the cycle of frequently occurring headaches.

Amitriptyline This is the drug of choice. It is important to explain that amitriptyline is not being used as an antidepressant, otherwise the patient may stop taking it. Start with 10 mg nocte and increase in 25-mg increments every 2 weeks to 75–100 mg. If tolerated, continue with this drug for 12 weeks before assessing efficacy, as it may take this long to work. If it has a beneficial effect, then continue for a further 6–9 months before withdrawing the drug.

Other agents Also consider the following.

- Other drugs such as Prothiaden and sodium valproate.
- Selective serotonin reuptake inhibitors seem to have little effect on chronic TTH, but may help if the patient is experiencing depression.
- Where chronic TTH and migraine coexist, in addition to the above measures the migraine may require symptomatic treatment (see Section 2.6.1), but on no more than 2 days per week.

Analgesic overuse, typically with paracetamol- or codeine-based compounds, requires that the appropriate drugs are withdrawn over 2–4 weeks if possible. It is wise to warn the patient that the headaches are likely to get worse before they get better, but unless the offending analgesics are withdrawn, the headache will not improve.

FURTHER READING

Dodick DW. Clinical practice: chronic daily headache. *N. Engl. J. Med.* 2006; 354: 158–65.

2.7 Epilepsy

Definition

Epilepsy is a condition characterised by recurrent (two or more) epileptic seizures, unprovoked by any immediate identified cause.

An epileptic seizure is a clinical manifestation presumed to result from an abnormal and excessive discharge from a set of neurons in the brain. The clinical manifestation consists of sudden and transitory abnormal phenomena which may include alterations in consciousness and motor, sensory, autonomic or psychic events perceived by the patient or an observer.

Pathophysiology

Pathological studies, increasingly from postoperative studies of resected foci, have shown a wide range of abnormalities, in particular the characteristic mesial temporal sclerosis seen in temporal lobe epilepsy, implying that these focal lesions may be epileptogenic. Diffuse cortical microdysgenesis may similarly play a part in the pathogenesis of idiopathic generalised epilepsy.

Aetiology

In childhood-onset seizures, there is a strong association with congenital, developmental and genetic abnormalities.

In elderly patients, stroke is the commonest association (in 50% of first-time seizures in the over-sixties). At any age, head trauma, central nervous system infection and tumours have strong associations with epilepsy.

In general, there are likely to be multifactorial aetiologies. A genetic predisposition to epilepsy could lower the susceptibility to other aetiological factors.

Epidemiology

- Incidence: 40–70 per 100,000 per year in developed countries.

- Prevalence: 0.5–1.0% of the general population have active epilepsy.

- Lifetime prevalence: 2–5% of the general population.

Clinical presentation

A witness account is essential, and a hand-held video recording of an attack would be extremely useful, as the diagnosis of epilepsy is a clinical one.

Epilepsy may be most usefully classified according to seizure types (Table 45). The classification of epilepsy as syndromes is less useful clinically at present, partly because future classifications will change as more is learned about the underlying, possibly genetic, aetiologies.

Generalised seizures

Tonic–clonic Features include the following.

- Sudden-onset loss of consciousness often associated with an audible cry, followed by a fall to the ground.

- Tonic stiffening phase lasts 10–30 seconds, during which time respiration may be impaired, leading to cyanosis.

- Followed by clonic phase, in which there is low-amplitude jerking of all four limbs. As the seizure progresses, its frequency slows and its amplitude increases. Lasts 30–60 seconds.

- Flaccidity of muscles with slow recovery of consciousness over 2–30 minutes.

- Associated with incontinence, tongue biting and autonomic features.

- May be more tonic or clonic.

- Does not imply pathological type, unless preceded by clear partial onset.

Typical absence Features include the following.

- Sudden loss of consciousness and motor activity without warning, resulting in a blank stare.

- Attacks end suddenly and patients may continue with what they were doing, unaware of what has just happened.

- Short attacks: <30 seconds.

- Automatisms, slight clonic movements or eyelid fluttering may occur in longer attacks.

- These seizures occur as part of idiopathic generalised epilepsy.

Atypical absence Features include the following.

- Blank stare.

- Onset and cessation are more gradual.

- Consciousness is only partially impaired.

- Focal signs are more prominent.

- Occurs in patients with diffuse cerebral damage.

Myoclonic Features include the following.

- Brief jerk either in single muscle or generalised, which is of rapid onset and cessation.

- No loss of consciousness.

- Often part of idiopathic generalised epilepsies.

Partial seizures

Simple Features include the following.

TABLE 45 CLASSIFICATION OF EPILEPTIC SEIZURES

Seizure type	Characteristics
Partial seizures	*Simple* Motor: either limb or adversive head turning (frontal) Sensory or special sensory, eg visual: symptoms usually positive (pins and needles) rather than negative (numbness) Autonomic: rising epigastric sensation and changes in skin colour, BP, heart rate and pupil size may all indicate a temporal lobe origin Psychic: dysphasia/speech arrest, déjà vu, sensations of unreality or depersonalisation, fear, anger, elation, illusions or structured hallucinations may all originate from a temporal lobe focus *Complex* Simple partial onset followed by impairment of consciousness With impaired consciousness at onset Partial seizures evolving to secondary generalised seizures

Generalised seizures	Absence seizures
	   Typical
	   Atypical
	Myoclonic seizures
	Clonic seizures
	Tonic seizures
	Atonic seizures
	Tonic–clonic seizures

Unclassifiable seizures	

- No alteration in consciousness, and no amnesia.

- Sudden onset and cessation.

- Symptoms depend on site of underlying cortical lesion (Table 45).

- The seizure lasts for only seconds.

Complex Features include the following.

- Often preceded by simple partial seizure (aura).

- Alteration in consciousness associated with blank staring, and often with motor signs such as unilateral dystonic posturing (temporal lobe).

- Automatism: this is a more or less co-ordinated involuntary motor activity occurring during a clouding of consciousness that occurs during or after an epileptic seizure, usually followed by amnesia. They may take many forms (Table 46).

- About 60% of complex partial seizures arise from the temporal lobes and 30% from the frontal lobes. Automatisms may occur as part of a complex partial seizure from any location.

Juvenile myoclonic epilepsy

Juvenile myoclonic epilepsy is a syndromic diagnosis worth knowing about because:

- it is common, causing 5–10% of all cases of epilepsy;
- it has an extremely good prognosis if treated correctly.

Clinical features

- Myoclonic jerks, generalised tonic–clonic seizures, with or without absences, and precipitated by sleep deprivation and alcohol.
- Clear diurnal variation, attacks frequently occurring within an hour of waking. Ask specifically about early morning twitching as this may not be reported.
- Of patients with juvenile myoclonic epilepsy, 90% become seizure-free when on sodium valproate, although high relapse rates occur off medication.
- Linked to chromosome 6.

Physical signs

- Uncommon unless seizures are due to an underlying cortical structural lesion.

- Epilepsy may occur as part of a wider phenotype in some neurodegenerative diseases.

- Consider the neurocutaneous syndromes.

Investigation

- Routine biochemical and haematological profiles.

- Electroencephalography (EEG).

- MRI.

- A hand-held video recording is very useful, especially if the diagnosis is not clearly epilepsy.

Electroencephalography

In practice, most patients require EEG as part of their initial evaluation. However, note the following.

- A normal interictal EEG does not exclude epilepsy. An abnormal EEG may support a primary idiopathic process and provide evidence of photosensitivity.

- EEG is a poor guide to seizure control, with the exception of 3 Hz spike-and-wave changes which are sensitive to treatment (Fig. 39).

- Minor asymmetries are not diagnostic.

MRI

Structural imaging is indicated as follows:

- partial seizures on history (Fig. 40);

- deficit revealed on neurological or psychological examination;

- difficult seizure control with antiepileptics;

- generalised seizures, onset before 1 or after 20 years of age.

The last point is debated. The reason for suggesting it is that a generalised seizure with no suggestion of partial onset is extremely likely to be a primary idiopathic type of epilepsy

TABLE 46 CLINICAL FEATURES OF AUTOMATISMS

Type	Feature
Oro-alimentary	Lip smacking Chewing Swallowing
Gestural	Fiddling with hands Picking at clothing Tidying
Ambulatory	Walking Running Circling Purposeless complex movement
Verbal	Humming Whistling Grunting
Mimicry	Displays of laughter, fear, anger, excitement

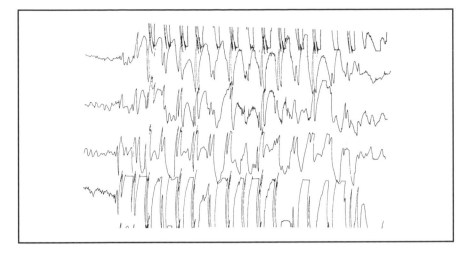

▲**Fig. 39** 3 Hz spike-and-wave.

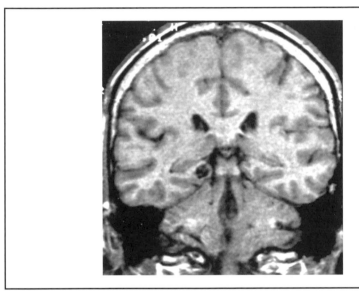

▲**Fig. 40** Right parahippocampal angioma in a patient with temporal lobe epilepsy seen on a coronal MRI scan.

in this age range. Some specialists will scan all new presentations.

Differential diagnosis

Half of new epilepsy referrals may have an alternative diagnosis. The distinction between an epileptic attack and a non-epileptic attack is discussed in Table 47, but it should be remembered that they may coexist.

Treatment

Emergency

For management of status epilepticus see Section 1.4.4.

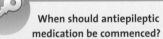

When should antiepileptic medication be commenced?

To answer this, one needs an appreciation of the risks of seizure recurrence to balance against the risk of antiepileptic medication.

- The risk of recurrence is highest in the first few days and weeks, then falls with time.
- 30% of patients will have a recurrent seizure by 3 months, 67% by 12 months and 78% by 36 months. Antiepileptic medication reduces but does not abolish this risk.
- At 12 months the risk of recurrence in those with a partial seizure is

94%. In those with seizures precipitated by an acute illness it is much lower at 40%.

On the basis of these figures you can see that it might be desirable to treat some patients after one seizure rather than wait for the customary two seizures, as the risk of recurrence may be high (about 80% with time overall). If a patient presents having had a single seizure 12 months before, then the subsequent risk of recurrence may be lower and one may choose to wait.

The decision to initiate antiepileptic treatment is based on the risk of recurrent seizures versus the risks of the drug itself, not on arbitrarily waiting for two seizures to occur.

Natural history of epilepsy on treatment

- Reassure the patient that 70–80% of newly diagnosed patients treated with a single antiepileptic drug will eventually be seizure-free.

- If remission is defined as 5 years seizure-free, then about 40% of patients enter remission in the first year, 20% in the next 9 years and 10% in the next 10 years.

Once the decision to initiate treatment has been made, follow these general principles.

- Start the drug at a low dose, then titrate up slowly until the seizures are abolished or the maximum tolerated dose has been reached.

- First-line drugs are usually carbamazepine for partial seizures or secondary generalised seizures (start at 100 mg daily, increasing by 200 mg every 2 weeks up to 600–1800 mg total daily dose), and sodium valproate for most generalised or idiopathic epilepsies (start at 200 mg daily,

TABLE 47 DIFFERENTIATION BETWEEN AN EPILEPTIC AND A NON-EPILEPTIC ATTACK

	Epileptic attack	Non-epileptic attack
Precipitant	Rare	Commonly stress related
Onset	Short	May be short or prolonged
Movement	Synchronous small-amplitude jerks if clonic	Asynchronous flailing of limbs, pelvic thrusting, opisthotonus
Injury	Tongue biting (sides) and falls, but directed violence rare	May bite tongue (tip), cheeks, lip and hands, and may throw themselves to ground; also, directed violence occurs
Consciousness	Complete or incomplete depending on type	Variable, but may be inconsistent with seizure type
Response to stimuli	None unless it is complex partial seizure	May terminate the attack. Suggestible
Incontinence	Common	Sometimes
Duration	Minutes	May be prolonged
Recovery	Few minutes, but may be prolonged confusion	Rapid or very prolonged

increasing by 200 mg every week up to 1000–2500 mg total daily dose).

- If seizures continue, reconsider the diagnosis, check compliance and review or obtain neuroimaging.

- If epilepsy is still thought to be the diagnosis, then introduce another first-line agent, for example carbamazepine, lamotrigine or sodium valproate. When a reasonable dose is achieved, then the first drug can be withdrawn slowly.

- Adjust the dose of the second drug to optimum.

- If seizures continue, try both first-line drugs together. Thereafter add a second-line drug at the expense of the least well tolerated first-line drug. Consider other second-line drugs in a similar manner.

- Three drugs are rarely better than two.

'When can I come off my tablets, doctor?'

This question is likely to be asked by the patient when in some form of remission. The first two points that need to be highlighted are as follows.

- No guarantees can be made that seizures will not recur.
- Think about driving: if the loss of a driving licence would be a devastating blow to the patient, he or she may decide to stay on medication.

The decision must be made by the patient, informed by the information you provide.

- In patients in remission for 2 years or more, the chance of a seizure in the subsequent 2 years are 43% if the drug is withdrawn, compared to 10% in those maintaining therapy.
- This figure may alter with the presence or absence of certain risk factors (Table 48).
- Within 10–15 years after the onset of epilepsy at least 70% of patients have been in remission for 5 years and 50% are off all drugs, so the prognosis is actually quite good.

Surgical treatment
Focal resections Consider surgical options in patients with seizures of partial onset that are refractory to intensive medical therapy over at least 2–3 years.

- Presurgical evaluation includes a detailed clinical assessment, EEG and video telemetry to obtain ictal EEG, high-resolution structural MRI (epilepsy protocol), a positron emission tomography scan if structural imaging is unclear, and neuropsychological and neuropsychiatric evaluation.

- One is looking for a convergence of data, implying one epileptogenic area. If these data are concordant, then the chance of seizure freedom postoperatively is approximately 60–70%. Data suggesting multiple foci indicates less chance of success.

- The commonest site of resection is the temporal lobe. The risk of serious morbidity or mortality during surgical resection is approximately 1%.

Other operations Remember the following.

- Division of the corpus callosum is reserved for patients with severe intractable seizures and drop attacks. The operation is aimed at reducing the number and severity of attacks, especially the drop attacks.

- Hemispherectomy is reserved for children or adolescents with medically intractable seizures due to severe unilateral hemisphere damage.

Management of the pregnant patient with epilepsy
General information Preconception counselling is very important.

- The background risk of major fetal malformations in developed

TABLE 48 FACTORS AFFECTING RISK OF RECURRENT SEIZURE FOLLOWING DRUG WITHDRAWAL

Risk	Factor
Increased risk	Age over 16 Taking more than one antiepileptic drug History of seizures after starting antiepileptic drugs History of tonic–clonic seizures History of myoclonic seizures Abnormal EEG in the previous year
Decreased risk	Risk of seizures declines the longer the seizure-free period

Occupational aspects

Driving

Patients may apply for a driving licence if they have been seizure-free for 1 year, or if they have an established pattern of seizures occurring only during sleep for the previous 3 years. Stricter rules apply to drivers of heavy goods vehicles (HGVs) and passenger-carrying vehicles (PCVs).

It is recommended, but not covered by legislation, that driving be suspended from the start of antiepileptic drug withdrawal until 6 months afterwards.

countries is 1–2%, and this is thought to rise to 3% in mothers with epilepsy on no medication, 4–6% with one antiepileptic drug and up to 15% with two or more. There is some evidence that this risk is dose dependent.

- The background risk of neural-tube defects is 0.2–0.5%, being increased to 1% by carbamazepine and 1–2% by sodium valproate.

Principles of drug management
Remember the following.

- If possible, maintain the patient on as few drugs and at as low a dose as possible.

- Consider withdrawing drugs prior to pregnancy if the patient has been seizure-free for 2 years.

- Advise folic acid 5 mg daily for 12 weeks before and after conception to reduce the risk of neural-tube defects.

- Serum alpha-fetoprotein measurement and high-resolution fetal ultrasound should be carried out at 16–18 weeks to screen for neural-tube defects, especially in those taking sodium valproate or carbamazepine.

- Oral vitamin K (20 mg/day) should be given to the mother if she is taking an enzyme-inducing drug (phenytoin, carbamazepine,

phenobarbital or primidone) in the last month of pregnancy to protect the baby from haemorrhagic disease of the newborn. The risk lasts for a week or so after birth and so some suggest that oral vitamin K be given to the baby for a further week to cover this period. However, vitamin K is still usually given by intramuscular injection to newborn babies. Fears still exist over the risk of childhood neoplasia with the injectable form, although more recent trials have failed to find this link.

Prognosis
Epilepsy carries an increased risk of death, mainly attributable to the underlying disease, accidents or suicide.

Patients with epilepsy are at risk of SUDEP (sudden unexplained deaths in epilepsy) at a rate of 1 per 200–1,000 per year. Young patients and those with frequent generalised seizures and learning disability have higher risk. The cause and strategies for prevention are not clear, although there is some evidence to suggest that either cerebrogenic cardiac arrhythmias or ictal apnoea may be responsible.

Employment
Recruitment is barred in the armed forces, the fire brigade, London Regional Transport, the merchant navy and diving. For many other occupations no specific legislation exists but employment is unlikely.

Leisure
To a large extent, this depends on the individual's particular seizure pattern, but in general adequate supervision for activities such as swimming, cycling and rock climbing is needed, together with an acceptance that risk is not something that can be eliminated from all activities.

FURTHER READING

Nashef L. From mystery to prevention: sudden unexplained death in epilepsy, time to move on. *J. Neurol. Neurosurg. Psychiatry* 1999; 67: 427.

- - - - - - - - - - - - - - - -

Sander JW and Shorvon SD. Epidemiology of the epilepsies. *J. Neurol. Neurosurg. Psychiatry* 1996; 61: 433–43.

- - - - - - - - - - - - - - - -

Sander JW, Hart YM, Johnson AL and Shorvon SD. National General Practice Study of Epilepsy: newly diagnosed epileptic seizures in a general population. *Lancet* 1990; 336: 1267–71.

2.8 Cerebrovascular disease

2.8.1 Stroke

The most widely accepted definition of a stroke is a clinical syndrome characterised by:

- rapidly developing clinical symptoms;

- signs of focal, and at times global (applied to patients with coma or subarachnoid haemorrhage), loss of cerebral function;

- symptoms lasting for more than 24 hours or leading to death with no apparent cause other than being of vascular origin.

The classification of stroke is broadly into ischaemic and haemorrhagic (Table 49). Ischaemic stroke is dealt with in this section, and intracerebral haemorrhage and subarachnoid haemorrhage are discussed in Section 2.8.4 and *Acute Medicine*, Section 1.2.30.

Aetiology

An ischaemic stroke can be classified according to its mechanism using the TOAST (Trial of Org 10172 in Acute Stroke Treatment) classification. Strokes are divided into five categories:

- thromboembolism from the heart;

- thromboembolism from major vessels;

- occlusion of small penetrating vessels, found predominantly in the basal ganglia, internal capsule or pons (lacunar stroke) (Fig. 41);

- other (ie not one of the above but a definite mechanism identified);

- unknown.

Occlusion of vessels may occur as a result of thrombosis and local occlusion, or subsequent to embolisation and distal occlusion.

Thrombosis is attributable to any element of Virchow's triad:

- abnormality of the vessel wall [atherosclerosis (especially if ulcerated), dissection or vasculitis in large vessels and lipohyalinosis in the small perforating vessels];

- abnormality of the blood (eg polycythaemia);

- disturbances of blood flow (eg atrial fibrillation).

> The main constituents of thrombi are:
>
> - platelets (form in fast-flow areas such as the internal carotid artery as a result of atheromatous plaque);
> - fibrin and red blood cells (form in slow-flow areas such as the cardiac atria in atrial fibrillation).

> This explains the theoretical rationale for the use of secondary preventive agents: antiplatelet drugs in atherothrombosis and warfarin in atrial fibrillation and heart failure.
>
> Risk factors for vascular disease (see below), eg hypertension, are responsible for the underlying pathological disease of blood vessels, particularly atherosclerosis.

Main modifiable risk factors for stroke

- Hypertension.

- Atrial fibrillation.

- Cigarette smoking.

- Previous transient ischaemic attack.

- Heart failure.

- Ischaemic heart disease.

- Diabetes mellitus.

- Excess alcohol.

- Hyperlipidaemia.

- Obesity.

- Inactivity.

- Elevated haematocrit.

Pathophysiology

Reduction in cerebral blood flow (CBF) below the normal (>50 mL/min per 100 g of tissue) sets off a cascade of events that ultimately leads to cell death if not reversed. As CBF falls below about 20 mL/min per 100 g, there is loss of electrical neuronal function, a potentially reversible stage. Below 10 mL/min per 100 g, irreversible damage starts to occur. The increased energy demands of the cell cannot be met and adenosine triphosphate becomes depleted. Consequently, energy-dependent ion homeostasis fails, leading to equilibration of all ions across the cell membrane (anoxic

TABLE 49 CLASSIFICATION OF STROKE TYPES	
Pathology	Mechanism
Ischaemic (85%)	Large-vessel atherothrombotic disease
	Small-vessel thrombotic disease/lacunar infarcts
	Embolic disease from cardiac source
	Other
	Unknown
Haemorrhagic (15%)	Primary intracerebral haemorrhage
	Subarachnoid haemorrhage

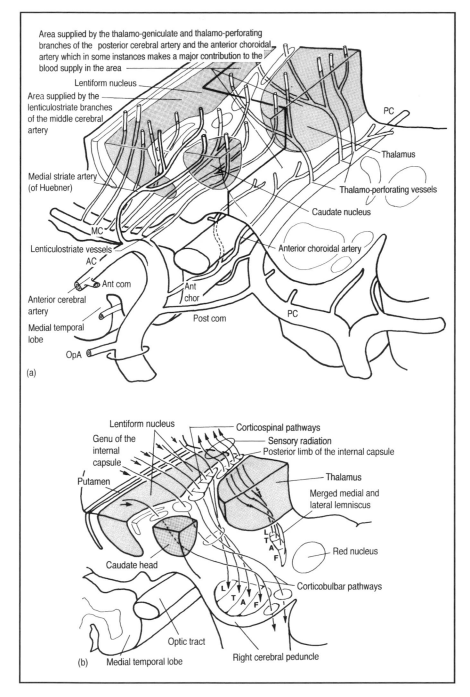

▲ **Fig. 41** (a) Schematic representation of the blood supply to the region of the internal capsule. Note that the main motor pathways at capsular level are supplied by the middle cerebral branches, and the main sensory pathways are mainly supplied by the posterior cerebral-derived vessels. This explains why capsular strokes tend to be primarily motor or sensory. The blood supply of the sublenticular visual pathways, the optic tract and the lateral geniculate body is derived from anterior choroidal or posterior cerebral-derived vessels. (b) Key diagram of pathway anatomy in the internal capsule. The right internal capsule is shown from above and anteriorly to indicate the motor and sensory rotations between the internal capsule and upper midbrain. A, arm; F, face; L, leg; T, trunk.

depolarisation) and the release of potentially toxic levels of glutamate and calcium influx. Several processes interact leading to an ischaemic cascade and, ultimately, cell death.

Epidemiology

- The annual incidence is 312 per 100,000 in those aged 45–84 years (200 per 100,000 in the overall population).

- Of all deaths in industrialised countries, 12% are due to stroke.

- Stroke is the commonest cause of severe physical disability and accounts for 5% of NHS hospital costs.

Physical signs

The neurological examination should enable one to identify the site of the lesion accurately, but in routine clinical practice this degree of accuracy has no value over and above a bedside system of classification such as the Oxfordshire Community Stroke Study classification (see Table 21). In the case of evolving signs this simple analysis is more likely to be incorrect, but it is used in some units and is worth being aware of. The immediate assessment of an acute stroke patient is discussed fully in *Acute Medicine*, Section 1.2.30.

Investigation

The most important specific investigation is a CT scan to exclude haemorrhage and enable early treatment with antiplatelet agents (and consideration of thrombolysis in active centres) and to exclude other possible diagnoses such as space-occupying lesions. In ischaemic stroke CT scans may initially appear normal, but remember that early signs of ischaemia are subtle and easily missed (Fig. 42).

At presentation patients should also have:

- ECG;

- CXR;

- FBC, erythrocyte sedimentation rate, urea and electrolytes, and glucose.

Differential diagnosis

Misdiagnosis of ischaemic stroke occurs in up to one-quarter of cases,

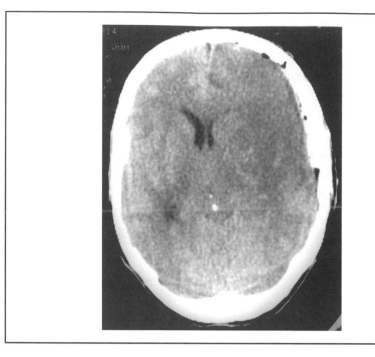

▲**Fig. 42** CT scan showing acute changes of cerebral infarction due to occlusion of left middle cerebral artery.

usually when a clear history is not available. Intracerebral haemorrhage is the most important differential diagnosis, and can only reliably be differentiated on CT scan. Other alternatives include brain tumour, subdural haematoma, cerebral venous thrombosis, focal cerebral infection, hypoglycaemia and postictal Todd's paresis. In a young person, consider multiple sclerosis.

> Stroke is a clinical diagnosis, but the most important distinction, between ischaemia and haemorrhage, requires special investigation, ie a CT scan. This has an impact on subsequent management, and will become ever more important with the advent of acute therapies for ischaemic stroke.

Treatment

Short term

General care Important points to consider in the investigation/management of an acute case are as follows.

- Early treatment is supportive in order to prevent complications.

- Careful monitoring of neurological status, BP, oxygenation, glycaemic control, hydration, nutrition, swallowing function, temperature control and bladder function are all crucial, and proper management in these areas will have an enormous impact on the mortality and morbidity of stroke patients.

- Management of stroke patients in a designated stroke unit reduces mortality and long-term dependency. Much planning needs to go into the ongoing care of patients, often elderly, whose stroke has left them dependent.

Acute therapies designed to minimise the size of infarct
Specific early treatments designed to reduce the size of infarct include thrombolysis and neuroprotective agents.

- Thrombolysis: the National Institute of Neurological Disorders and Stroke (NINDS) trial demonstrated that compared

with placebo, patients treated within 3 hours of onset of stroke with intravenous recombinant tissue plasminogen activator (rtPA) had a favourable outcome at 3 months. There was a significant increase in the number of treated patients suffering from symptomatic intracranial haemorrhage, but importantly there was no overall increase in mortality at 3 months. Subsequent trials using rtPA have failed to show significant benefit in terms of functional outcome. However, a meta-analysis of 12 thrombolysis trials demonstrated significant improvements in functional outcome in those patients treated with thrombolysis up to 6 hours after stroke, although there was an increase in overall mortality in this group. Patients treated up to 3 hours after stroke also gained benefit in functional outcome, without the increased mortality seen in the 0–6 hours treatment group. Hence it appears that rtPA given up to 3 hours after stroke seems to have some benefit, but it is not clear how many patients will present early enough to be treated within this window.

- Neuroprotection: neuroprotective agents have been disappointing to date, but it is likely that they will need to be given in combination with thrombolysis so that cerebral tissue preserved in this manner will benefit from reperfusion.

Agents used to reduce stroke recurrence in the acute setting
These include antiplatelet therapy and anticoagulants.

- Antiplatelet therapy: aspirin prevents 10 deaths or recurrent strokes per 1,000 patients treated in the first 2 weeks following acute ischaemic stroke and should be commenced, once haemorrhage has been excluded, at a dose of 300 mg daily. It is then usual to switch to long-term prophylaxis at a dose of 75 mg daily.

- Anticoagulants: warfarin and heparin are not associated with any overall benefit in the treatment of stroke because of an increase in haemorrhagic complications and so cannot be recommended for acute treatment. Heparin is used occasionally for 'stroke in evolution' and basilar artery thrombosis, and frequently for carotid or vertebral artery dissection (but without supportive evidence from randomised controlled trials).

Long term

The diagnosis has been made and treatment initiated. Subsequent management is directed at establishing the underlying cause of the stroke, initiating secondary preventive measures and managing the consequent impairment.

Further investigations In appropriate circumstances the following are likely to be helpful in determining cause and identifying factors important in secondary preventive treatment.

- Electrocardiography should have been performed acutely but it is critical to ensure that it is reviewed. The diagnosis of atrial fibrillation will have a significant impact on further management.

- Carotid Doppler and magnetic resonance angiography to look for symptomatic internal carotid artery stenosis in a case of carotid territory ischaemia. If these two investigations are in agreement, they should avoid the need for intra-arterial angiography.

- Transthoracic echocardiography if an embolic source is suspected. In a young stroke patient in whom an embolic source is

considered, transoesophageal echocardiography should be performed to rule out patent foramen ovale.

- Serum cholesterol.

- Thrombophilia screen: at present the significance of these tests is not clear, so reserve for cases with no other clear aetiological risk factors, young patients and those with a strong family history. Similarly, a sickle cell screen is crucial when appropriate.

Secondary preventive treatment: risk factor reduction Most of the evidence is from primary prevention studies, but removal of as many risk factors as possible is sensible.

Secondary preventive treatment: antiplatelet therapy Consider the following.

- Aspirin is beneficial in secondary prevention of all vascular events, as demonstrated by the Antiplatelet Trialists' Collaboration, and it seems to reduce subsequent vascular events by about 23%. It should be commenced as soon as possible (ie after haemorrhage excluded), as established by both the International Stroke Trial (IST) and the Chinese Acute Stroke Trial (CAST).

- Dipyridamole modified release (MR) 200 mg bd should be added if further events occur on aspirin monotherapy.

- If the patient has multiple vascular risk factors, start with combination therapy (aspirin plus dipyridamole MR).

- If the patient is genuinely aspirin intolerant, use clopidogrel. Alternatively, dipyridamole MR monotherapy could be considered in patients with low vascular risk factors, but not in those

with high vascular risk factors as dipyridamole MR alone seems to have no effect on non-stroke vascular events.

Secondary preventive treatment: anticoagulants Warfarin should be prescribed for most patients who have had an ischaemic stroke with atrial fibrillation. It is not clear exactly when to start this, but after major stroke wait at least 2 weeks (possibly less in minor strokes) to reduce the chances of haemorrhagic conversion.

Secondary preventive treatment: carotid surgery Two trials, the North American Symptomatic Carotid Endarterectomy Trial (NASCET) and the European Carotid Surgery Trial (ESCT) studied patients with a recent transient ischaemic attack or minor stroke, and found a beneficial effect of carotid endarterectomy in those with a stenosis of ≥70%.

Secondary preventive treatment: carotid endovascular treatment Endovascular treatment (angioplasty and stenting) is a less invasive alternative to surgery for internal carotid artery stenosis. The most obvious advantages are the avoidance of a surgical incision and its ability to be performed under local anaesthesia, thus avoiding the effects of anaesthetic drugs and intubation. Because of this, the risk of potentially fatal complications such as myocardial infarction and pulmonary embolism is also reduced. The use of local anaesthesia also means a faster recovery for patients treated endovascularly, reducing the length of hospital stay and potentially reducing costs. The potential pitfalls of endovascular treatment of carotid stenosis include the fact that there are very few interventionists with extensive experience of angioplasty and stenting in the carotid artery.

NEUROLOGY: **DISEASES AND TREATMENTS**

This is likely to mean that at centres with little endovascular experience, angioplasty and stenting is initially less safe than surgery, with the major risk being distal embolisation to the brain during passage of a catheter through a tight stenosis. A meta-analysis that examined the safety and efficacy of endovascular treatment of carotid stenosis compared with endarterectomy in randomised trials found no significant difference in the major risks of treatment (stroke or death). Patients suitable for carotid endarterectomy should only be offered stenting within the ongoing randomised trials of stenting versus surgery.

Secondary preventive treatment: cholesterol Raised cholesterol is an important risk factor for coronary artery disease (CAD), but its association with cerebrovascular disease is less clear. CAD is a major cause of death in stroke patients, and so it seems reasonable to treat a cholesterol level over 5 mmol/L (and some would say even lower) after a stroke or transient ischaemic attack with a statin. This is particulary important in patients with diabetes mellitus.

Complications

Complications of acute stroke include the following.

- Cerebral oedema: the commonest cause of death, usually at 4–5 days.
- Haemorrhagic transformation.
- Seizures complicate 10% of infarcts or haemorrhages, but do not influence mortality.
- Depression occurs in 50% of those who suffer acute strokes, particularly with left anterior lesions.
- Deterioration in glycaemic control.

- Syndrome of inappropriate antidiuretic hormone secretion, peaking at 7–9 days.
- Pressure sores.
- Pulmonary embolism.
- Aspiration.

Prognosis

- 20% of cases result in death in the first month, 30% in first year.
- In those alive at 1 year, the annual death rate is 8.5%.
- The annual risk of recurrence is 13% in the first year, 5% thereafter.
- The risk of stroke or cardiac event by 5 years is 40%.
- It is very important to remember not only the risk of recurrent stroke but also of cardiac events.

Occupational aspects

Following stroke, patients often report reduced exercise tolerance and increased fatigue, which may continue beyond good functional recovery. This has implications for the timing of return to work when appropriate.

Driving is discouraged for 3 months.

FURTHER READING

Adams HP Jr, Bendixen BH, Kapelle LJ *et al.* Classification of subtype of acute ischemic stroke: definitions for use in a multicenter clinical trial. TOAST (Trial of Org 10172 in Acute Stroke Treatment). *Stroke* 1993: 24: 35–41.

Bronner LL, Kanter DS and Manson JE. Primary prevention of stroke. *N. Engl. J. Med.* 1995; 333: 1392–400.

Coward LJ, Featherstone RL and Brown MM. Safety and efficacy of endovascular treatment of carotid artery stenosis compared with carotid endarterectomy: a Cochrane systematic review of the randomized evidence. *Stroke* 2005; 36: 905–11.

Davenport R and Dennis M. Neurological emergencies: acute stroke. *J. Neurol. Neurosurg. Psychiatry* 2000; 68: 277–88.

McCabe DJ and Brown MM. Prevention of ischaemic stroke: antiplatelets. *Br. Med. Bull.* 2000; 56: 510–25.

Pulsinelli W. Pathophysiology of acute ischaemic stroke. *Lancet* 1992; 339: 533–6.

Wardlaw JM, Warlow CP and Counsell C. Systematic review of evidence on thrombolytic therapy for acute ischaemic stroke. *Lancet* 1997; 350: 607–14.

2.8.2 Transient ischaemic attacks

A transient ischaemic attack (TIA) is an episode of acute loss of focal cerebral or monocular function with symptoms lasting less than 24 hours, which is thought to be due to inadequate cerebral or ocular blood supply as a result of an arterial, cardiac or haematological cause.

The clinical significance of a TIA is no different to that of a minor stroke. Patients make a good recovery from both (TIAs usually recover within 30–60 minutes, despite the definition), and the challenge for the clinician is how to prevent a major stroke occurring. Investigation and secondary prevention are as detailed in Section 2.8.1. The distinct characteristics of TIAs are discussed below.

Clinical presentation

The diagnosis is made on a history of focal neurological symptoms (Table 50), as physical signs will almost certainly have disappeared by the time of assessment. The vascular territory involved, carotid or vertebrobasilar, is suspected on the same basis as for ischaemic

TABLE 50 SYMPTOMS RAISING THE POSSIBILITY OF TIAS

Carotid	Vertebrobasilar
Contralateral paresis, heaviness or clumsiness in the leg, arm/hand and face	Bilateral, unilateral or alternating paresis (may be contralateral and ipsilateral in face/limbs)
Contralateral and predominantly negative sensory symptoms in the leg, arm/hand and face	Sensory loss, unilateral or bilateral (may be contralateral and ipsilateral in face/limbs)
Contralateral homonymous hemianopia	Diplopia
Unilateral monocular visual loss	Bilateral visual loss
Aphasia	Dysphagia
Dysarthria	Dysarthria
Combination of the above	Combination of the above

strokes. Isolated dysarthria or homonymous hemianopia are more difficult to interpret, as they may be caused by TIAs in either territory.

- Non-focal symptoms such as loss of consciousness, dizziness, mental confusion, generalised weakness and incontinence are unacceptable as evidence of a TIA.
- Some focal symptoms occurring in isolation should also not be interpreted as TIAs (see below).

The symptoms below are not acceptable as evidence of a TIA if they occur in isolation:

- vertigo;
- diplopia;
- dysphagia;
- loss of balance;
- tinnitus;
- scintillating scotomas;
- amnesia;
- drop attacks;
- sensory symptoms confined to one part of limb or face.

Physical signs

Examine for the following.

- Cardiovascular abnormalities: the examination is usually normal but it is necessary to exclude predisposing factors.

- Carotid bruits: not always present even if there is a very tight stenosis.
- Cholesterol embolus: if visualised on fundoscopy this may indicate that the aetiology is atheromatous plaque in the aortic arch or internal carotid artery in a case of amaurosis fugax.

Consider subclavian steal syndrome

Vertebrobasilar symptoms brought on by exercise of the ipsilateral arm may be the result of stenosis of the proximal subclavian artery or aortic arch, leading to retrograde flow down the vertebral artery (Fig. 43). On examination there may be a bruit in the supraclavicular fossa with reduced BP and pulse pressure in the ipsilateral arm.

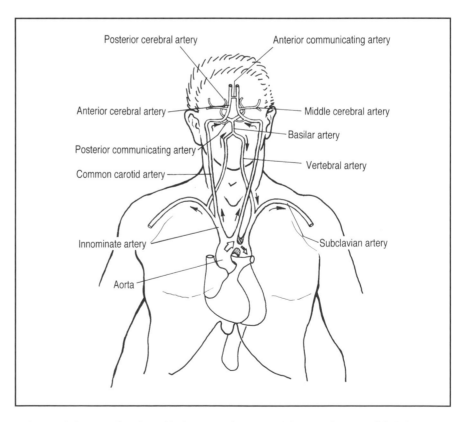

▲ **Fig. 43** Subclavian steal syndrome. The lesion is in the aortic arch between the origin of the left common carotid artery and the left subclavian artery. The blood therefore tends to flow up both carotids and the right vertebral artery and then flows back down the left vertebral artery, ultimately rejoining the subclavian artery to supply the left arm.

Differential diagnosis

Migraine and epilepsy are two of the commonest differential diagnoses encountered and the differential diagnosis of TIA includes:

- partial epilepsy;
- migraine with aura;
- migraine equivalents;
- multiple sclerosis;
- intracranial space-occupying lesions;
- intracranial vascular malformations;
- cardiac dysrhythmia;
- vestibular disorders;
- peripheral nerve or root lesions;
- anxiety and hyperventilation;
- hypoglycaemia;
- transient global amnesia.

Migraine

The difficulty arises when considering migraine equivalents, ie migraine without headache. The following points are helpful.

- Migrainous symptoms are usually positive (tingling and scintillating scotoma), whereas TIA symptoms are usually negative representing a loss of function (numbness, reduced vision and weakness).

- The spread of symptoms in migraine tends to be slow, ie over several minutes.

- After a migraine patients often feel generally unwell for hours, which is not usually the case after a TIA.

Partial epilepsy

- Symptoms are usually positive (jerking and tingling) and are brief compared with a TIA.

- Very frequent attacks are usually epileptic.

Note that occasionally focal lower limb shaking, occurring on standing, has been associated with severe contralateral carotid artery stenosis.

Prognosis

The risk of stroke following a TIA is increased:

- 13 times in the first year, and by seven times in each year subsequent to that one;
- 4% in the first month;
- 9% in the first 6 months;
- 12% in the first 12 months;
- 4% per annum thereafter.

Most strokes occur in the same territory as the previous TIA. Possibly for this reason, amaurosis fugax has a much lower chance of leading to a stroke.

> Patients with TIA have arterial disease, and as such have a higher risk of heart disease. In fact, the risk of myocardial infarction and sudden cardiac death is about 4% per annum, which emphasises the point that you must consider heart disease in TIA and stroke patients.

2.8.3 Intracerebral haemorrhage

Aetiology

Almost all cases of intracerebral haemorrhage (ICH) are caused by one of the following:

- primary hypertensive ICH (at least 50%);
- ruptured saccular aneurysms and arteriovenous malformations (30%);
- ICH associated with bleeding disorders (10%).

In addition, cerebral amyloid angiopathy (CAA) is recognised as a common cause in the elderly.

Other causes include:

- tumours;
- haemorrhagic infarction;
- trauma;
- sympathomimetic drugs;
- cerebral vasculitis.

And rarely:

- mycotic aneurysm (endocarditis);
- haemorrhagic leucoencephalopathy;
- herpes simplex encephalitis.

Pathology

Chronic hypertension causes a vasculopathy in the small perforating arteries, characterised by lipohyalinosis, fibrinoid necrosis and the formation of Charcot–Bouchard microaneurysms. Rupture of these results in haemorrhage in predominantly deep areas of the brain (Table 51).

Small haematomas dissect along white matter tracts, but large haematomas rupture into the parenchyma, causing destruction of tissue and elevation of intracranial pressure. Death occurs due to hemisphere and/or brainstem compression.

TABLE 51 SITES OF HYPERTENSIVE ICH

Site	Frequency (%)
Putamen	35–50
Subcortical (lobar)	30
Cerebellum	16
Thalamus	10–15
Pons	5–12

Epidemiology

- ICH occurs in 10–15% of all strokes.

- It is twice as common as subarachnoid haemorrhage.

Clinical presentation

An ICH is clinically indistinguishable from ischaemic stroke, but headache, vomiting and seizures at onset suggest ICH. A large haemorrhage will cause death or coma within hours, whatever the location. The onset may be rapid, but an ICH associated with anticoagulant therapy may evolve slowly.

> An ICH cannot reliably be distinguished from ischaemia on clinical grounds. A CT scan is essential to make the diagnosis.

Physical signs

Smaller haematomas may have distinguishing physical signs depending on the site.

Supratentorial

- Putamen: predominantly hemiplegia, and also aphasia, homonymous hemianopia, hemineglect and deviation of eyes away from the affected side.

- Thalamic: predominantly hemisensory deficit, and also hemiparesis, aphasia (dominant side) and neglect (non-dominant side). Ocular signs may be prominent, with forced downward deviation of the eyes, skew deviation (vertical separation of gaze) and ipsilateral Horner's syndrome.

- Lobar: depends on the site of the lesion.

Infratentorial

- Cerebellar: may be slow to develop, so the patient is unlikely to be comatose at onset. There will be deviation of the eyes away from the haemorrhage, ipsilateral cranial nerve V–VII palsies and ipsilateral Horner's syndrome. Hemiplegia and aphasia are absent, as are cerebellar signs

early on. Progresses to coma as a result of brainstem compression.

- Pontine: total paralysis, decerebrate rigidity (extension to pain), pinpoint reactive pupils and absent doll's eyes response.

Investigation

A CT scan will be diagnostic (Figs 44–46). If the patient is under

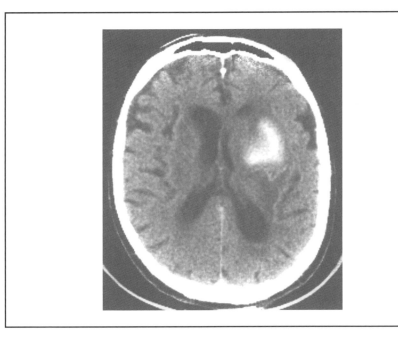

▲ **Fig. 44** Putaminal haemorrhage on CT scan.

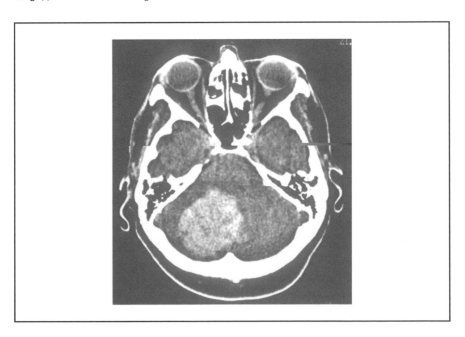

▲ **Fig. 45** Cerebellar hemisphere haemorrhage on CT scan. (Courtesy of Professor M. Brown, Institute of Neurology, University of London.)

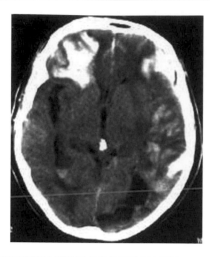

▲**Fig. 46** Multiple superficial haemorrhages of different ages seen on CT head scan. This patient was presumed to have cerebral amyloid angiopathy. (Courtesy of Professor M. Brown, Institute of Neurology, University of London.)

40 years old with no history of hypertension, it may be wise to enhance the scan to look for an underlying lesion.

An angiogram is warranted when there is significant suspicion of an underlying lesion. Factors that increase the likelihood of finding an abnormality include:

- age under 45 years old;

- absence of hypertension;

- lobar haemorrhage, unless the patient is over 65 years old as CAA would then be a more likely aetiology.

Consider cerebral amyloid angiopathy

- A common cause of ICH in the elderly; it is sporadic but there are a few autosomal dominant families.
- Subcortical, often multiple, haemorrhage, particularly in occipital and parietal lobes.
- Pathological changes found in 10% of septuagenarians and in 60% of those aged over 90 years.
- If there is any association between CAA and an Alzheimer-type pathology.
- 10–30% of those with CAA will have progressive dementia.

Differential diagnosis
See Section 2.8.1.

Treatment

Medical management
See Table 52.

Surgical
Trials have not shown benefit for surgical intervention in ICH. However, selected patients may benefit from surgery as follows.

- Patients with a cerebellar haemorrhage over 3 cm, because of the risk of hydrocephalus and brainstem compression. Remember, these patients may deteriorate slowly. Do not wait for brainstem signs to occur as it will be too late to reverse any deficit.

- Young patients who were initially stable but subsequently deteriorate may benefit from surgery, especially if there is superficial lobar haemorrhage.

Surgery is not indicated if:

- the patient's Glasgow Coma Scale score is 4 or less (unless cerebellar) (see Section 1.4.5);

- there is only a small lesion or minimal deficit.

For other types of ICH, surgery is less likely to result in a beneficial outcome.

Complications
- Death.

- Hydrocephalus.

- Disability.

TABLE 52 PRINCIPLES OF MEDICAL MANAGEMENT OF PATIENTS WITH ICH

Priorities	Action
Immediate priorities (first few hours)	Protect and maintain airway Prevent hypoxia: give oxygen if saturation is <95% on pulse oximetry Regular monitoring and neurological observations: review if condition deteriorates Nursing: bed-rest, elevate head of bed by 30° and protect pressure areas
Later priorities (first few days)	Maintain hydration: intravenous fluids if the patient cannot drink safely Consider nutrition: nasogastric (later via percutaneous endoscopic gastrostomy tube) if the patient cannot swallow safely
Other aspects	Hypertension: treat if BP is extremely high (>200/120 mmHg), but with caution Agitation: give the minimum sedation possible (often a difficult judgement) Pain: use paracetamol or codeine Bowels: use stool softeners to prevent straining

Prognosis

- 35–50% of patients will die by 1 month.

- 10% are independent at 1 month, 20% by 6 months.

FURTHER READING

Hankey GJ and Hon C. Surgery for primary intracerebral haemorrhage: is it safe and effective? A systematic review of case series and randomized trials. *Stroke* 1998; 28: 2126–32.

Miller JH, Wardlow J and Lammie GA. Intracerebral haemorrhage and cerebral amyloid angiopathy: CT features with pathological correlation. *Clin. Radiol.* 1999; 54: 422–9.

2.8.4 Subarachnoid haemorrhage

Aetiology

Ruptured saccular (berry) aneurysms are the cause of 80% of cases of non-traumatic subarachnoid haemorrhage (SAH). These are usually found at bifurcations and branchings of the arteries of the circle of Willis or its major branches. The reason why some aneurysms rupture and others do not is not known, but the risk is greater for larger aneurysms than for smaller.

Epidemiology

The incidence of SAH is 8–12 per 100,000 per year and is the diagnosis in 1–4% of patients presenting to emergency departments with headache. Risk factors include hypertension, cigarette smoking, heavy alcohol consumption (particularly binge drinking), adult polycystic kidney disease and some connective tissue disorders.

Clinical presentation

SAH can present with relatively minor symptoms, devastating neurological dysfunction or be a cause of sudden death.

The typical presentation is with the sudden onset of a severe headache, usually described as 'the worst headache I've ever had' or 'like being hit on the back of the head with a hammer'. This usually occurs when the patient is active, rather than asleep, and often during exertion. There is frequently a transient loss of consciousness, and also vomiting.

Between 20 and 50% of patients with documented SAH report a distinct and unusually severe 'warning headache' in the days or weeks prior to the episode of bleeding.

Physical signs

Many patients will have some or all of the following features:

- Impaired conscious level: Glasgow Coma Scale (GCS) score can vary from 3 (minimum) to 15 (maximum).

- Focal neurological signs, in particular third nerve palsy (posterior communicating artery aneurysm), sixth nerve palsy (posterior fossa aneurysm, but also a false localising sign with raised intracranial pressure), bilateral leg weakness (anterior communicating aneurysm), nystagmus or ataxia (posterior fossa aneurysm), and aphasia, hemiparesis and hemianopia (middle cerebral artery aneurysm).

- Neck rigidity.

- Retinal haemorrhages, which are thought to result from an acute increase in intracranial pressure that causes obstruction to the venous outflow from the eye.

Patients may be hypertensive, have cardiac dysrhythmias and have ECG patterns mimicking myocardial infarction, all of which can lead to diagnostic confusion. Those whose SAH has led to syncope may have sustained a head injury, which can also make diagnosis difficult.

Investigation

Immediate

The investigation of choice in suspected SAH is an immediate CT scan without contrast, taking very thin cuts through the base of the brain to optimise the chances of seeing small collections of blood (see Fig. 24). The sensitivity of modern scanners for detecting SAH is very high: 98–100% if scanning is performed within 12 hours of onset of symptoms, and 93% within the first 24 hours.

Lumbar puncture should be performed in suspected cases of SAH if the CT scan is negative, equivocal or technically unsatisfactory. 'Traumatic taps' occur in up to 20% of procedures and need to be distinguished from true haemorrhages: the 'three tube' method, which looks for decreasing numbers of erythrocytes in successively collected specimens, is not entirely reliable. The diagnosis of SAH is established by centrifuging the cerebrospinal fluid (CSF) specimen without delay and demonstrating the presence of xanthochromia (due to the presence of oxyhaemoglobin and bilirubin) by spectrophotometry (Fig. 47). Note, however, that xanthochromia may not be present if the CSF is examined within 12 hours of haemorrhage occurring. Hence in the face of a normal CT scan, lumbar puncture should be delayed until 24 hours after the ictus.

Subsequent

In cases of proven SAH where intervention (radiological or

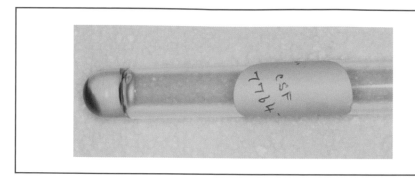

▲**Fig. 47** Test tube of blood-stained CSF after centrifugation to reveal xanthochromic supernatant in a case of SAH.

surgical) is contemplated (see Treatment section), imaging of the cerebral vessels by four-vessel angiography is required.

Differential diagnosis

Many studies have shown that about 30% of patients with SAH are misdiagnosed at presentation. The differential diagnosis includes infective causes of headache (meningitis, encephalitis and viral infections such as influenza), other causes of headache (migraine, cluster or tension headache, and sinus-related headache), neck pain and psychiatric disorder.

Complications

The patient may present with neurological deficit, recover, but then develop hemiplegia or other focal signs 4–10 days after rupture because of delayed cerebral ischaemia.

Rebleeding is the most feared complication. Series of patients admitted to hospital with SAH in the 1960s showed that about 10% died of the original haemorrhage, but 50% rebled, with 80% mortality in this group. Therefore, the overall mortality was about 50%, with many survivors remaining neurologically disabled.

Treatment

General measures

Bed-rest and monitoring for hypertension. High BP does not need treatment unless there are signs of end-organ damage.

Specific measures

Nimodipine is used for the prevention and treatment of ischaemic neurological deficit due to vascular spasm after SAH: for prevention at a dose of 60 mg po every 4 hours, and for treatment by intravenous infusion at a rate of 0.5–2 mg/hour. Once volume resuscitation (when necessary) has been completed, preventive treatment should be given to all patients with SAH who are not hypotensive. Intravenous nimodipine should only be administered in the setting of a neurological intensive care unit because hypotension is a common and serious problem.

In appropriately selected patients, surgery prevents rebleeding and improves their outcome. Indications for surgery are proven intracranial aneurysms in the following:

- patients with GCS ≥12;
- patients with GCS <12 who have space-occupying intracranial

haemorrhage associated with an aneurysm, or with hydrocephalus;

- age alone is not a contraindication to surgery.

After surgery, patients typically remain in hospital for 2 weeks. They should be treated for general vascular risk factors (hypertension, cholesterol, diabetes and they should stop smoking) and they must inform the Driver and Vehicle Licensing Agency (DVLA) regarding driving (if they make a full recovery their licence is usually returned after 3 months). There are no long-term lifestyle restrictions (except smoking).

Prognosis

With modern medical and surgical management, a poor outcome (death or severe disability) occurs in 20% of all those with SAH admitted to hospital. However, many of the worst affected do not ever reach hospital, so that the true mortality from SAH is nearer 50%. A good clinical outcome is expected in 90–95% of those admitted in good clinical condition (GCS of 14 or 15).

Prevention

Incidental aneurysms occur in up to 1% of the population. Any such patient should be referred for specialist advice, but the majority (aneurysms <10 mm in diameter) do not require surgery.

FURTHER READING

Edlow JA and Caplan LR. Avoiding pitfalls in the diagnosis of subarachnoid haemorrhage. *N. Engl. J. Med.* 2000; 342: 29–36.

- - - - - - - - - - - - - - - - - -

International Study of Unruptured Intracranial Aneurysms Investigators. Unruptured intracranial aneurysms: risk of rupture and risks of surgical intervention. *N. Engl. J. Med.* 1998; 339: 1725–33.

2.9 Brain tumours

Pathology

Brain tumours can arise within the brain parenchyma or adjoining structures (eg meninges), or invade by direct or haematological metastatic spread. Tumours can be benign or malignant, malignancy implying rapid growth, poor differentiation, high mitotic rate, necrosis and vascular proliferation.

Metastasis to extracranial sites is rare. A benign tumour may be as devastating as a highly malignant tumour by virtue of its position, its ability to infiltrate locally or its propensity to transform to malignancy. The classification of brain tumours is shown in Table 53, and their age distribution in Table 54.

Epidemiology

Benign and malignant primary brain tumours are uncommon. Overall, the incidence is about 6–14 per 100,000 annually. Malignant tumours of the brain are a rare occurrence, accounting for approximately 2% of all cancers in adults. Approximately 4,400 people are newly diagnosed with a brain tumour each year in the UK compared with over 40,000 women with breast cancer and approximately 25,000 men with prostate cancer. The most common brain tumours in adults are benign meningioma and glioblastoma multiforme. Generally, the tumours that tend to occur in adults become more common with increasing age. Secondary ('metastatic') brain tumours are more common than primary brain tumours and are more likely to occur than primary tumours in the elderly.

Clinical presentation

The nature of the clinical presentation will reflect the site of the tumour (Figs 48 and 49) and its rate of expansion.

General symptoms

Rapidly expanding tumours or those blocking the flow of cerebrospinal fluid and causing obstructive hydrocephalus will present with symptoms (postural headache, nausea and vomiting, diplopia) and signs (papilloedema and sixth nerve palsy) of raised intracranial pressure. Headaches tend to be worse in the morning and coughing, sneezing and stooping may make the headaches worse. Seizures (partial or generalised) sometimes occur and are one of the most common presenting symptoms in patients with meningiomas. Impairment of consciousness may occur as the tumour enlarges. A stroke-like presentation with sudden-onset symptoms usually reflects bleeding into a tumour.

TABLE 53 CLASSIFICATION OF BRAIN TUMOURS

Type	Site	Diagnosis
Primary	Intraparenchymal	Gliomas 　Astrocytoma, many types 　Glioblastoma multiforme 　Oligodendroglioma 　Mixed glioma, eg oligoastrocytoma 　Ependymal tumours Neuronal tumours, eg gangliocytomas Primitive neuroectodermal tumours, eg medulloblastoma
	Extraparenchymal (extrinsic/extra-axial)	Meninges: meningioma Cranial nerve sheath: schwannomas/neuromas Pituitary gland: microadenomas, macroadenomas Bone: osteomas Blood vessel: haemangioblastomas
Secondary	Direct extension	Nasopharyngeal Chordoma Glomus jugulare tumours
	Metastasis	
	Haematological	Primary CNS lymphoma

CNS, central nervous system.

TABLE 54 AGE DISTRIBUTION OF BRAIN TUMOURS BY SITE

Location	Adult	Childhood
Supratentorial	(70% of adult brain tumours) Glioma Meningioma Pituitary Metastasis (commonest)	Craniopharyngioma Pinealoma Gliomas (mainly astrocytomas of optic nerve and thalamus)
Infratentorial	(Mainly cerebellar; occurrence in brainstem is rare) Metastasis Acoustic neuroma Cerebellar haemangioblastoma	Medulloblastoma (infancy) Cerebellar astrocytoma Ependymoma of fourth ventricle

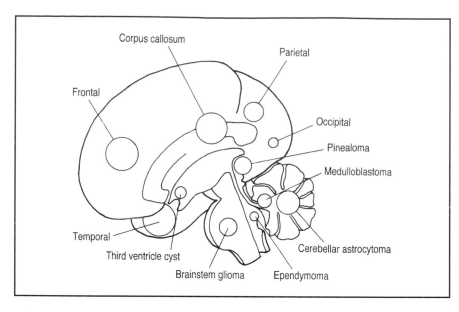

▲ **Fig. 48** Main intracerebral tumour sites.

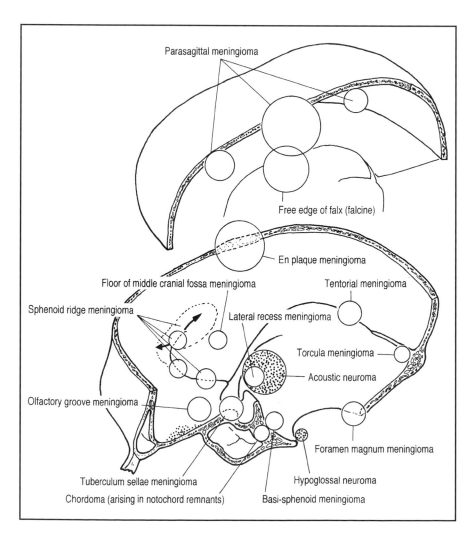

▲ **Fig. 49** Main locations of extracerebral intracranial tumours.

Symptoms due to the location in the brain

As a tumour grows it can damage nearby brain tissue. This may lead to:

- limb numbness or weakness;

- cerebellar signs;

- visual field defects (eg bitemporal hemianopia in pituitary tumours);

- hearing defects (acoustic neuromas);

- dysphasia;

- dysphagia;

- anosmia;

- personality changes;

- symptoms of hormone imbalance (pituitary tumours).

Common presentations are shown in Table 55. Rarely, patients may present with paraneoplastic syndromes (see Section 2.11).

Investigation

The most important investigation is CT or MRI scan. CT is particularly good if there is a stroke-like presentation in order to rule out haemorrhage. If a tumour is suspected, it is important that contrast is used as some tumours may be isodense to brain tissue and therefore do not show up without it. MRI is preferable for:

- posterior fossa tumours;

- detecting multiple lesions, which are more suggestive of metastases.

The high incidence of metastases compared with primary brain tumours makes a CXR and blood tests (FBC, erythrocyte sedimentation rate, urea and electrolytes, liver function tests, calcium and phosphates) essential. Further investigation of a patient with cerebral metastases will be

TABLE 55 BRAIN TUMOURS: COMMON PRESENTATIONS

Site	Common symptoms and signs
Frontal	Personality change Contralateral motor signs Dysphasia (dominant hemisphere) (NB Foster Kennedy syndrome: ipsilateral optic atrophy and contralateral papilloedema)
Parietal	Contralateral sensory change/cortical sensory loss Visual field defect (optic radiation) Neglect Apraxias (NB Gerstmann's syndrome: agraphia, left/right disorientation, acalculia and finger agnosia)
Occipital	Homonymous hemianopia ± macular sparing
Temporal	Memory and behavioural disturbance
Parasagittal	Gait abnormality (small steps) Spastic paraparesis (consider in the differential diagnosis of spinal cord compression)
Posterior fossa	Raised intracranial pressure Ataxia and nystagmus Cranial nerve lesions
Pituitary	Bitemporal hemianopia (pressure on optic chiasm) Endocrine disturbance (see *Endocrinology*, Section 2.1) Cranial nerve III, IV, Va, Vb and VI (lateral extension to cavernous sinus) (NB pituitary apoplexy: sudden blindness and subarachnoid haemorrhage)

guided by clinical symtoms and signs, eg anaemia may lead to oesophago-gastroduodenoscopy and colonoscopy in search of a gastrointestinal malignancy.

Pituitary function tests are perfomed if a mass is seen in the pituitary fossa on a CT or MRI scan. Lumbar puncture is unlikely to be safe and has a low positive yield.

Cerebral biopsy should be performed in most patients to exclude potentially treatable causes and also to classify and grade the tumour. Four malignancy grades are recognised by the World Health Organisation system, with grade I tumours the biologically least aggressive and grade IV the biologically most aggressive tumours. The histological criteria for malignancy grading are not uniform for all tumour types and thus all tumours must be classified before

the malignancy grade can be determined.

Differential diagnosis

The important conditions to consider in the differential diagnosis of a space-occupying lesion are as follows.

- Vascular causes such as haematoma with mass effect, giant aneurysm, arteriovenous malformation, cerebral infarct with oedema and venous thrombosis.

- Trauma resulting in haematoma/contusion.

- Infection of the CNS including abscess, tuberculosis, herpes simplex encephalitis and hydatid cysts.

- Many inflammatory conditions that may cause focal signs, particularly multiple sclerosis and neurosarcoidosis.

Treatment

In some cases, treatment aims for a cure. If a benign tumour can be removed by surgery, then cure is likely. In other cases a cure is unrealistic and treatment aims to control progression of the tumour by reducing the bulk or by limiting the growth or spread of the tumour so that it progresses less rapidly. The main treatments used for brain tumours are surgery, chemotherapy, radiotherapy and medication to control the symptoms. The treatment or combination of treatments used in each case depends on the following factors:

- type of tumour (benign or malignant);

- grade of tumour if it is malignant;

- exact site of the tumour;

- patient's general health.

Symptomatic treatment

Consider steroids in the acute setting for the symptomatic treatment of oedema: dexamethasone 12 mg iv, followed by 4 mg qds orally or intravenously for no more than 1 week (it loses efficacy after this). The patient may require anticonvulsant medication for seizures (phenytoin or sodium valproate are most often used). Analgesia is a very important part of symptomatic treatment and strong analgesics such as morphine may be required. Nausea and vomiting can be controlled with antiemetics such as cyclizine and prochlorperazine.

Surgery

Surgery is usually the main treatment option for benign tumours. Aggressive surgical resection for malignant lesions is impossible because the lesions are widely invasive beyond the macroscopic margins, and large-volume resections are associated with unacceptable morbidity. Surgery may be attempted if the lesion is situated in the frontal lobe or occipital pole.

Radiotherapy

Radiotherapy is not curative, but some tumours are sensitive. In the treatment of malignant cerebral glioma, radiotherapy offers a survival benefit of approximately 6 months. Radiotherapy is sometimes used instead of surgery when an operation is not possible for a malignant brain tumour. It may be used as an adjunct to surgery if it is not possible to remove all the tumour with surgery, or to kill cancerous cells that may be left behind following surgery.

Chemotherapy

The benefits of chemotherapy in the treatment of primary malignant brain tumours are not clear but it is sometimes used as an adjunctive treatment to surgery and radiotherapy depending on various factors such as the type of tumour.

Prognosis

The length of survival following diagnosis of a brain tumour is dependent on the age of the patient, the histologic subtype and grade of the tumour, and the presenting symptoms. Survival chances have improved gradually over the last 30 years but remain poor; for all adults diagnosed with a malignant brain tumour in England and Wales during 1986–90, 30% survived to 1 year and 15% to 5 years. A patient with a grade 1–2 glioma may survive for years, whereas a patient with a grade 4 tumour will survive for a maximum of a few months if treated with surgery alone. The prognosis for metastatic disease is poor.

Disease associations

Neurocutaneous syndromes

The vast majority of brain tumours are sporadic. However there are a number of familial syndromes that are well documented as being associated with an increased incidence of brain tumours. Even in the most common of these (neurofibromatosis types 1 and 2), the precise relative risk is difficult to define. The prevalence of neurocutaneous syndromes is higher in the medical examination setting (such as PACES) than in real life. Beware the patient with skin lesions and neurological signs! Table 56 summarises these syndromes.

FURTHER READING

Allcutt DA and Mendelow AD. Presentation and diagnosis of brain tumours. *Br. J. Hosp. Med.* 1992; 47: 745–52.

- - - - - - - - - - - - - - - - -

Collins VP. Brain tumours: classification and genes. *J. Neurol. Neurosurg. Psychiatry* 2004; 75 (Suppl. 2): ii2–ii11.

- - - - - - - - - - - - - - - - -

DeAngelis LM, Burger PC, Green SB and Cairncross JG. Malignant glioma: who benefits from adjuvant chemotherapy? *Ann. Neurol.* 1998; 44: 691–5.

- - - - - - - - - - - - - - - - -

TABLE 56 BRAIN TUMOURS AS PART OF NEUROCUTANEOUS DISORDERS

Syndrome	Genetics	Features
Von Hippel–Lindau disease	Autosomal dominant, 3p26–25	Brain: haemangioblastoma (cerebellar, less common in cerebral hemispheres and brainstem) Eyes: retinal angioma Skin: hamartomas Visceral organs: tumours and cysts Phaeochromocytoma
Neurofibromatosis 1	Autosomal dominant, 17q11.2	CNS: optic and chiasmatic nerve glioma, neurofibroma and plexiform neurofibroma Eyes: Lisch nodules Skin: café-au-lait spots (numerous), axillary and/or inguinal freckles
Neurofibromatosis 2	Autosomal dominant, 22q11–13.1	Brain: bilateral acoustic neuromas. Less commonly, meningioma, glioma and other neuromas. Schwannomas compress cranial or spinal roots in their foramina Eye: presenile cataracts Skin: cutaneous neurofibromas, café-au-lait spots (less numerous)
Tuberous sclerosis	Autosomal dominant, 9q34.1–34.2 (some families)	Brain: cortical tubers, subependymal nodules, astrocytoma Eye: hamartomas Skin: shagreen plaques, ungual fibroma, facial angiofibromas (adenoma sebaceum) Other: widespread hamartomatosis

Delattre JY and Uchuya M. Radiotherapy and chemotherapy for gliomas. *Curr. Opin. Oncol.* 1996; 8: 196–203.

McKinney PA. Brain tumours: incidence, survival and aetiology. *J. Neurol. Neurosurg. Psychiatry* 2004; 75 (Suppl. 2): ii12–ii17.

2.10 Neurological complications of infection

2.10.1 New variant Creutzfeldt–Jakob disease

Aetiology
There is increasing evidence supporting a causal association between bovine spongiform encephalopathy (BSE) and new variant Creutzfeldt–Jakob disease (nvCJD).

- Glycosylation patterns of the disease-associated prion protein (PrP) in nvCJD resembles that in BSE-infected cattle, but is not seen in sporadic CJD.
- In mice, the characteristics of the agents responsible for nvCJD and BSE were identical, but different from those in sporadic CJD.

The only environmental risk factor for nvCJD that has been identified is UK residence, although several cases have now been described in other European countries, especially France. The size of the potential problem in the UK is difficult to predict as the time and source of exposure to BSE in current cases of nvCJD is unknown. Genetic analysis indicates that BSE is transmitted only to humans who have the prion protein gene (*PRNP*) codon 129 methionine homozygous genotype.

Clinical presentation
In nvCJD, the mean age of onset is 29 years and mean disease duration is 14 months, compared with 60 years and 5 months, respectively, in sporadic CJD. As of 6 March 2006, there have been a total of 160 cases of definite or probable nvCJD in the UK.

⚠ Psychiatric or sensory symptoms are prominent early features in nvCJD compared with rapidly progressive dementia in sporadic CJD.

Physical signs
Cerebellar signs are prominent early in the course of the disease. Up-gaze paresis, which is uncommon in sporadic CJD, often occurs in nvCJD. Pyramidal signs, primitive reflexes (such as grasp and pout reflexes) and myoclonus may also be seen.

Investigation
The following may be helpful.

- Electroencephalography may show slow waves, but not the periodic spike-and-wave complexes typical of sporadic CJD.
- Elevated levels of the neuronal protein 14.3.3 in cerebrospinal fluid may be found.
- An MRI brain scan often demonstrates the characteristic 'pulvinar sign' that is high signal in the posterior thalami or 'pulvinar'.
- Post-mortem neuropathological examination is the only way of confirming the diagnosis, although tonsillar biopsy may demonstrate involvement and can be helpful in making a diagnosis of 'probable' nvCJD in patients with normal MRI scans who do not undergo a post-mortem.

Complications
Several cases of nvCJD are now felt to be transmitted from infected blood products. There is concern that levels of PrP in the lymphoreticular tissue of patients with nvCJD may be higher than in those with sporadic CJD. Therefore, blood and blood products from those confirmed as having been affected by nvCJD have now been withdrawn in the UK and donated blood is depleted of white cells ('leucodepletion').

FURTHER READING

Hill AF, Butterworth RJ, Joiner S, *et al.* Investigation of variant Creutzfeldt–Jakob disease and other human prion diseases with tonsilar biopsy samples. *Lancet* 1999; 353: 183–9.

Llewelyn CA, Hewitt PE, Knight RS, *et al.* Possible transmission of variant Creutzfeldt–Jakob disease by blood transfusion. *Lancet* 2004; 363: 417–21.

Peden AH, Head MW, Ritchie DL, Bell JE and Ironside JW. Preclinical vCJD after blood transfusion in a PRNP codon 129 heterozygous patient. *Lancet* 2004; 364: 527–9.

Stewart GE and Ironside JW. New variant Creutzfeldt–Jakob disease. *Curr. Opin. Neurol.* 1998; 11: 259–62.

Zeidler M, Stewart GE, Barraclough CR, *et al.* New variant Creutzfeldt–Jakob disease: neurological features and diagnostic tests. *Lancet* 1997; 350: 903–7.

2.11 Neurological complications of systemic disease

2.11.1 Paraneoplastic conditions

Non-neurological malignancies can affect the nervous system in many ways. This can be by infiltration or compression, either by direct spread of the primary tumour or by haematogenous metastatic spread. However, a wide range of non-metastatic remote complications are also described. Many of these can be attributed to cachexia, to competition between a tumour and body tissues for substances such as glucose and tryptophan, or to the adverse affects of chemotherapy such as vincristine and cisplatin. Others appear to have an immunological basis. It is this latter group that will be discussed as paraneoplastic conditions.

> • Paraneoplastic syndromes can occur up to several years prior to detection of the underlying tumour. In some cases, the tumour is not identified until post-mortem.
> • The tumour is usually small, suggesting that it is being held at bay by the immune response.
> • An immune response is directed against a tumour antigen also expressed on neural tissue (onconeural antigen). Paraneoplastic disorders are therefore autoimmune in nature.
> • The pathogenesis of certain paraneoplastic conditions is antibody mediated (Lambert–Eaton myasthenic syndrome) whereas in others it may be cytokine or T-cell mediated.
> • Identification of a particular associated antineuronal antibody will direct the hunt for the underlying tumour.
> • None of the paraneoplastic syndromes is invariably associated with malignancy.

Clinical presentation

Numerous neurological paraneoplastic syndromes are described. Given the broad range of symptoms, what is it that makes the clinician consider a diagnosis of paraneoplastic syndrome?

- Conditions that progress rapidly over weeks to months before reaching a plateau.

- Patients are usually significantly disabled at the time of presentation, and mild waxing and waning symptoms are unlikely to be paraneoplastic in origin.

- Presentations are usually stereotyped as described below.

Paraneoplastic conditions involving the central nervous system

- Paraneoplastic encephalomyelitis includes the following conditions.

  (a) Limbic encephalitis: symptoms are anxiety, depression, impairment of recent memory and fluctuating confusion. More than 70% are associated with small-cell lung carcinoma (SCLC). This is also described in Hodgkin's disease (HD).

  (b) Brainstem encephalitis: there are variable brainstem signs and there may be corticospinal tract involvement. Mainly associated with SCLC.

  (c) Myelitis/anterior horn cell disease: this can mimic motor neuron disease. Any sensory signs are due to associated subacute sensory neuronopathy. Often associated with brainstem encephalitis.

- Paraneoplastic cerebellar degeneration causes ataxia, dysarthria and nystagmus. There may be associated paraneoplastic encephalomyelitis. Described with SCLC, gynaecological tumours and HD.

- Paraneoplastic opsoclonus/ myoclonus syndrome: in affected children, 50% have neuroblastoma, whereas in adults it is associated with cerebellar and brainstem signs and encephalopathy. Clonazepam may offer relief.

- Necrotising myelopathy mimics transverse myelitis or cord compression.

Paraneoplastic conditions involving the eye

Cancer-associated retinopathy is a triad of photosensitivity, ring scotomatous visual field loss and attenuated calibre of retinal arterioles.

Paraneoplastic conditions involving the neuromuscular junction

- Stiff man syndrome: stiffness of proximal limbs and trunk. Described with breast cancer and HD. In association with breast cancer, antibodies to amphiphysin have been described.

> Stiff man syndrome is also associated with organ-specific autoimmune diseases and insulin-dependent diabetes mellitus. Of those affected, 60% have antibodies to glutamic acid decarboxylase.

- Lambert–Eaton myasthenic syndrome: weakness of proximal muscles, mainly in the legs, and autonomic dysfunction. There is also post-tetanic stimulation of deep tendon reflexes and antibodies to the presynaptic voltage-gated calcium channel. Usually in association with SCLC.

- Myasthenia gravis: muscle fatiguability, ptosis and

TABLE 57 ONCONEURAL ANTIGENS

Antibody	Antigen	Associated cancer	Syndrome
Anti-Hu	All neuronal nuclei	Sickle cell lung disease and neuroblastoma	PEM, SSN
Anti-Yo	Purkinje cell cytoplasm	Gynaecological and breast	PCD
Anti-Ri	Neuronal nuclei	Breast, gynaecological, SCLC	PCD, opsoclonus
Anti-amphiphysin	Synaptic vesicles	Breast	PEM, stiff man syndrome
Anti-VGCC	Presynaptic VGCC	SCLC	LEMS
Anti-AchR	AchR	Thymoma	Myasthenia gravis
Anti-Tr	Neuronal cytoplasm, Purkinje cells, spiny dendrites	HD	PCD

AchR, acetylcholine receptor; HD, Hodgkin's disease; LEMS, Lambert–Eaton myasthenic syndrome; PCD, paraneoplastic cerebellar degeneration; PEM, paraneoplastic encephalomyelitis; SCLC, small-cell lung carcinoma; SSN, subacute sensory neuronopathy; VGCC, voltage-gated calcium channel.

ophthalmoplegia. Affects antibodies to the acetylcholine receptor and is associated with thymoma.

Paraneoplastic conditions involving the nerve

- Subacute sensory neuronopathy: rapid progressive loss of all sensory modalities, especially proprioception, may result in pseudoathetosis. This may be associated with myelitis, but is usually in association with SCLC. The differential diagnosis of this striking neuropathy includes Sjögren's syndrome.

- Motor neuronopathy: affects legs more than arms, often in a patchy distribution, but spares bulbar musculature. Associated with HD and other lymphomas.

- Paraneoplastic vasculitic neuropathy: a mononeuritis multiplex associated with SCLC, endometrial cancer and others.

- Brachial neuritis: asymmetric pain, weakness and wasting in the muscles of the shoulder girdle is usually idiopathic, but can occasionally be associated with malignancy.

- Autonomic neuropathy: may rarely be paraneoplastic.

Paraneoplastic conditions involving muscle

- Dermatomyositis: associated with cancer in 10% of cases (see *Rheumatology and Clinical Immunology*, Section 2.3.5).

- Necrotising myopathy: necrosis without inflammation; rare.

Investigations

Cerebrospinal fluid (CSF) analysis may show an increased level of protein and a mild pleocytosis. Associated anti-neuronal antibodies may be identified in both serum and CSF, but this is an emerging field. Table 57 summarises our knowledge of onconeural antigens.

Treatment

This is a difficult issue. There is limited evidence that complete cure of the malignancy driving the immune response leads to either partial or complete resolution of the paraneoplastic condition. However, there is growing evidence that immunosuppressive therapies administered in an attempt to control the neurological symptoms

may remove immunological control of the tumour, leading to more rapid growth and increased chance of metastasis.

FURTHER READING

Newsom-Davis J. Paraneoplastic neurological disorders. *J. R. Coll. Physicians Lond.* 1999; 33: 225–7.

- - - - - - - - - - - - - - - -

Dalmau JO and Posner JB. Paraneoplastic syndromes. *Arch. Neurol.* 1999; 56: 405–8. (An up-to-date account of the onconeural antigens.)

- - - - - - - - - - - - - - - -

Cher LM, Henson JW, Das A and Hochberg FH. Paraneoplastic syndromes. In: Vinken PJ and Bruyn GW, eds. *Handbook of Clinical Neurology, Vol. 71. Systemic Diseases, Part 3.* Amsterdam: Elsevier, 1998: 673–704. (Thorough, with historical perspective and an in-depth review of therapies.)

2.12 Neuropharmacology

Failure of the neuronal signalling process is responsible for a wide variety of symptoms in disorders such as Parkinson's disease (PD), depression, dementia, schizophrenia, mania and epilepsy. Drugs used in the treatment of these disorders modulate neuronal signalling in the defective pathway to restore, as far as possible, normal neurotransmission. This section focuses on the fundamental processes of chemical neurotransmission modulated by centrally acting drugs (Fig. 50).

For a centrally acting drug to have clinical utility, it must selectively target a specific neurotransmitter at a specific set of interneuronal connections. However, because a relatively small number of major neurotransmitters mediate chemical signalling in diverse central neuronal pathways, absolute selectivity of drug action is rarely achieved. The result is that side effects are particularly common with these agents.

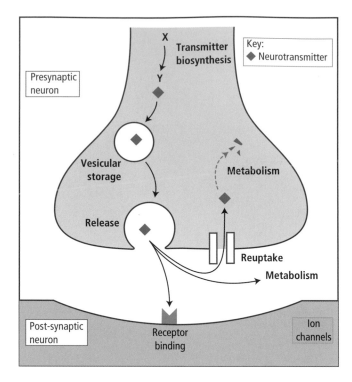

▲**Fig. 50** Processes in neurotransmission susceptible to modulation by centrally acting drugs.

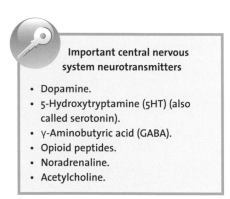

Important central nervous system neurotransmitters

- Dopamine.
- 5-Hydroxytryptamine (5HT) (also called serotonin).
- γ-Aminobutyric acid (GABA).
- Opioid peptides.
- Noradrenaline.
- Acetylcholine.

Dopamine

Dopaminergic neurons (Fig. 51) are found in the following places within the central nervous system (CNS).

- Nigrostriatal pathways: where deficient dopaminergic neurotransmission is responsible for PD.

- Mesolimbic and mesocortical pathways: where excess dopaminergic neurotransmission has been implicated in schizophrenia.

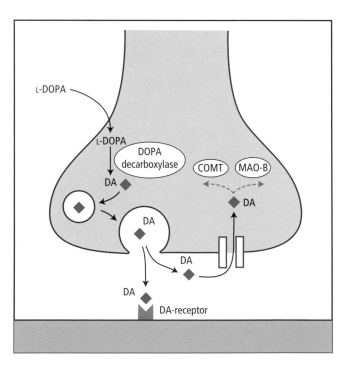

▲**Fig. 51** Dopaminergic neurotransmission. COMT, catechol *O*-methyltransferase; DA, dopamine; MAO-B, monoamine oxidase B.

- Tuberoinfundibular neurons: from where dopaminergic activity results in tonic inhibition of prolactin secretion.

- Chemoreceptor trigger zone (outside the blood–brain barrier):

where dopaminergic function is involved in emesis.

Dopamine receptors

There are two main families, D_1 and D_2, but also a number of receptor subtypes. Most known functions are mediated by D_1- and D_2-like receptors.

Dopamine receptor agonists

These include bromocriptine, lisuride, pergolide, ropinirole, apomorphine (used in the treatment of PD), and cabergoline and quinagolide (used to treat hyperprolactinaemia). Dyskinesias are less common with dopamine receptor agonists than with levodopa (L-DOPA) in the treatment of PD, but hallucinations and confusion are common in the elderly.

Dopamine receptor antagonists

These are used in the treatment of schizophrenia (eg chlorpromazine, thioridazine, flupentixol and haloperidol) and to treat nausea and vomiting (prochlorperazine, metoclopramide and domperidone). Side effects of long-term dopamine receptor blockade in schizophrenia include depression, akathisia, parkinsonism, tardive dyskinesia and neuroleptic malignant syndrome. Shorter-term treatment can result in hyperprolactinaemia and galactorrhoea. Acute dystonia and oculogyric cases are recognised side effects of dopamine receptor blockade.

Atypical antipsychotics (eg clozapine, olanzapine, risperidone and quetiapine) have actions on some dopamine receptor subtypes, but also on other central neurotransmitters.

Levodopa

Levodopa is the precursor for dopamine synthesis used in the treatment of PD. It is given in combination with a peripheral DOPA decarboxylase inhibitor to prevent its metabolism in the gut wall and to enhance oral bioavailability. The long-term use of L-DOPA is

associated with the development of dyskinesia.

Inhibitors of metabolism

Dopamine is metabolised by MAO-B and COMT. Selegiline, an inhibitor of MAO-B, is used in the treatment of PD, as is entacapone, an inhibitor of COMT.

5HT (serotonin)

5HT-containing neurons are found in the midline raphe nuclei, with widespread projections to the cortex, limbic system, hypothalamus and cord (Fig. 52). 5HT is involved in the control of sleep, mood and emotion, appetite, sexual arousal and vomiting. Drugs that modulate the 5HT system are used in the treatment of migraine, depression, schizophrenia, to suppress appetite and to treat vomiting. Certain drugs of abuse, including amphetamines, LSD and MDMA (ecstasy), promote 5HT neurotransmission.

5HT receptors

There are many 5HT receptor subtypes. All, with the exception

of the $5HT_3$ receptor, are G protein-coupled seven-transmembrane-domain receptors that activate an intracellular second messenger cascade that reduces intracellular cyclic adenosine monophosphate levels.

5HT receptor agonists

The major 5HT agonists used clinically are the triptans (sumatriptan, zolmitriptan and naratriptan), which are used in the acute treatment of migraine. Side effects include nausea and vomiting and, rarely, cardiac ischaemia caused by 5HT receptor-induced coronary vasospasm. LSD is a partial agonist at the $5HT_2$ receptor and is a hallucinogen.

5HT receptor antagonists

The 5HT receptor antagonist pizotifen is used in the long-term prophylaxis of migraine. The $5HT_3$ receptor antagonists ondansetron and granisetron block the $5HT_3$ receptor in the chemoreceptor trigger zone and vagus nerve, and are particularly effective for treating

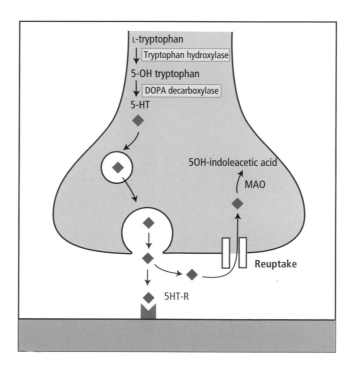

▲ **Fig. 52** Serotonergic neurotransmission.

the nausea and vomiting associated with cancer chemotherapy.

Drugs affecting 5HT release

Fenfluramine and dexfenfluramine promote 5HT release and have been used as appetite suppressants. These drugs have been associated with the development of cardiac valve fibrosis and pulmonary hypertension. MDMA also promotes 5HT release.

Drugs blocking 5HT reuptake

Selective serotonin reuptake inhibitors (SSRIs) such as fluoxetine, paroxetine and sertraline potentiate 5HT neurotransmission by blocking reuptake (Fig. 52). They have equivalent efficacy in the treatment of depression to tricyclics, but are associated with a lower incidence of side effects and have a better safety profile in overdose. Nefazodone and venlafaxine are newer antidepressants classified as serotonin–noradrenaline reuptake inhibitors whose clinical efficacy and side-effect profile appears similar to SSRIs.

Inhibitors of metabolism

MAO inbibitors reduce 5HT metabolism and are used in the management of depression. Non-selective MAO inhibitors such as phenelzine and tranylcypromine are associated with significant dietary and drug interactions. Selective and reversible MAO inhibitors such as moclobemide are somewhat safer.

5HT₄ receptors

5HT₄ receptors in the enteric nervous system are involved in modulation of gut motility, and a variety of agonists and antagonists are under development for motility disorders.

GABA

GABA is a widely distributed inhibitory neurotransmitter in the

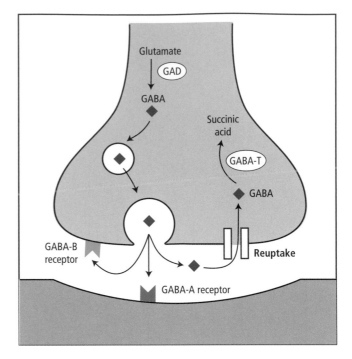

▲**Fig. 53** GABAergic neurotransmission. GAD, glutamic acid decarboxylase; GABA-T, GABA transaminase.

CNS. Drugs which potentiate GABAergic neurotransmission (Fig. 53) in the CNS include benzodiazepines, vigabatrin and valproate, all of which are used to treat epilepsy.

GABA$_A$ receptor

The GABA$_A$ receptor is a multi-subunit, ligand-gated, chloride ion channel that hyperpolarises the postsynaptic membrane when activated. GABA effects at this membrane are potentiated by benzodiazepines and barbiturates, which have distinct binding sites (Fig. 54).

GABA receptor modulators

Benzodiazepines potentiate the action of GABA at the GABA$_A$ receptor, as do the barbiturates which are much less selective. Benzodiazepines are useful as sedatives, anxiolytics and anticonvulsants.

Inhibitors of metabolism

Vigabatrin is an inhibitor of GABA transaminase that enhances GABAergic neurotransmission by preventing GABA metabolism. It is used as add-on therapy in seizures resistant to monotherapy that are being treated with first-line drugs.

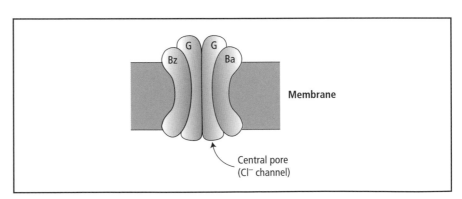

▲**Fig. 54** GABA$_A$ receptor. G, GABA-binding site; Bz, benzodiazepine-binding site; Ba, barbiturate-binding site.

The action of sodium valproate may be mediated in part by the inhibition of GABA transaminase.

Other GABA-like drugs

Gabapentin was synthesised to mimic the structure of GABA with the intention that it might be useful as an antiepileptic agent. However, it is not believed to act on GABA receptors in the brain, but rather to bind to voltage-dependent calcium channels in the CNS. It has found its main therapeutic use in the management of neuropathic pain.

Opioid peptides

The endogenous opioid peptides (enkephalins, endorphins and dynorphins) are derived from three distinct gene products (preproopiomelanocortin, preproenkephalin and preprodynorphin) by sequential peptide cleavage. Neurons containing these peptides are distributed widely in the CNS where they modulate the perception of pain.

Opioid receptors

Three main classes of opioid receptor are recognised: μ, δ and κ. The μ receptors are thought to be responsible for most of the analgesic effects of opioid receptor activation and also for respiratory depression, sedation and dependence. All three receptors are coupled to G proteins and the inhibition of adenylate cyclase (see Fig. 55 and *Cell Biology*, Receptors and Intracellular Signalling).

Opioid receptor agonists

These include the pure agonists morphine and pethidine, and the partial agonists pentazocine, nalorphine and buprenorphine. All are used as analgesics. Heroin (diamorphine) has therapeutic use, but like all opioid agonists it is also a drug of abuse.

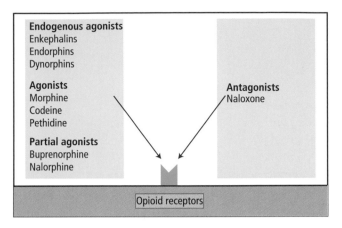

▲ **Fig. 55** Opioid peptides.

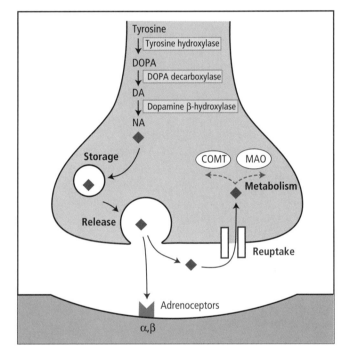

▲ **Fig. 56** Noradrenergic neurotransmission.

Opioid receptor antagonists

Nalaxone is a competitive antagonist at μ, δ and κ opioid receptors. It reverses opioid-induced analgesia, sedation and respiratory depression and is used in the treatment of opioid overdose.

Noradrenaline

In the CNS noradrenergic neurotransmission (Fig. 56) is involved in the control of mood, wakefulness and BP regulation. A functional deficiency in noradrenergic neurotransmission is thought to underlie some forms of depression and many drugs used to treat depression potentiate noradrenergic neurotransmission.

Interference with synthesis

α-Methyldopa is an antihypertensive that is metabolised by DOPA decarboxylase and dopamine β-hydroxylase to yield α-methylnoradrenaline, a 'false transmitter'. Depression is a recognised side effect of this agent.

Inhibitors of metabolism

Classical MAO inhibitors (eg pargyline and isocarboxazid) are irreversible, non-competitive inhibitors of MAO-A and MAO-B. Moclobemide, a newer antidepressant, is a reversible competitive inhibitor of MAO-A.

Inhibitors of reuptake

Amphetamines and cocaine are stimulant drugs of abuse that inhibit noradrenaline uptake. Inhibition of noradrenaline reuptake underlies the antidepressant effect of reboxetine, a new class of antidepressant noradrenaline reuptake inhibitor.

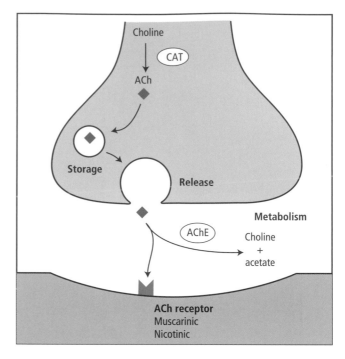

▲ **Fig. 57** Cholinergic neurotransmission. CAT, choline acetyltransferase; AChE, acetylcholinesterase.

The 'tyramine effect'

Dietary tyramine, found in some cheeses, red wine and Marmite, is normally metabolised in the bowel wall and liver by MAO-A. Patients taking classical MAO inhibitors are at risk of severe hypertensive reactions if they consume such foods because the tyramine is absorbed systemically, where it provokes noradrenaline release from sympathetic nerve terminals. Such hypertensive crises can be treated with α-adrenoreceptor antagonists (eg phentolamine) or calcium channel blockers.

To mitigate the 'tyramine effect' produced by the MAO inhibitor selegiline, this drug has now been produced in a transdermal patch formulation.

Acetylcholine

Cholinergic neurons (Fig. 57) are widely distributed in the CNS, particularly in the basal forebrain, striatum and nucleus accumbens. Functional overactivity of cholinergic neurotransmission is seen in PD and a loss of cholinergic neurons is seen in Alzheimer's dementia.

Acetylcholinesterase inhibitors

Centrally acting acetylcholinesterase inhibitors (donepezil, rivastigmine and galantamine) have been used to treat Alzheimer's disease. Short-term improvement in objective measures of cognition has been shown, but the long-term value of these agents is unclear.

Muscarinic acetylcholine receptor antagonists

Blockade of the muscarinic acetylcholine receptor with trihexyphenidyl (benzhexol), benzatropine or orphenadrine is of limited therapeutic use in patients with PD, in particular where tremor is the prominent symptom. Side effects of these agents include confusion, blurred vision, urinary retention and dry mouth. Muscarinic acetylcholine receptor antagonists are also used in the treatment and prevention of drug-induced extrapyramidal disorders.

FURTHER READING

Cooper JR, Bloom FE and Roth RH. *The Biochemical Basis of Neuropharmacology*, 8th edn. Oxford: Oxford University Press, 2002.

——————————————

Nester EJ, Hyman SE and Malenka R. *Molecular Basis of Neuropharmacology: A Foundation for Clinical Neuroscience.* New York: McGraw-Hill, 2001.

3.1 Neuropsychometry

An organised and thorough cognitive examination performed by the clinician is important both in the initial assessment and diagnosis of a patient's condition and in the subsequent follow-up. The most routinely used test is the Folstein Mini-Mental State Examination, which records a score out of 30. However, use of this test does have its limitations: because it is heavily weighted toward verbal tasks, false 'normals' occur. A wider battery of tests enables for more sensitivity and specificity.

Orientation and attention

Is the patient orientated in place, person and time? Disorientation in person is seldom organic. Poor orientation should prompt examination of attention. This can be done by testing immediate recall of a string of digits. The normal forward digit span is five to six digits, and backwards it is three to four digits. Patients who perform poorly in recalling digits usually perform poorly on subsequent tests that require concentration. These areas are particularly impaired in acute confusional states.

Language

Listen carefully to the patient's general conversation. See Section 1.2.17 for assessment of language.

Alzheimer's disease

Speech is fluent, but with semantic or anomic errors. There are also errors on naming objects, and the more severe the dementia, the less obscure the objects that are named incorrectly (high-frequency words). Also look for preservation of repetition.

Memory

Memory is divided into episodic memory (recollection of events) and semantic memory (our working knowledge of the world). Episodic memory is further divided into antegrade or retrograde, depending on its relation to the onset of a disease.

Episodic memory

Ask the patient to relate his or her life history from early childhood to the present day and have this verified by a relative. Antegrade episodic memory can be tested by the patient's ability to remember a name and address 5 minutes after being told it. Impairment of antegrade episodic memory is characteristic of Alzheimer's disease.

Semantic memory

Naming and describing objects.

Frontal lobe dysfunction

This includes executive function: our ability to plan and reason.

Letter fluency

Ask the patient to give as many words (not proper nouns) beginning with a certain letter within 1 minute. Then ask them to name as many animals as possible within a further minute (beginning with any letter). Normal individuals will name approximately 20 words and slightly more animals. In frontal lobe dysfunction, there is a decrease in letter frequency more than category (animal) frequency. This pattern of impairment is reversed in Alzheimer's disease.

Concrete thinking

Cognitive estimates Ask the patient to estimate/guess the answers to the following questions.

- How high is the Post Office tower?
- How far is it to New York?
- How tall is the average man?
- How long is the average woman's spine?
- How many camels are there in Holland?

Patients' answers may be both fixed and wildly out.

Proverbs Enquire as to the meaning of 'People in glass houses should not throw stones'. The patient may translate such proverbs literally.

Visuospatial

Test the following.

- Ask a patient to draw a clock face and to set the hands to ten-to-two. Look for signs of neglect.
- Copying of geometric figures.
- Line bisection.

Impairment in the ability to perform the above usually reflects non-dominant parietal lobe dysfunction.

Cortical and subcortical dementias

Dementias can be divided into those in which the pathology is predominantly subcortical or cortical. Good examples of subcortical dementia are progressive supranuclear palsy and Huntington's disease. Typically, the patients are lethargic and withdrawn with slow thought processing. Memory impairment reflects frontal dysfunction, with recollection aided by cues. Cortical dementia, as seen in Alzheimer's disease, is more rapid and the amnesia more severe. Dysphasia, dyspraxia and agnosia may be present. The lack of motivation and attention that characterise subcortical dementias are not usually seen, but as neurodegenerative diseases progress there is an overlap of symptoms between cortical and subcortical dementias.

FURTHER READING

Folstein MF, Folstein SE and McHugh PR. 'Mini-mental state': a practical method for grading the cognitive state of patients for the clinician. *J. Psychiatr. Res.* 1975; 12: 189–98.

Pasquier F. Early diagnosis of dementia: neuropsychology. *J. Neurol.* 1999; 246: 6–15.

Savage CR. Neuropsychology of subcortical dementias. *Psychiatr. Clin. North. Am.* 1997; 20: 911–31.

3.2 Lumbar puncture

Principle

Analysis of the cerebrospinal fluid (CSF) can yield valuable diagnostic information in a wide range of clinical circumstances.

Normal findings

- Pressure 80–200 mmH$_2$O (CSF).

- Lymphocytes or mononuclear cells: no more than 5/μL.

- No red blood cells.

- Total protein 0.15–0.5 g/L.

- Glucose 60–80% of blood glucose concentration.

- No xanthochromia (see Section 2.8.4).

A 'bloody tap' is not uncommon: if the patient has a normal blood count, then the ratio of white cells to red cells is approximately 1:1,000. Hence, if the red cell count is 10,000/μL, the expected white cell count in the CSF sample will be 10/μL.

Indications

Inflammatory conditions

- Central nervous system: multiple sclerosis, acute demyelinating encephalomyelitis and neurosarcoid.

- Peripheral nervous system: Guillain–Barré syndrome and chronic inflammatory demyelinating neuropathy.

Neoplastic

Particularly malignant meningitis (diffuse meningeal infiltration). In this instance at least 5–10 mL of fresh CSF should be sent for cytological evaluation. Repeat sampling may be necessary.

Infective

Bacterial, viral and fungal.

Other indications

- Subarachnoid haemorrhage.

- Benign intracranial hypertension.

- Rapidly progressive dementia.

Contraindications

- Symptoms or signs of raised intracranial pressure without imaging.

- Focal neurological signs without imaging.

- Local infection (skin, bone and pustular acne).

- Thrombocytopenia or a clotting disorder.

Practical details

Performed properly this should not be the painful terrifying experience that patients expect. As in all invasive procedures, allow adequate time for the local anaesthetic to work. Positioning of the patient is absolutely crucial to success, and without it failure is inevitable. Although routinely performed with the patient lying on the left side (for a right-handed operator), knees drawn up to the chest and the uppermost shoulder vertically over the other (Fig. 58), it is equally acceptable for the patient to be sat on the bed and leaning forward onto a chair or table. The latter position is often easier if the subject is obese.

A common mistake is to insert the needle too low. Remember that the L3/4 space is located between the iliac crests (Fig. 59). Remember also that the spinal cord ends at approximately L1, so it is quite difficult to go too high.

After injection of a small amount of local anaesthetic into the skin, massage it with finger or thumb in order to disperse the 'bleb'. This enables you to remain confident about the 'feel' of your anatomical landmarks, which is crucial to success.

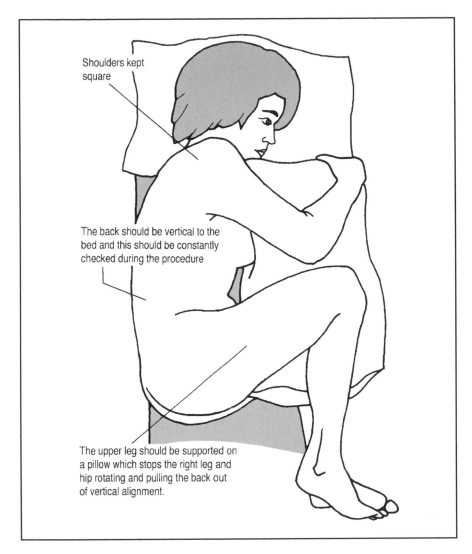

Fig. 58 The correct position for lumbar puncture.

Shoulders kept square

The back should be vertical to the bed and this should be constantly checked during the procedure

The upper leg should be supported on a pillow which stops the right leg and hip rotating and pulling the back out of vertical alignment.

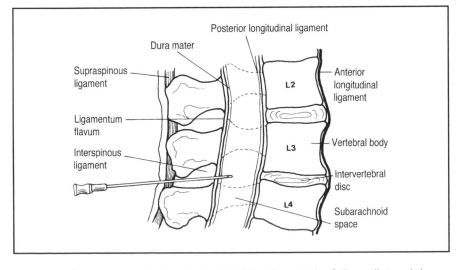

Posterior longitudinal ligament

Dura mater

Supraspinous ligament

Ligamentum flavum

Interspinous ligament

L2

Anterior longitudinal ligament

L3

Vertebral body

Intervertebral disc

L4

Subarachnoid space

Fig. 59 Lumbar puncture needle shown *in situ* at L3/4 (often the easiest level). The needle is angled slightly headwards. If inserted at 90°, it tends to hit the upper surface of the arch of L4, producing a very characteristic grating sensation and an appropriate response from the patient.

If anatomical landmarks cannot be discerned (scoliosis, etc.), lumbar puncture should be performed under radiological guidance. A pressure reading should be obtained with the patient relaxed, legs uncurled and breathing normally. If the patient starts in a sitting position it is possible, after insertion of the needle into the subarachnoid space, to carefully move the patient into a lying position to enable pressure recording.

After the procedure the patient need rest for no more than 30 minutes. Enforced bed-rest has not been shown to reduce the incidence of post-lumbar puncture headache (PLPH, see below).

Complications

Post-lumbar puncture headache
This occurs in some degree in about 10% of procedures. It is not related to the amount of CSF taken but is likely to be due to continuous leak of CSF from the hole made in the dura. Incidence of PLPH is therefore related to the size of the hole, and hence predictors of PLPH include:

- gauge of the needle;
- angle the bevel is inserted (if inserted horizontally the dural fibres will be parted, but if vertical the fibres will be sliced through);
- number of attempts.

The headache is a typical low-pressure headache, worse on standing and ameliorated by lying down. Patients should be reassured. Symptoms normally resolve in a matter of days and, with the exception of bed-rest, adequate fluid intake (occasionally intravenous) and simple analgesia, no further treatment is required.

Cerebral herniation

This is catastrophic and can be avoided by imaging prior to lumbar puncture.

FURTHER READING

Patten J. *Neurological Differential Diagnosis*, 2nd edn. London: Springer, 1996: 273–81.

3.3 Neurophysiology

Neurophysiological investigation uses a variety of techniques to aid the diagnosis of disease processes affecting both the central and peripheral nervous systems.

3.3.1 Electroencephalography

Principle

It is thought that electroencephalography (EEG) signals reflect extracellular current flow from the summation of excitatory and inhibitory postsynaptic potentials.

Normal findings

The waking EEG pattern consists of mainly alpha (8–12 Hz) and beta (>12 Hz) activity, with minimal gamma (4–7 Hz) activity.

In sleep, there is increasing delta (1–3 Hz) activity as the depth of sleep becomes greater. In drowsiness, there is disappearance of alpha activity with increased beta and gamma activities.

Indications

To evaluate suspected epilepsy and altered consciousness (eg brain death), and to detect structural lesions (eg tumour) and certain diseases such as herpes simplex encephalitis or Creutzfeldt–Jakob disease (CJD).

In epilepsy, the EEG is used to distinguish partial from generalised seizures, localise the epileptic focus in partial seizures and characterise epilepsy syndromes, eg 3-Hz spike-and-wave activity in absence attacks. Prolonged EEG monitoring or video-telemetry improves diagnostic accuracy in epilepsy. The EEG is not useful in aiding the diagnosis of a patient presenting with 'funny turns'. Minor asymmetries should not be considered pathological.

The typical sign of a focal cerebral lesion is polymorphic focal activity. In herpes simplex encephalitis, the EEG shows slowing with periodic sharp-wave complexes over the temporal lobe. EEG changes in CJD are discussed in Section 2.11.

3.3.2 Evoked potentials

Principle

Evoked potentials measure electrical conduction through the nervous system in response to sensory stimulation.

Visual-evoked potentials (VEPs) are elicited by monocular visual stimulation with a chequerboard pattern. Normally, a response is recorded from the visual cortex approximately 100 ms after eye stimulation, the P100 latency.

Brainstem auditory-evoked potentials (BAEPs) are elicited by monoaural stimulation with repetitive clicks, which generate waves in cranial nerve VIII and the brainstem. Normally, five waveforms occur (I–V) within 10 ms of the stimulus, representing sequential activation of structures of the auditory pathway.

Somatosensory-evoked potentials (SSEPs) are generated by electrical stimulation of a peripheral nerve, with recordings over the spine and scalp to assess central sensory

processing. Responses depend on which nerves are stimulated.

Indications

- VEPs: abnormal (delayed P100 latency) in optic neuritis in multiple sclerosis (MS), tumours compressing the optic nerve, ischaemic optic neuropathy, toxic amblyopias, glaucoma and Leber's hereditary optic atrophy.

- BAEPs: abnormal (as indicated by the presence, latency and interpeak intervals of waveforms I–V) in VIII nerve and brainstem lesions (eg MS), acoustic neuromas and brainstem gliomas.

- SSEPs: conduction delay or block arises in any disease affecting the central nervous system sensory pathways, eg MS. Abnormally large SSEPs may be seen in myoclonus of cortical origin.

3.3.3 Electromyography

Principle

Electromyography (EMG) records electrical activity of motor units from resting and voluntary muscle activity. Relaxed muscle normally shows no spontaneous electrical activity, except in the end-plate area where neuromuscular junctions are found. All voluntary muscle activity is recorded as motor unit potentials. A motor unit potential is the sum of muscle fibre potentials innervated by a single anterior horn cell.

Indications

- EMG is commonly used to evaluate anterior horn cell diseases, inflammatory muscle diseases, muscular dystrophies, myotonic disorders, neuromuscular junction disorders, axonal peripheral neuropathies and chronic radiculopathies.

- Single-fibre EMG is mainly used to diagnose myasthenia gravis and other neuromuscular junction transmission disorders by the detection of jitter (see Section 2.2.5).

3.3.4 Nerve conduction studies

Principle

Motor nerve conduction studies (NCS) record the compound muscle action potential (CMAP) of a muscle to stimulation of its motor nerve (Fig. 60).

Sensory NCS are done by recording sensory action potentials in sensory fibres when these fibres are stimulated. Supramaximal stimulation is used. Conduction velocity and amplitude of responses are measured.

F-waves can also be recorded in the muscle after the CMAP. Its latency represents conduction retrogradely up the motor nerve to the anterior horn cell and back to the muscle. Increased latency with normal motor conduction may be seen in radiculopathies (ie proximal disease).

Indications

NCS are used to determine the presence and extent of peripheral nerve damage in entrapment neuropathies; whether the pathological process is axonal or demyelinating; or whether conduction block is present.

- Demyelination slows conduction velocities markedly; axonal loss reduces the amplitude of response although conduction velocity remains relatively normal.
- NCS are also used to evaluate neuromuscular junction disorders, eg myasthenia gravis where there is a decremental response to repetitive nerve stimulation.

FURTHER READING

Daube JR, ed. *Clinical Neurophysiology*, 2nd edn. Oxford: Oxford University Press, 2002.

3.4 Neuroimaging

3.4.1 Computed tomography and computed tomography angiography

Principle

CT images are produced by detecting X-rays that have been directed through tissue. The images depend on how much of the original beam has managed to pass through the tissue, known as X-ray attenuation. Contrast agents improve the sensitivity and specificity of CT. Enhancement occurs when the blood–brain barrier is compromised, eg in inflammatory lesions or tumours.

CT angiography (CTA) is based on detecting enhancement of arterial

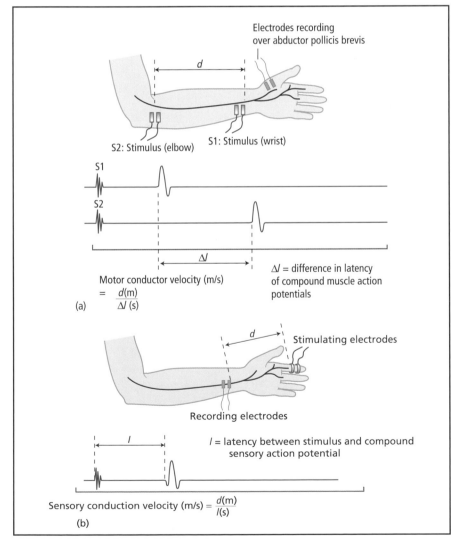

▲ **Fig. 60** Principles of NCS. (**a**) Measurement of motor conduction velocity in the median nerve. (**b**) Measurement of sensory conduction velocity in the median nerve.

vessels after the injection of contrast using fast helical CT scanners.

Indications

CT is best used to detect acute bleeding and calcium (bone). It is the initial investigation of choice in stroke, subarachnoid haemorrhage (SAH) and head trauma. It is also used to assess bony pathology, eg bony erosion from tumours, and when MRI is contraindicated, In stroke, CT may not reveal an infarct within the first 48 hours. MRI will detect an infarct within a few hours of a stroke. However, CT is preferred because it detects intracranial haemorrhage better than MRI in the first 48 hours. In head trauma, CT is indicated because it detects bony injuries and traumatic intracerebral or subarachnoid haemorrhage.

> ⚠ If SAH is strongly suspected a lumbar puncture must be performed, even if a CT scan is normal.
>
> CTA may be used in patients who decline catheter angiography and have contraindications for magnetic resonance angiography (MRA) in order to detect carotid artery stenosis, carotid dissection, arteriovenous malformations and cerebral aneurysms. However, CTA is inferior to angiography or MRA.

Contraindications

Contrast agents are contraindicated in patients with asthma or who are allergic to the contrast itself. Renal failure is a relative contraindication. In pregnancy, the fetus must be shielded from the harmful radiation.

3.4.2 Magnetic resonance imaging and magnetic resonance angiography

Principle

A magnetic resonance image is obtained when a radiofrequency pulse excites the protons in the tissue, producing radio wave emissions. The signal intensity depends on the mobile hydrogen nuclei concentration of tissues. T1 (spin-lattice) and T2 (spin-spin) relaxation time constants depend on the physical properties of the tissue. As in CT, contrast enhancement is due to disruption of the blood–brain barrier.

Magnetic resonance angiography (MRA) is performed using the time-of-flight (TOF) or phase-contrast (PC) techniques. In TOF MRA, vessels are detected because of the inflow of unsaturated spins into the imaging plane. In PC MRA, vessels are detected because moving protons within them accumulate phase shifts proportional to their velocity as they cross a magnetic gradient (Fig. 61).

Indications

MRI is best for soft tissue and vascular abnormalities, and is superior to CT for detecting posterior fossa or spinal cord (eg syrinx and epidural abscess) lesions. Indications for MRI include stroke, tumour, degenerative diseases, multiple sclerosis, vascular lesions (eg aneurysm and vascular malformation), epilepsy, myelopathy and cerebral infections (eg abscess),

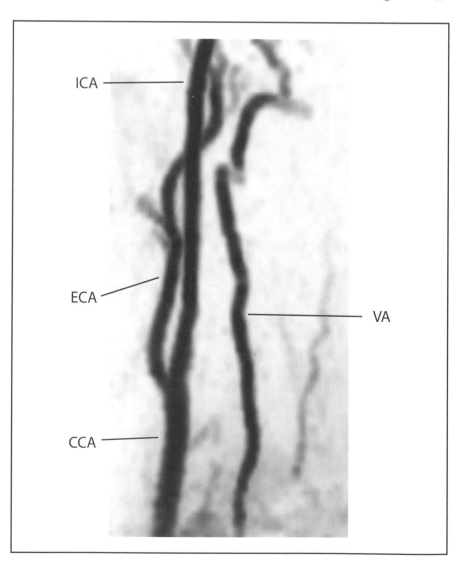

▲ **Fig. 61** Normal MRA of right-sided carotid and vertebral artery systems. CCA, common carotid artery; ICA, internal carotid artery; ECA, external carotid artery; VA, vertebral artery.

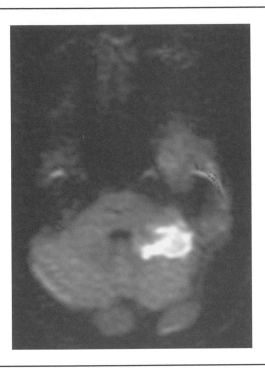

▲**Fig. 62** DWI scan demonstrating acute infarction in the right cerebellar hemisphere. (Courtesy of Professor M. Brown, Institute of Neurology, University of London.)

herpes simplex encephalitis and meningitis.

In stroke, after taking into account the advantages of CT, note that haematomas of more than 2–3 days old are better seen with MRI.

Diffusion-weighted MRI (DWI) is exquisitely sensitive to acutely infarcted tissue (Fig. 62) and perfusion-weighted MRI (PWI) detects cerebral tissue that is underperfused in the setting of acute stroke. If the defect in PWI is greater than that seen on DWI, it may be that this tissue is under threat from ischaemia, but is not infarcted. Therefore it would survive if perfusion could be reinstated, for example using thrombolytic therapy.

Indications for MRA are similar to CT angiography, but the former provides better-quality images. In the investigation of carotid artery stenosis, arterial angiography (which carries a risk of stroke) should not

be required if MRA and carotid Dopplers are concurrent.

Contraindications

Metallic objects, eg shrapnel in eyes, intracranial clips and pacemakers are contraindications for MRI.

3.4.3 Angiography

Principle

Angiography is performed by introducing a catheter via the femoral or brachial artery, up the aorta, into the carotid or vertebral arteries and injecting radio-opaque contrast to enable detailed visualisation of vessels.

Indications

Angiography is used to diagnose aneurysms, arterial stenosis (eg thromboembolism, dissection, vasculitis and atherosclerosis), arteriovenous malformations and cerebral venous sinus thrombosis. Therapeutic interventional

procedures can also be carried out, eg embolisation of aneurysms, arteriovenous malformations or blood supply to tumours, arterial thrombolysis and angioplasty.

Complications

These include local haematoma or bleeding, infection, pseudoaneurysm formation, vessel damage, renal failure, contrast reaction, stroke or transient ischaemic attack and death. In experienced hands, diagnostic angiography carries a risk of stroke of less than 1%. However, interventional procedures carry a risk of major complications of up to 10%, including vessel perforation.

FURTHER READING

Edelman RR and Warach S. Magnetic resonance imaging (1). *N. Engl. J. Med.* 1993; 328: 708–16.

Edelman RR and Warach S. Magnetic resonance imaging (2). *N. Engl. J. Med.* 1993; 328: 785–91.

Gilman S. Imaging the brain: first of two parts. *N. Engl. J. Med.* 1998; 338: 812–20.

Gilman S. Imaging the brain: second of two parts. *N. Engl. J. Med.* 1998; 338: 889–96.

3.5 Single-photon emission computed tomography and positron emission tomography

Single-photon emission computed tomography (SPECT) and positron emission tomography (PET) are two methods by which functional, rather than conventional structural, neuroimaging can be performed. Functional neuroimaging can be divided into techniques that demonstrate synaptic activity or regional activation (called functional mapping) based on the close association between blood flow and neuronal activation/synaptic activity, and techniques that enable the detection of particular neurotransmitter or neurochemical substances. Tracer design is therefore based on physiological molecules involved in metabolic turnover (eg oxygen, glucose and amino acids) and enzyme activation, or on neurotransmitters and their receptors. The specific tracers are labelled with γ-emitting radioisotopes for SPECT and positron-emitting radionuclides for PET.

Single-photon emission computed tomography

Gamma-emitting radionuclides are commercially available and images are taken with a routine nuclear medicine camera. This makes SPECT less expensive and more widely available compared with PET. The disadvantages are inferior spatial resolution and less quantification than are possible with PET.

Positron emission tomography

PET depends on radionuclides labelled with positrons (positively charged electrons). Positrons have a short half-life and are generated by a cyclotron, and thus PET can only be performed in a centre with a cyclotron. Commonly used positron-labelled radionuclides include oxygen (^{15}O), carbon (^{11}C) and nitrogen (^{13}N). Fluorine (^{18}F) is used to replace hydrogen. The image gathered represents the distribution of the emitted positrons. The increased sensitivity of PET over SPECT enables patients to undergo less radioactive exposure.

Functional imaging

Functional imaging techniques are concerned with describing activity of neurons in the brain associated with a given physiological, cognitive or pathological state, ie function of the brain as opposed to structure. Studies using PET may be steady-state or activation studies, in which a physical or cognitive task is associated with changes in cerebral blood flow in discrete brain regions.

Steady-state studies

- A characteristic pattern of impaired metabolism in parietal and posterior temporal regions is seen in early Alzheimer's disease.

- Patchy abnormalities, particularly in the distribution of the middle cerebral artery, are seen in vascular dementia.

- Reduced uptake of ^{18}F-DOPA is seen in the basal ganglia in Parkinson's disease.

- Hypometabolism is seen in the striatum in Huntington's disease.

Activation studies

- Localisation of cerebral function in normal volunteers, eg language, memory, attention and motor control.

- Studies of the reorganisation of the brain in the recovery of function following brain injury, eg after stroke (Fig. 63).

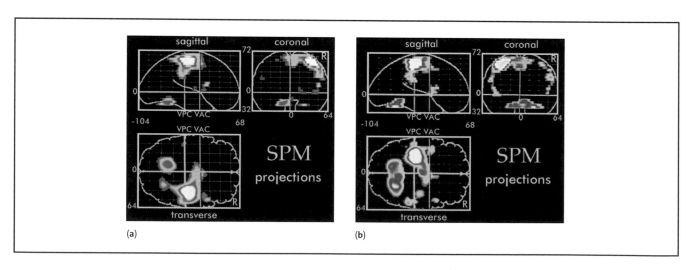

▲ **Fig. 63** Statistical parametric map (SPM) of brain areas activated (in comparison with rest) by a paced, sequential, finger-to-thumb opposition task in patients with lesions of left internal capsule using (**a**) left hand and (**b**) recovered right hand. SPMs are presented as projections through the brain seen from side (sagittal), back (coronal) and top (transverse) views. The frontal pole is on the right side of the transverse section. Highly significant changes of activity between active and resting states are shown in colour, coded to represent levels of significance (white being the greatest significance). In comparing (**b**) with (**a**), it can be seen that the same task has led to activations that are not only bilateral but more extensive, reflecting recruitment of other motor areas not normally activated by simple motor tasks. (Reproduced from Chollet *et al. Ann. Neurol.* 1991; 29: 63–71 with permission of Lippincott, Williams and Wilkins Inc.)

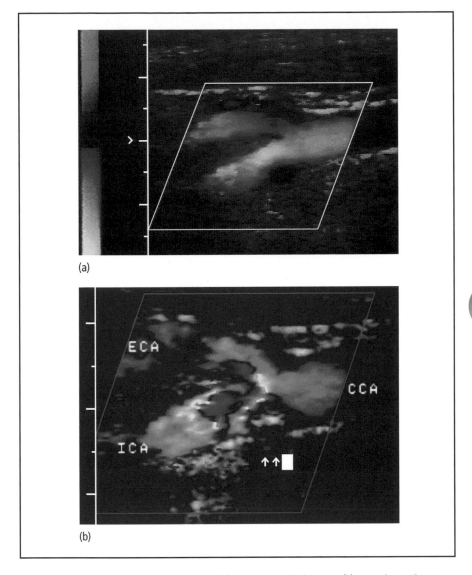

(a)

(b)

▲ **Fig. 64** Colour flow Doppler ultrasound scans: (**a**) normal carotid bifurcation; (**b**) internal carotid artery stenosis causing turbulent blood flow (seen in blue). CCA, common carotid artery; ICA, internal carotid artery; ECA, external carotid artery. (Courtesy of Professor M. Brown, Institute of Neurology, University of London.)

3.6 Carotid Dopplers

Principle

The technique utilises the fact that sound waves reflected off red blood cells give an indication of the flow velocity within the vessel (Fig. 64). A stenosed vessel gives a high flow velocity. The accuracy of the test compared with angiography (the gold standard) is operator dependent, but should approach at least 90% in good centres.

> Carotid Dopplers cannot distinguish between an absence of flow (complete occlusion) and very low flow (tight stenosis with a patent vessel).

Indications

To screen for carotid artery stenosis when clinically suspected. If this technique is used in conjunction with magnetic resonance angiography and the results are in agreement, then arterial angiography (and its risk of stroke) should not be required.

NEUROLOGY: SECTION 4
SELF-ASSESSMENT

4.1 Self-assessment questions

Question 1

Clinical scenario

A 67-year-old woman presents to the neurology clinic with a 6-month history of tingling and numbness in her feet and hands. In the last 2 months, she has developed a left foot drop and is now complaining that her right hand feels weak.

Question

Which is the *least* likely diagnosis to cause the above?

Answers

A Guillain–Barré syndrome
B Lead poisoning
C Vasculitis
D Diabetes mellitus
E Hypothyroidism

Question 2

Clinical scenario

A 29-year-old woman complains of a 6-month history of a burning sensation over the lateral aspect of the right thigh down to, but not, below the knee.

Question

Which of the following is most likely to help the patient?

Answers

A Pulsed cyclophosphamide and methylprednisolone
B Intravenous immunoglobulin
C Amitriptyline

D Plasmapheresis
E Beta interferon

Question 3

Clinical scenario

A 30-year-old man presents with a history of muscle pain and weakness developing after prolonged exercise. He also complains of having episodes of dark urine after exercise.

Question

Which of the following is the most likely diagnosis?

Answers

A Carnitine palmitoyltransferase deficiency
B Inclusion body myositis
C Acid maltase deficiency
D McArdle's disease
E Myasthenia gravis

Question 4

Clinical scenario

A 65-year-old woman presents with dysphagia.

Question

Which of the following is *unlikely* to indicate motor neuron disease?

Answers

A Brisk jaw jerk
B Spastic tongue movement
C Wasting of small hand muscles
D Optic atrophy
E Foot drop

Question 5

Clinical scenario

A 25-year-old man presents with a right foot drop.

Question

Which of the following would *not* indicate a common peroneal nerve palsy?

Answers

A Normal right ankle jerk
B Weakness of ankle dorsiflexion
C Weakness of ankle eversion
D Weakness of ankle inversion
E Numbness over the web of the first and second toes of the right foot

Question 6

Clinical scenario

A 50-year-old woman complains of pain radiating through the knee and down the medial side of the calf to the medial malleolus.

Question

Which one of the following nerve roots would give rise to such pain?

Answers

A L2
B L3
C L4
D L5
E S1

Question 7

Clinical scenario

A patient presents with weakness of dorsiflexion of the right big toe.

Question

Which nerve root would you expect to be affected in this case?

Answers

A L2
B L3

C L4
D L5
E S1

Question 8

Clinical scenario
A patient with back pain is noted to have an absent right ankle jerk.

Question
Which of the following would cause the above?

Answers
A A nerve root lesion of L4 only
B A nerve root lesion of L5 only
C A nerve root lesion of S1 only
D A nerve root lesion of either L4 or L5
E A nerve root lesion of either L5 or S1

Question 9

Clinical scenario
A 48-year-old man presents with a history of excruciating pain in his left shoulder that woke him early one morning 2 weeks ago. Since then, he has noticed difficulty abducting the right shoulder due to weakness. There was wasting of his right deltoid when he was examined.

Question
What is the most likely diagnosis?

Answers
A Neuralgic amyotrophy
B Guillain–Barré syndrome
C Cervical disc prolapse
D Syringomyelia
E Polymyalgia rheumatica

Question 10

Clinical scenario
A patient presents with weakness of elbow extension.

Question
Which of the following nerve roots is likely to be affected?

Answers
A C5
B C6
C C7
D C8
E T1

Question 11

Clinical scenario
A patient presents with weakness of elbow and wrist extension

Question
In which of the following distributions would you expect sensory loss to be detected?

Answers
A Shoulder tip
B Lateral aspect of the wrist, flexors, forearm and thumb
C Middle finger
D Little and ring fingers
E Medial aspect of forearm

Question 12

Clinical scenario
A 40-year-old man is referred to you with muscle weakness. Examination confirms the presence of proximal upper and lower limb weakness, with minimal distal limb weakness.

Question
Which of the following is the *least* likely diagnosis?

Answers
A Statin myopathy
B Dermatomyositis
C Cushing's disease
D Myotonic dystrophy
E Limb girdle muscular dystrophy

Question 13

Clinical scenario
A 30-year-old previously fit and well woman presents with a 2-day history of progressive leg weakness and bladder dysfunction. Examination reveals a spastic paraparesis.

Question
What is the most important investigation for this patient?

Answers
A Cerebrospinal fluid examination
B MRI scan of the spine
C Electromyography and nerve conduction studies
D Anti-ganglioside antibodies
E Creatine kinase

Question 14

Clinical scenario
A 73-year-old man is admitted with a 3-day history of paraesthesiae in his hands and feet followed by progressive symmetrical ascending weakness in his lower limbs. One week prior to his current symptoms he had several days of diarrhoea. He appears breathless when you examine him.

Question
Which of the following parameters is most useful in monitoring this patient's respiratory function?

Answers
A Forced vital capacity
B Peak expiratory flow rate
C Peak inspiratory flow rate
D Diffusing capacity of the lung for carbon monoxide
E Total lung capacity

Question 15

Clinical scenario
A 73-year-old man is admitted with a 3-day history of paraesthesiae in his hands and feet followed by progressive symmetrical ascending weakness in his lower limbs. One week prior to his current symptoms he had several days of diarrhoea.

Question
Which of the following treatments should be started if the patient continues to deteriorate?

Answers

A   Intramuscular human tetanus
     immunoglobulin
B   Intravenous immunoglobulin
C   Intravenous methylprednisolone
D   Intravenous antibiotics
E   Thrombolysis

Question 16

Clinical scenario

A 30-year-old man presents to
clinic with a 5-year history of
fasciculations, mainly in his calf
muscles. These tend to be more
prominent after exercise.
Neurological examination is
completely normal.

Question

What is the most likely diagnosis?

Answers

A   Motor neuron disease
B   Myasthenia gravis
C   Benign fasciculation syndrome
D   Polymyositis
E   Becker's muscular dystrophy

Question 17

Clinical scenario

A 60-year-old man presents
to clinic with muscle weakness
and mild dysphagia. On
examination, he is noted to
have disproportionate weakness
in his finger flexors relative to
the corresponding extensors,
and disproportionate weakness
of knee extensors compared to
hip flexors.

Question

What is the most likely diagnosis in
this case?

Answers

A   Polymyositis
B   Motor neuron disease
C   Oculopharyngeal muscular
     dystrophy
D   Inclusion body myositis
E   Myasthenia gravis

Question 18

Clinical scenario

A 38-year-old woman is referred to
you with muscle weakness.

Question

Which two of the following features
would *not* be compatible with a
diagnosis of myasthenia gravis?

Answers

A   Pupillary dilatation
B   Ptosis
C   Hoarse voice
D   Internuclear ophthalmoplegia
E   Fatiguable muscle weakness
F   Facial weakness
G   Normal deep tendon reflexes
H   Dysphagia
I   Nasal speech
J   Normal sensory examination to
     pinprick

Question 19

Clinical scenario

A 45-year-old man presents with
progressive leg weakness.

Question

Which two features would *oppose* a
diagnosis of Guillain–Barré
syndrome?

Answers

A   Severe back pain
B   Recent chest infection
C   Urinary incontinence at the
     beginning of the illness
D   Fluctuating BP
E   Sluggish pupillary reactions
F   Normal arm and leg reflexes
G   Marked fatiguability of leg
     movement
H   Subjective sensory disturbance
I   Dysarthria
J   Shortness of breath on exertion

Question 20

Clinical scenario

A 65-year-old man presents with a
4-month history of dysarthria and

progressive difficulty in swallowing.
Examination reveals a weak
fasciculating tongue, a brisk
gag reflex, and jaw jerk.

Question

What is the most likely diagnosis?

Answers

A   Basilar artery thrombosis
B   Multiple sclerosis
C   Miller Fisher syndrome
D   Amyotrophic lateral sclerosis
E   Wernicke's encephalopathy

Question 21

Clinical scenario

A 64-year-old man was referred
to the outpatient clinic with a
6-month history of episodes of
loss of awareness without collapse.
A witness account mentioned the
occurrence of chewing movements
during the attacks. He also has
diabetes mellitus and hypertension.

Question

What one of the following is the
most likely diagnosis?

Answers

A   Hypoglycaemia
B   Transient ischaemic attack
C   Postural hypotension
D   Cardiac arrhythmia
E   Complex partial seizure

Question 22

Clinical scenario

A 38-year-old woman presents with a
2-day history of fever, headache and
a 40-minute period of continuous
convulsive seizures.

Question

Which one of the following is *not*
appropriate in the management of
her condition?

Answers

A   Immediate administration of
     4 mg of intravenous lorazepam
B   Arterial blood gas measurement

C Neuroimaging (CT or MRI brain scan) and lumbar puncture

D Intravenous phenytoin at a dose of 15–20 mg/kg, given at a rate of 150 mg/min

E Immediate commencement of broad-spectrum antibiotics and antiviral agents

Question 23

Clinical scenario
A 24-year-old woman was referred to the outpatient clinic with recurrent and frequent episodes of falling asleep during the day.

Question
Which one of the following does *not* support the diagnosis of narcoleptic syndrome?

Answers
A A history of recurrent episodes of transient paralysis on awakening

B Low hypocretin levels in her cerebrospinal fluid

C Human leucocyte antigen allele DQB1 0602

D Epworth Sleepiness Score of 14

E Feeling unrefreshed after each brief episode of sleep

Question 24

Clinical scenario
A 38-year-old woman with a long history of migraine is receiving prophylactic treatment with amitriptyline 100 mg at night. She is referred to the outpatient clinic with worsening migraine control despite good compliance with her medication. Her GP had recently started another medication for an unrelated condition.

Question
Which one of the following may cause a reduction in plasma amitriptyline levels when co-prescribed?

Answers
A Warfarin

B Sodium valproate

C Fluoxetine

D St John's wort

E Trimethoprim

Question 25

Clinical scenario
A 24-year-old woman is seen in the Emergency Department with a 5-day history of visual impairment in one eye.

Question
Which one of the following features does *not* support the diagnosis of optic neuritis?

Answers
A Reduced colour appreciation in the affected eye

B Flame-shaped haemorrhages around the macula

C Relative afferent pupillary defect

D Cecocentral scotoma

E Normal optic disc appearances

Question 26

Clinical scenario
A 76-year-old man presents to clinic with a 6-month of slowness and stiffness.

Question
Which of the following would *not* be compatible with a diagnosis of idiopathic Parkinson's disease?

Answers
A Unilateral bradykinesia and rigidity

B Prominent falls

C Lack of tremor

D Reduction in up-gaze

E Asymmetrical resting tremor in the hand only

Question 27

Clinical scenario
A 78-year-old woman with known idiopathic Parkinson's disease for 10 years attends clinic with severe visual hallucinations and episodes of increasing confusion. She normally takes one Sinemet Plus (100 mg levodopa/25 mg carbidopa) five times daily, 200 mg entacapone five times daily, selegiline 10 mg mane and cabergoline 4 mg nocte.

Question
What should be the first action to improve the hallucinations?

Answers
A Prescribe a new atypical neuroleptic such as olanzapine

B Prescribe a traditional antipsychotic such as haloperidol

C Gradually reduce the Sinemet Plus

D Gradually reduce the entacapone

E Gradually reduce the cabergoline

Question 28

Clinical scenario
A 46-year-old woman with a marked change in personality over the last 2 years is referred to the neurology clinic. She has become increasingly sexually flirtatious, exhibiting inappropriate behaviour in social situations. Impairment of her abstract thinking, memory and planning has become increasingly obvious. However, the ability to perform arithmetic tasks is relatively preserved. Her speech output is diminished. There is no motor impairment. Physical examination is unremarkable except for the presence of grasp reflexes.

Question
What is the clinical diagnosis?

Answers
A Alzheimer's disease

B Normal pressure hydrocephalus

C Frontotemporal dementia

D Dementia with Lewy bodies

E Huntington's disease

Question 29

Clinical scenario

A 58-year-old man presents with progressive imbalance over the past month.

Question

Which two of the following symptoms and signs would be inconsistent with a cerebellar lesion?

Answers

A Horizontal gaze-evoked nystagmus
B Finger–nose dysmetria
C *Marche à petit pas*
D Titubation
E Rebound phenomenon
F Poor tandem walking
G Papilloedema
H Headache
I Dizziness on turning over in bed
J Symptoms worse in the dark

Question 30

Clinical scenario

A 78-year-old woman presents to clinic with forgetfulness and failure to look after herself at home. She recently got lost at her local shops and had to be taken home by a friend. She feels there is very little the matter. Her Mini-Mental State Examination score is 22/30.

Question

What is the most likely diagnosis?

Answers

A Bilateral subdural haemorrhages
B Normal pressure hydrocephalus
C Alzheimer's disease
D Vascular dementia
E Pseudo-dementia

Question 31

Clinical scenario

An 84-year-old man presents to clinic with a 6-month history of increasing confusion, visual hallucinations, reduced mobility and falls.

Question

What is the most likely cause for his problems?

Answers

A Alzheimer's disease
B Frontotemporal dementia
C Dementia with Lewy bodies
D Parkinson's disease with dementia
E Vascular dementia

Question 32

Clinical scenario

A 30-year-old man who is otherwise well presents with a tremor that is worst when he tries to write or drink. He has had it for several years, but recently it has become worse and is now socially embarrassing. He finds it improves when he has had a relaxed meal with wine. His father has a similar tremor, but he also has a tremor of his head.

Question

What is the most probable diagnosis?

Answers

A Early-onset idiopathic Parkinson's disease
B Wilson's disease
C Spinocerebellar ataxia type 6
D Huntington's disease
E Benign essential tremor

Question 33

Clinical scenario

An 82-year-old man has suffered from severe depression for most of his life and has recently been treated with quetiapine for psychosis. His psychiatrist has noticed that he has been parkinsonian for several years and had put this down to his current and previous neuroleptics. Recently, the man is failing to mobilise, is becoming even slower and is starting to shake.

Question

What clinical feature would be most suggestive that he has developed super-added idiopathic Parkinson's disease?

Answers

A His tremor is most disabling when he drinks his tea
B The glabellar tap is positive
C He has marked orofacial dyskinesias
D He has a marked left-sided arm, chin and leg tremor at rest
E He has severe symmetrical bradykinesia

Question 34

Clinical scenario

A 23-year-old is admitted with a heroin overdose. After treatment with a naloxone infusion he wakes up, but says that he cannot get out of bed because his legs are weak and he is unable to walk. On examination he has marked weakness of all movements at the ankles and of knee flexion. He has preserved knee jerks, but the ankle jerks are absent. He has sensory loss to pinprick in the distal legs, but it is difficult to clarify the exact distribution. A lumbosacral MRI scan demonstrates mild degenerative changes only.

Question

What is the most probable diagnosis?

Answers

A Diffuse cortical ischaemia
B Bilateral lumbosacral plexopathy
C A thoracic cord lesion
D Bilateral sciatic nerve palsies
E Myopathy due to rhabdomyolysis

Question 35

Clinical scenario

A 72-year-old diabetic smoker presents to the Emergency

Department with immobility. His right leg has been weak for several months, but over the past 2 weeks he has developed progressive left leg weakness as well. Recently he has struggled to pass urine, but this morning he was incontinent without any awareness. On examination he smells of alcohol and is dishevelled, but he is fully cooperative and alert. He has flaccid leg weakness, worse on the right than the left, which mainly affects hip flexion and dorsiflexion. His knee reflexes are brisk but his ankle jerks are absent. He has a sensory level to pinprick at T5 and has lost vibration sense to the hips and joint position sense to the knees. His plantar responses are extensor. His cranial nerve and upper limb examinations are normal.

Question

What are the two most probable diagnoses?

Answers

A Motor neuron disease
B Bilateral subdural haematomas
C Cervical spondylosis
D Thoracic cord metastases
E Subacute combined degeneration of the spinal cord
F Tertiary syphilis
G Intrinsic thoracic cord lesion
H Spinal neurofibroma
I Anterior spinal artery occlusion
J Bilateral strokes

Question 36

Clinical scenario

You are asked to see a 35-year-old man, a heavy smoker, who is currently being treated with clozapine by the psychiatrists for a major depressive illness. He has had several other neuroleptics in the past. The psychiatrists have noticed that over the past 4 months he has developed a strange jerking of his arms and neck. He never knew his father, who died in a psychiatric hospital when he was only 2 years old, and his paternal grandfather was also said to be 'twitchy', although he died of a heart attack in his sixties. He has lost contact with his two sons and is divorced.

Question

What is the likely diagnosis

Answers

A Tardive dyskinesia
B Huntington's chorea
C Inherited Creutzfeldt–Jakob disease with myoclonus
D Wilson's disease
E Sydenham's chorea

Question 37

Question

Levodopa, used in the treatment of Parkinson's disease, exerts its therapeutic effect by/as:

Answers

A A precursor for dopamine synthesis
B An inhibitor of DOPA decarboxylase
C Stimulating dopamine release
D Binding to the dopamine receptor
E Preventing reuptake of dopamine

Question 38

Question

Most 5-hydroxytryptamine (5HT) receptors are:

Answers

A Ligand-gated ion channels that activate an intracellular second messenger cascade that increases intracellular cyclic adenosine monophosphate (cAMP) levels
B Ligand-gated ion channels that activate an intracellular second messenger cascade that reduces intracellular cAMP levels
C Ligand-gated ion channels that increase intracellular calcium concentration
D G protein-coupled seven-transmembrane-domain receptors that activate an intracellular second messenger cascade that increases intracellular cAMP levels
E G protein-coupled seven-transmembrane-domain receptors that activate an intracellular second messenger cascade that reduces intracellular cAMP levels

Question 39

Question

Which one of the following is *not* an important central nervous system neurotransmitter?

Answers

A Dopamine
B 5-hydroxytryptamine (serotonin)
C γ-Aminobutyric acid
D Adrenaline
E Acetylcholine

Question 40

Question

Gabapentin exerts its therapeutic effect by/as:

Answers

A A precursor for γ-aminobutyric acid (GABA) synthesis
B An inhibitor of GABA transaminase
C Stimulating GABA release
D Binding to the GABA receptor
E Binding to voltage-dependent calcium channels

Question 41

Question

Patients who are taking monoamine oxidase (MAO) inhibitors (MAOIs) are at risk of severe hypertensive reactions if they eat certain foods because:

Answers

A MAOIs inhibit breakdown of dopamine

B MAOIs inhibit breakdown of 5-hydroxytryptamine

C MAOIs inhibit breakdown of noradrenaline

D Dietary tyramine is normally metabolised by MAO in the brain

E Dietary tyramine is normally metabolised by MAO in the bowel wall and liver

4.2 Self-assessment answers

Answer to Question 1

B

Lead poisoning causes a motor neuropathy and could not explain the presence of sensory signs.

Answer to Question 2

C

The patient is likely to have meralgia paraesthetica, which will benefit from drugs such as pregabalin, gabapentin, carbamazepine, lamotrigine and amitriptyline.

Answer to Question 3

A

In carnitine palmitoyltransferase (CPT) deficiency, patients typically develop symptoms after prolonged exercise, whereas in McArdle's disease patients develop symptoms within minutes of starting exercise and may also describe a 'second wind' phenomenon. Myoglobinuria secondary to rhabdomyolysis is more common in CPT deficiency than in McCardle's disease.

Answer to Question 4

D

In motor neuron disease there are no sensory, sphincter or visual pathway disturbances.

Answer to Question 5

D

Weakness of ankle inversion would be indicative of an L5 root lesion rather than a common peroneal nerve palsy.

Answer to Question 6

C

The description is that of L4 nerve root pain. L2 and L3 pain radiates to the anterior thigh; L5 pain radiates through the buttock, down the posterolateral aspect of the thigh and lateral aspect of the calf, and across the dorsum of the foot to the big toe; and S1 pain radiates through the inner buttock to the posterior aspect of the thigh, and then through the posterolateral aspect of the calf to the lateral border of the foot.

Answer to Question 7

D

An L5 root lesion causes weakness of ankle dorsiflexion, inversion and eversion, and dorsiflexion of the great toe. L2 weakness affects hip flexion and thigh adduction; L3 weakness affects thigh adduction and knee extension; L4 weakness affects knee extension and ankle inversion; and S1 weakness affects plantar flexion, eversion and knee flexion.

Answer to Question 8

C

The ankle jerk is supplied by S1 only. The knee jerk is supplied by L3 and L4.

Answer to Question 9

A

The history of sudden onset of excruciating arm (usually shoulder) pain, followed by shoulder and/or parascapular muscle weakness several days later is typical of neuralgic amyotrophy. The pain is so severe it is often confused with the pain of a myocardial infarction.

Answer to Question 10

C

C7 supplies triceps and wrist extensors. A lesion of C5 causes weakness of the deltoid (shoulder abduction) and infraspinatus; of C6 weakness of biceps (elbow flexion) and brachioradialis; and of C8 and T1 weakness of intrinsic hand muscles.

Answer to Question 11

C

C7 supplies triceps and wrist extensors (motor), and the middle finger (sensory).

Answer to Question 12

D

Myotonic dystrophy causes predominantly distal muscle weakness. Also note other features of this condition, including frontal balding, myopathic facies, cataracts, cardiac conduction abnormalities, gonadal atrophy, glucose intolerance and mental retardation.

Answer to Question 13

B

It is important to exclude acute spinal cord compression with an MRI scan of the spine with this history and examination findings.

Answer to Question 14

A

The patient is likely to have Guillain–Barré syndrome. Forced vital capacity, and not peak respiratory flow rate, is useful in monitoring respiratory function. The patient is also at risk of arrhythmia because of autonomic instability, hence cardiac monitoring is also required.

Answer to Question 15

B

The patient is likely to have Guillain–Barré syndrome. Intravenous immunoglobulin or plasmapheresis is the treatment of choice. Supportive measures such as intubation and ventilation may be needed as well.

Answer to Question 16

C

Fasciculations are virtually never the sole presenting feature of motor neuron disease. The long history and lack of physical signs make benign fasciculations the most likely cause in a young person.

Answer to Question 17

D

The pattern of weakness described is characteristic of inclusion body myositis.

Answer to Question 18

A and D

Internuclear ophthalmoplegia results from lesions in the medial longitudinal fasciculus, which connects the third cranial nerve nucleus on one side to the sixth cranial nerve nucleus on the contralateral side. A lesion in the right medial longitudinal fasciculus produces weakness of the right medial rectus and therefore diminished or slow adduction of the right eye, as well as a jerky nystagmus in the abducting left eye when the patient attempts to look to the left. It is commonly seen in multiple sclerosis.

Answer to Question 19

C and F

The bladder and bowel can be affected in Guillain–Barré syndrome, but early involvement would be more suggestive of a conus lesion. Reflexes are depressed early in the illness.

Answer to Question 20

D

Amyotrophic lateral sclerosis is characterised by a combination of upper and lower motor neuron signs as described in this scenario.

Answer to Question 21

E

The diagnosis of transient ischaemic attack (TIA) should only be made if there is a clear history of focal neurological deficit. 'Positive' symptoms, such as chewing movements, would not be expected in TIA or any of the other diagnoses listed.

Answer to Question 22

D

The obvious concern is that this woman has meningitis or encephalitis as a cause of her status epilepticus. Intravenous lorazepam is an appropriate first-line antiepileptic agent in this circumstance. Intravenous phenytoin is a second-line drug, but not at a rate of 150 mg/min; the maximum rate of infusion should be 50 mg/min.

Answer to Question 23

E

Patients who feel that their sleep does not refresh them ('non-restorative' sleep) are likely to have obstructive sleep apnoea, a central sleep disorder (brainstem lesions or degenerative brain conditions) or a mixed pattern (sometimes seen in myotonic dystrophy).

Answer to Question 24

D

St John's wort is proven to be effective in mild to moderate depression, but it induces the cytochrome P450 3A4 enzyme system and the P-glycoprotein transporter and thereby reduces the plasma levels of drugs metabolised via these pathways. These include HIV protease inhibitors, HIV non-nucleoside reverse transcriptase inhibitors, the immunosuppressants ciclosporin and tacrolimus, and amitriptyline.

Answer to Question 25

B

In optic neuritis the optic disc may be swollen and uncommonly the peripheral retinal veins are sheathed, but retinal haemorrhages are not a feature.

Answer to Question 26

B

Idiopathic Parkinson's disease is almost always asymmetrical at onset. The posture becomes more stooped and the steps shorter, but falls are not prominent in the early stages of the disease.

Answer to Question 27

E

The development of hallucinations and confusion is a common and difficult clinical problem in patients who have long-standing Parkinson's disease. It may be drug-related or due to an underlying Parkinson's disease-associated dementia. Cabergoline is a dopamine agonist with a side-effect profile similar to levodopa, but it is less well tolerated and hence should be the first drug to reduce in this scenario.

Answer to Question 28

C

The presentation is typical of frontotemporal dementia. Patients with Alzheimer's disease tend to present much less dramatically with forgetfulness for recent events and a tendency to repeat conversations; normal-pressure hydrocephalus should be suspected if there is disturbance of gait or urinary incontinence at an early stage; and dementia with Lewy bodies should be considered in cases with fluctuating symptoms, visual hallucinations and extrapyramidal signs.

Answer to Question 29

C and I

Marche à petit pas is a feature of Parkinson's disease. Dizziness on turning over in bed suggests a vestibular problem.

Answer to Question 30

C

This presentation would be absolutely typical of Alzheimer's disease where forgetfulness is a common early feature, as is the patient's belief that there is nothing wrong. Gait disturbance (apraxia) and urinary incontinence would suggest normal-pressure hydrocephalus; stepwise progression of symptoms would be typical of vascular dementia.

Answer to Question 31

C

The presentation, particularly visual hallucinations, is typical of dementia with Lewy bodies. Patients with Alzheimer's disease tend to present with forgetfulness for recent events and a tendency to repeat conversations, but early motor impairment would be unusual. Visual hallucinations would be less usual for the other diagnoses.

Answer to Question 32

E

The history of an intention tremor that is improved by alcohol in a patient with a family history of tremor is typical of benign essential tremor. In Parkinson's disease the tremor is most marked at rest. Tremor can be a feature of Wilson's disease, but this is a rare condition and a family history would not be expected. Huntington's disease presents with choreiform movements.

Answer to Question 33

D

Parkinson's disease is almost always asymmetrical at onset. A tremor that is worse while drinking tea is an intention tremor; the glabellar tap is not a useful sign; and orofacial dyskinesias are features most likely due to neuroleptics in this case.

Answer to Question 34

D

The sciatic nerves supply all the muscles below the knee and the knee flexors, and they also provide sensory innervation of the lateral border of the lower leg and entire foot, except the medial malleolus, which is supplied by the saphenous nerve. The femoral nerve is responsible for the knee jerk.

Answer to Question 35

D and H

The history suggests a gradually developing pathological process and the signs indicate that this must be in the spinal cord rather than the brain. Motor neuron disease is excluded by the sensory findings.

Answer to Question 36

B

The family history suggests an autosomal dominant disease with anticipation, meaning that the condition presents earlier and more severely in succeeding generations. Huntington's is the only one of the diagnoses listed that is plausible.

Answer to Question 37

A

Levodopa is a precursor for dopamine synthesis. It is given in conjunction with a peripheral DOPA decarboxylase inhibitor to prevent its metabolism in the gut wall and to enhance oral bioavailability.

Answer to Question 38

E

The $5HT_3$ receptor is a ligand-gated ion channel; all other 5HT receptors are G protein-coupled seven-transmembrane-domain receptors.

Answer to Question 39

D

Noradrenaline is an important central nervous system neurotransmitter, but not adrenaline.

Answer to Question 40

E

Gabapentin was synthesised to mimic the structure of GABA,

but it is not believed to act on GABA receptors: it is thought to exert its therapeutic effect by binding to voltage-dependent calcium channels in the central nervous system.

Answer to Question 41

D

Monoamine oxidase inhibitors prevent the breakdown of monoamine neurotransmitters, including dopamine, 5-hydroxytryptamine and noradrenaline. But the basis of the 'cheese effect' is that dietary tyramine is normally metabolised by MAO in the bowel wall and liver, and when this is blocked by an MAOI, tyramine is absorbed systemically and provokes noradrenaline release from sympathetic nerve terminals.

OPHTHALMOLOGY

Author:

JD Firth

Based upon and containing material from the first edition of
Medical Masterclass by P Frith and H Towler

Editor:

JD Firth

Editor-in-Chief:

JD Firth

1.1 Clinical scenarios

1.1.1 Examination of the eye

Examination of the eye by the non-specialist requires the following assessments:

- visual acuity;
- visual fields;
- pupil responses;
- ocular media and fundus using the ophthalmoscope;
- ocular movements.

Testing of acuity, fields, pupil responses and ocular movements may be required during examination of the cranial nerves in Station 3 of PACES or as part of examination of the eye in Station 5: the necessary techniques are described in *Clinical Skills for PACES*. Ophthalmoscopy will be required only in Station 5. The following short notes emphasise important aspects about use of the ophthalmoscope and pharmacological methods of dilating the pupil.

How to use the direct ophthalmoscope

The direct ophthalmoscope provides an image that is magnified and upright but of a very limited area, so that the retina has to be 'scanned' to provide the observer with a composite view. It also lacks depth perception, and examination of the peripheral retina is restricted. Its advantages are its ease of use, relatively simple construction and

maintenance, and ability to examine the retina through an undilated pupil. When using the direct ophthalmoscope, remember the following.

- First, check that the batteries and bulb are satisfactory.

- It is always preferable to examine the eye through dilated pupils, although this may not always be possible (see below). Select the larger aperture if the pupil is dilated, the smaller if not.

- Stand about 1 m from the patient and rotate the lens dial to provide the sharpest image. You should remove spectacles if normally worn by you or the patient, unless either of you has a high error of focus.

- Shine the ophthalmoscope light at the patient's pupils and look for the normal red reflex from the retina (the same as the 'red eye' from flash photography). Any opacity within the media of the eye such as a cataract (Fig. 1) or vitreous haemorrhage (Fig. 2) will darken the red reflex. A subluxed lens may be evident, especially if the pupil is dilated (Fig. 3).

- Examine each eye in turn, using your right hand and eye for the patient's right eye and vice versa (if you can do so). Try to remain as upright as possible because this enables the patient to look beyond you and maintain fixation on a distant object. It is also important to approach from a slightly temporal direction, which means

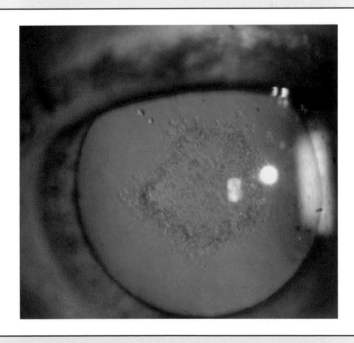

▲ **Fig. 1** Early cataract seen against the red reflex. The granular appearance in the centre of the pupil is typical of a posterior subcapsular cataract due to use of systemic corticosteroids.

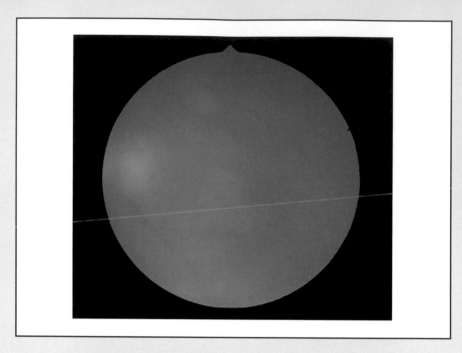

▲ **Fig. 2** Vitreous haemorrhage: the optic disc can just be seen through a diffuse vitreous haze caused by red cells. With a dense haemorrhage the red reflex may be entirely obscured.

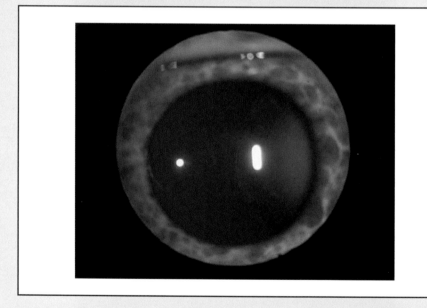

▲ **Fig. 3** A horizontally subluxed lens, which can be seen following blunt trauma, or in Marfan's syndrome (where the lens normally subluxes upwards) or homocystinuria (where it normally moves downwards).

that the optic disc is easily identified and sharp focus on it is possible. If you approach the eye straight on, the pupil will constrict and the rather featureless retina at the macula may be difficult to identify.

- Once the optic disc is identified it should be systematically assessed for colour, swelling, cupping, haemorrhage, venous pulsation (often present, so try to count the pulse), neovascularisation and pigmentation (Figs 4 and 5).

- Next follow the four main vascular arcades peripherally (temporal and nasal, above and below) assessing vessel calibre and regularity, and arteriovenous (AV) crossing changes for AV nipping, while also looking for neovascularisation or vascular occlusion. Cotton-wool spots are most frequently seen between vascular branches along the major arcades or close to the optic disc (Fig. 6).

- Next, examine the macula looking for the normal bright light reflex from the fovea, while also assessing any pigmentary change (Fig. 7), haemorrhage or hard exudates. Subtle macular changes may not be readily seen with the direct ophthalmoscope.

- Finally, examine the more peripheral retina in all quadrants by asking the patient to look up and down, and right and left.

Use the green filter ('red-free') on the ophthalmoscope to give better contrast, especially when examining for diabetic retinopathy or vascular changes: it will allow fine red structures to be more clearly defined.

Dilatation of pupils

Indications for dilatation of the pupils

Examination of the fundus of the eye is complete only if the pupil is dilated. It is possible to examine the optic disc through an undilated pupil, particularly if the room is dark, but the macula or more peripheral retina will not be seen adequately.

Contraindications to pupil dilatation for fundoscopy

- Patients with acute head injury or those in a coma, in whom it is important to observe serial neurological signs that include pupil size and reactivity.
- Patients at risk of acute angle-closure glaucoma if an inappropriate dilating agent is used (see below).

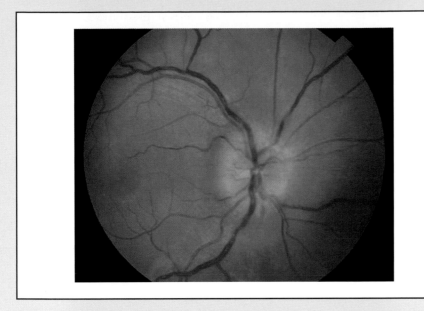

▲**Fig. 4** Optic disc swelling. If vision is normal, this may be papilloedema secondary to raised intracranial pressure; if vision is reduced, acute optic neuropathy is likely.

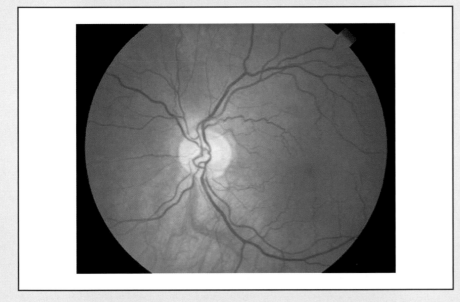

▲**Fig. 5** Optic disc atrophy. There are many causes, including previous neuritis or ischaemia, or optic nerve compression. Visual acuity will depend on the cause.

Before dilatation

Before dilating the pupils, assess and record the pupil reactions, including the relative afferent responses. Patients should be warned of the following.

- Near vision especially will be blurred for about 2 hours.
- Bright lights may be uncomfortable.
- Driving is not advisable.

- If they develop eye pain or discomfort, they should phone back immediately or attend an eye Emergency Department.

Choice of dilating agent

The various dilating agents that can be used are shown in Table 1. For diagnostic purposes, tropicamide drops are ideal: 1% for adults and 0.5% for children. Tropicamide blocks the parasympathetic

terminals in the pupillary constrictor muscle. A brown iris dilates more slowly than a blue one, and its dilatation is more prolonged; in very dark eyes, cyclopentolate 1% drops can be used but the patient should be warned to expect a more sustained blurring of vision. Phenylephrine 2.5% drops stimulate the sympathetic system and act synergistically with tropicamide to enable maximum pupil dilatation. However, phenylephrine should be used with caution in both children and adults with ischaemic heart disease because it may induce hypertension, exacerbate angina or cause arrhythmias as a result of its sympathomimetic action when absorbed.

The procedure

One or two drops are placed in the lower conjunctival fornix of each eye and 15–20 minutes allowed for the pupils to dilate. Tropicamide drops sting: if the child is reluctant to allow drops to be put directly into the eyes, lie the child down, place a drop at the inner corner of each closed eye and wait. The child will always open the eye and so the drop rolls in with minimum fuss.

Complications

Dilatation of the pupil can precipitate acute glaucoma in susceptible eyes, but this is rare, occurring in less than 1 in 1,000 patients and less frequently with tropicamide than cyclopentolate. The onset of acute glaucoma is during the recovery phase of pupil dilatation, usually several hours after the drops have been instilled. Eyes at risk are typically long-sighted (hypermetropic), with spectacle lenses that are convex and magnifying. These eyes have shallow anterior chambers and are predisposed to obstruction of the drainage angle between the iris and cornea when the pupil is mid-dilated.

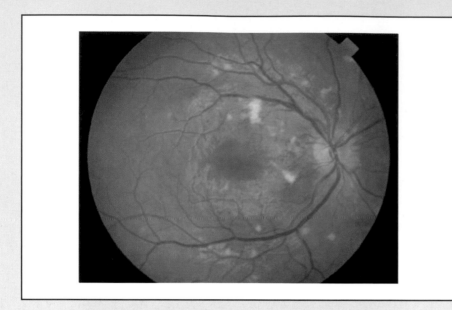

▲ **Fig. 6** Cotton-wool spots: retinal microinfarcts, scattered between branches of major retinal vessels.

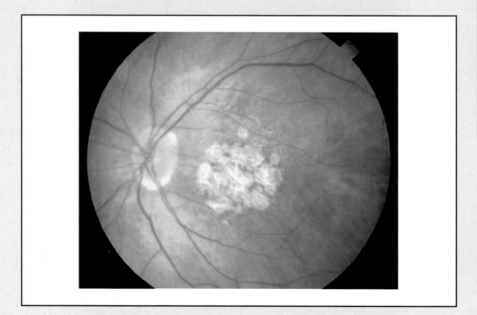

▲ **Fig. 7** Atrophy at the fovea in age-related macular degeneration. Pigmentation may also be found.

TABLE 1 DILATING DROPS			
Agent	Mode of action	Duration (hours)	When to use
Tropicamide 1%	Parasympathetic block	2–4	Adult
Tropicamide 0.5%	Parasympathetic block	2–4	Child
Cyclopentolate 1%	Parasympathetic block	6–8	Very dark iris
Phenylephrine 2.5%	Sympathomimetic	2–4	Full examination of peripheral retina, or photography
Phenylephrine 10%	Sympathomimetic	2–4	Very dark iris

Shallowing of the anterior chamber can also occur as a result of the progressive enlargement of the lens with age, particularly if there are any coexisting cataracts. Short-sighted (myopic) eyes are not predisposed to acute glaucoma. Patients with known common chronic glaucoma may be safely dilated.

1.2 Acute scenarios

1.2.1 An acutely painful red eye

> **Scenario**
>
> A 25-year-old man presents with a red eye that has become increasingly painful over the past 3 days. The eye aches badly, bright light makes the pain worse and his vision has become slightly blurred.

Introduction

There are many causes of a red eye (Table 2): most can be immediately discounted in this case as the association of redness with pain suggests that this is not merely an episode of conjunctivitis. The following are most likely.

- Iritis: inflammation of the front chamber of the eye, also known as anterior uveitis.

- A corneal lesion, such as an ulcer.

These are difficult to distinguish, except by slit-lamp examination, and both may give rise to photophobia and blurring of vision.

> Iritis is a prime cause of a painful red eye, especially if photophobia is also present.

⚠ Danger signals in the patient with a red eye are pain and visual blurring. These are *not* features of a benign condition: the patient requires urgent ophthalmological assessment, including slit-lamp examination.

History of the presenting problem

Significant signs to look for include the following.

- Change in vision: a distinct impairment of vision, as in this case, suggests a serious problem and must never be ignored (see Table 2).

- Discharge: a purulent discharge suggests bacterial conjunctivitis.

- Characteristics of pain: patients with conjunctivitis may complain of grittiness, but they do not have pain. Photophobia is common in corneal diseases and with intraocular inflammation. Pain made worse by reading, which requires accommodation, suggests iritis. Severe pain suggests scleritis (see Section 1.2.2).

Other relevant history

Ask specifically about the following.

- Previous similar episodes.

- Features to suggest a systemic disease: note particularly the presence of erythema nodosum, dysuria or urethral discharge, oral or genital ulceration, joint or back pain, shortness of breath or diarrhoea, and any signs of abnormality in immune status (AIDS) or intravenous drug use. See Sections 2.1 and 2.2 for further discussion of causes of iritis and scleritis.

- Soft contact lens wear: there is a risk of acute bacterial infections of the cornea, particularly if lenses are worn overnight.

Examination

Check the eye for the following.

- Where is it red? In conjunctivitis or diffuse scleritis the redness may involve the whole of the visible portion of the eye. Redness localised around the corneal limbus is suggestive of intraocular inflammation, and sectoral redness is commonly seen in conjunctival haemorrhage, nodular scleritis and episcleritis (see Section 1.2.2). The conjunctiva may show prominent follicles in chlamydial and viral conjunctivitis.

- Is it sticky? This would suggest conjunctivitis.

- Visual acuity: measure with the glasses normally worn and through a pinhole. Acuity worse than 6/9 may indicate serious ocular pathology.

- Size and shape of the pupil: in cases of iritis this may be irregular due to the formation of adhesions. In acute glaucoma it is characteristically mid-dilated and unreactive. A relative afferent pupillary defect always indicates serious retinal or optic nerve disease.

Specialist assessment will involve the following.

- Fluorescein staining: to reveal a corneal ulcer.

- Slit-lamp examination: to look for keratitic precipitates (see Section 2.1 and Fig. 8), although larger precipitates on the corneal surface can sometimes be seen with a direct ophthalmoscope.

- Measurement of intraocular pressure: it is mandatory to exclude secondary glaucoma in those with inflammatory disorders of the eye.

In the absence of systemic symptoms, general examination of the patient is unlikely to give valuable clues.

🔑 In assessing the patient with a red eye, always check the contralateral eye carefully. A systemic cause is more likely if there is simultaneous bilateral inflammation.

TABLE 2 DIFFERENTIAL DIAGNOSIS OF A RED EYE

	Disease	Discriminating clinical features
Common	Bacterial conjunctivitis	Sticky eye, normal vision
	Viral conjunctivitis	Less sticky eye, preauricular lymphadenopathy, upper respiratory tract infection, discomfort
	Chlamydial conjunctivitis	Conjunctival follicles, recurrent stickiness
	Allergic conjunctivitis	Itchy; sometimes with an atopic history
	Episcleritis	Discomfort, sectoral and self-limiting
	Iritis	Pain, photophobia, visual blurring, irregular pupil, keratitic precipitates
Unusual	Scleritis	Pain (may be worse at night), systemic associations (see Section 1.2.2)
	Corneal abscess	Soft contact-lens wear or trauma, white corneal infiltrate, pain, blurred vision
Rare	Endophthalmitis	Trauma or eye surgery, intravenous drug use, poor vision
	Acute glaucoma	Hazy cornea, mid-dilated unreactive pupil, hard eye

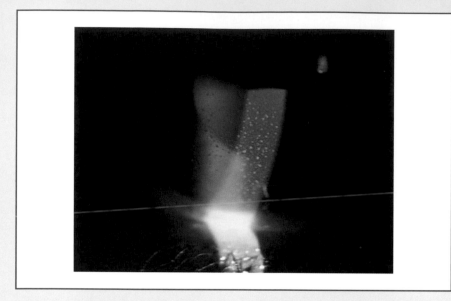

▲ **Fig. 8** Slit-lamp view shows multiple white keratitic precipitates characteristic of iritis. These are deposited in the front chamber from the aqueous, as a sediment onto the inner surface of the cornea.

Introduction

> The adult who presents with red eyes and severe ocular pain has scleritis until proved otherwise. This is much less common than iritis, but should prompt a search for an active underlying systemic vasculitis, especially rheumatoid arthritis or Wegener's granulomatosis.

Scleritis is an uncommon, capricious and sight-threatening condition, especially compared with the related but milder condition of episcleritis, which is usually self-limiting.

The degree of pain associated with scleritis is variable, but some characteristics are particular pointers to this diagnosis:

- pain interrupting sleep, which may even lead to pacing about or banging the head against a wall;

- pain worse on eye movement (but see also Section 2.5);

- pain that is so unbearable that the patient asks for the eye to be removed.

Other relevant history

This woman has constitutional, upper respiratory and joint symptoms, but you should take a full functional enquiry from anyone who may have scleritis, paying particular attention to the following.

- General symptoms: anorexia, malaise, fever and weight loss.

- Musculoskeletal: joint pain and muscle pain.

- Upper respiratory problems: especially sinusitis, epistaxis and deafness.

- Respiratory problems: breathlessness, stridor, haemoptysis and chest pain.

Investigation

In most patients with a unilateral red eye the diagnosis can be made on clinical grounds and confirmed by targeted investigation (see Table 2). Conjunctival infection can be confirmed by culture if a chlamydial or viral cause is suspected. A first uncomplicated attack of unilateral acute iritis does not require investigation. For iritis associated with systemic symptoms, initial investigations should be as follows.

- CXR, biochemistry (particularly serum calcium and angiotensin-converting enzyme level) or biopsy of involved tissue may suggest sarcoidosis.

- C-reactive protein may be raised in any active systemic inflammatory process.

- Look for human leucocyte antigen (HLA)-B27 positivity if ankylosing spondylitis is possible.

Management

Viral conjunctivitis is most commonly due to RNA viruses and is self-limiting. Herpes simplex corneal disease is treated with topical aciclovir. Acute iritis is treated with topical steroids and mydriatics, and the patient should be told that iritis can recur. This is much more likely if the patient is HLA-B27 positive, when there is a 50% chance of a further attack.

1.2.2 Two painful red eyes and a systemic disorder

Scenario

A 60-year-old woman has felt unwell for several weeks, with malaise, anorexia and joint swelling. For the first time in her life she has had sinus congestion, with some bleeding when blowing her nose and a feeling of her ears being blocked up. In the past week both her eyes have become very bloodshot and last night the pain around her eyes became severe enough to stop her from sleeping properly, which is the reason for her attending the Emergency Department today.

Patients presenting with a vasculitis will typically give a history of many months of ill-health.

Examination

The eye is red, although the pattern varies and often redness of the sclera is patchy (Fig. 9); there may also be swelling or thinning (Fig. 10).

Full-thickness loss of sclera, called scleromalacia perforans and usually associated with rheumatoid arthritis, is uncommon but sight-threatening (see Section 2.2).

Episcleritis causes a similar pattern of redness, but with much lesser intensity of symptoms and signs.

General examination of the patient will clearly be directed by the history, but should particularly focus on the nose (discharge/bleeding and septal perforation), ears (deafness), upper respiratory tract (stridor), lungs (any abnormal signs) and joints (in particular for signs suggestive of rheumatoid arthritis).

Investigation

General investigations are directed towards finding evidence of an autoimmune or vasculitic systemic disorder.

- Urine: dipstick and microscopy for proteinuria, haematuria and red cell casts.

- FBC, electrolytes, and renal and liver function tests: look in particular for anaemia of chronic disorders, neutrophilia and impaired renal function.

- Inflammatory markers: C-reactive protein.

- Serological tests for autoimmune or vasculitic conditions: in particular rheumatoid factor and antineutrophil cytoplasmic antibody.

- CXR.

Specialist assessment will involve ultrasonography of the eye coat, which should be done by an expert because both getting a reliable image and interpreting the results need care and experience; in scleritis the affected sclera is thickened.

Management

If scleritis is confirmed, treatment for the eye, as for systemic features, should be with systemic immunosuppression, usually initially wih corticosteroids in an oral dose of prednisolone 1 mg/kg per day. Threatened perforation may require a pulsed intravenous steroid regimen and other cytotoxics.

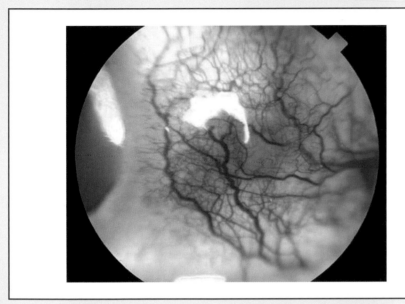

▲**Fig. 9** Anterior nodular scleritis before treatment. The episcleral vessels are markedly dilated and the underlying sclera swollen. There is scleral translucency with the underlying darker choroid visible in the centre of the nodule.

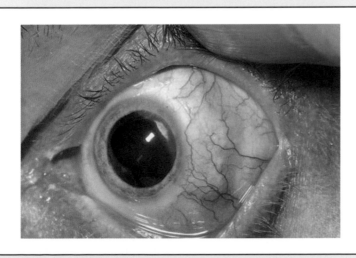

▲**Fig. 10** Healed anterior scleritis. After treatment with prednisolone and ciclosporin, the sclera has returned to normal thickness but is more translucent, allowing the darker choroid to show through.

1.2.3 Acute painless loss of vision in one eye

Scenario

A 60-year-old bricklayer reports that earlier this evening, as he was watching the television, he suddenly noticed 'something wrong with his vision'. He says that he 'found he could see nothing'.

Introduction

🔑 Abrupt painless loss of vision in one eye may be caused by a retinal arterial or venous occlusive event.

History of the presenting problem

Patients with acute loss of vision need to be talked through the event to unearth those exact details that will provide a diagnosis, and which can easily become garbled in the telling. Ask about the following points if the information does not emerge spontaneously.

- Has his vision recovered completely? Is it back to normal?

- Was the loss in one eye or both? Did he check each eye separately at the time or is there some doubt about this?

- Was the blindness complete (total loss of vision) or was it partial?

- If partial, which area was affected most?

- How long did the episode last? Was it for seconds, minutes or hours?

Beyond this, look for features to confirm one of the following diagnoses.

Arterial occlusion

If the loss of sight was complete, even if only in part of the field of vision and in one eye only (with vision in the other eye entirely normal), then this is likely to be an arterial event in the retina, either amaurosis fugax or a completed stroke. Retinal transient ischaemic attacks (TIAs), like others, are usually brief (<30 minutes) and are by definition strictly uniocular. They almost always imply an embolic event, most commonly from the ipsilateral carotid bifurcation. In contrast, the patient with a postchiasmal TIA affecting vision will rarely report the episode. Transient disturbances of vision with vague characteristics do not allow a definite diagnosis, although they may be regarded as possible TIAs.

Retinal vein occlusion

Occlusion of the retinal vein will present with an acute onset, often coming on overnight. However, the onset is not as abrupt as with an arterial event, nor is the loss of vision transient. Loss of vision, although pronounced, is less complete than with an arterial occlusion.

Other causes of acute painless loss of vision

The following must be considered.

- Vitreous haemorrhage: in which the patient may describe an acute onset of floaters.

- Acute optic neuropathy (see Section 1.2.5).

- Giant-cell arteritis: the visual loss may not be painful, but headaches and/or other systemic features are associated (see Section 1.2.5).

- Migraine equivalent: a possible homonymous loss, a geometric pattern, persistence with the eyes closed and scintillation all suggest a migraine equivalent even if a headache was not a feature.

Other relevant history

Cerebral TIAs, vascular events elsewhere in the body and vascular risk factors should be explored. Has the patient got multiple sclerosis or had any previous neurological episodes that might support this diagnosis?

Examination

Arterial occlusion

With a retinal TIA there may be no eye signs, although emboli should be sought after dilating the pupil with 1% tropicamide.

With a completed retinal stroke, in the acute event the fundus looks pale with narrowed arterioles and a 'cherry red spot' usually appears at the fovea as the underlying choroidal circulation shows through (Fig. 11). Emboli may be visible at the disc within the main retinal artery or at retinal arteriolar bifurcations (see Section 2.3). Later (within days) the fundus may look normal; optic atrophy supervenes within weeks as the nerve fibres die back. At all stages there will be a relative afferent pupillary defect.

🔑 Examination for a relative afferent pupillary defect is crucial in cases of acute visual loss. Move a bright light from one eye to the other, watching each direct pupil response: asymmetry suggests a defect on the side of the pupil that tends to dilate.

Retinal vein occlusion

The retinal appearance is of flame and blot haemorrhages in a global pattern if the central vein is blocked (Fig. 12), or wedge-shaped if a branch vein is occluded (Fig. 13).

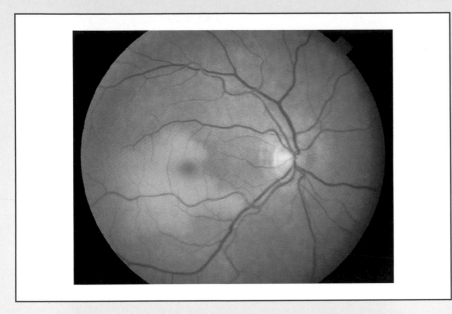

▲**Fig. 11** Retinal artery occlusion: the right eye shows inferotemporal branch retinal artery occlusion with a cherry red spot and surrounding retinal oedema and pallor. Visual loss is profound and may be total.

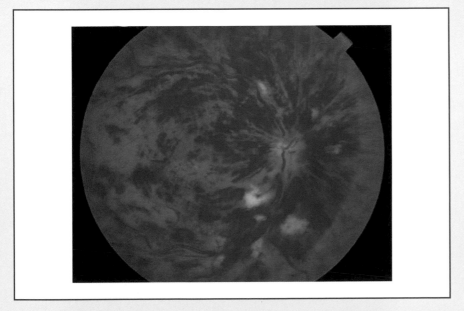

▲**Fig. 12** Central retinal vein occlusion with characteristic 'bloodstorm' appearance and cotton-wool spots.

Other causes of acute painless loss of vision

Consider retinal detachment, in which a uniocular visual field defect may be present corresponding to the site of the lesion, and vitreous haemorrhage, in which the red reflex may be obscured (see Fig. 2).

General examination

Has the patient got atheromatous vascular disease? Check for a bruit at the ipsilateral carotid bifurcation, listening with the diaphragm below the angle of the jaw and asking the patient to hold his breath; check also for vascular bruits elsewhere and for absent peripheral pulses.

Are there any abnormal cardiovascular findings? Is the patient in atrial fibrillation? What is the BP? Are there any murmurs? Are the temporal arteries thickened, tender or pulseless? (See Section 1.2.5.)

Investigation

In all cases check FBC, renal and liver function, inflammatory markers (erythrocyte sedimentation rate/C-reactive protein), blood sugar and lipids. Also check the ECG for myocardial ischaemia or even an occult myocardial infarction.

Carotid imaging is warranted if surgery is to be considered. Patients with bilateral episodes require particularly careful assessment, including an echocardiogram to look for a cardiac source of embolism.

Management

All patients need attention to cardiovascular risk factors such as smoking, diabetes, hyperlipidaemia and hypertension. Carotid endarterectomy should be considered for stenosis of 70% or more; otherwise daily aspirin is beneficial, if tolerated.

If this patient has a completed retinal arterial occlusion with permanent loss of vision in one eye, he may have difficulty laying bricks accurately for a week or so until he adjusts to judging depth monocularly. He is entitled to drive once he has adjusted to monocularity, because the good eye (if normal) provides the acuity and visual field that are legally necessary.

> Internal carotid stenosis of greater than 70% may warrant endarterectomy as well as control of other vascular risk factors. Otherwise consider aspirin.

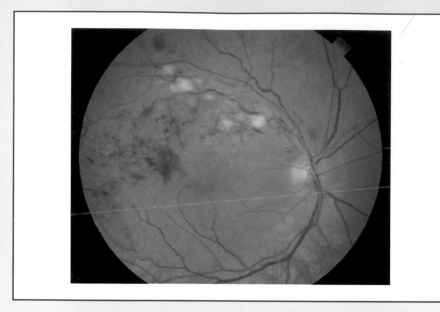

▲**Fig. 13** Branch retinal vein occlusion in a sector above the fovea. Vision may be affected, depending on changes at the fovea itself, such as haemorrhage or oedema.

1.2.4 Acute painful loss of vision in a young woman

Scenario

A 25-year-old woman reports that the vision in one of her eyes has become blurred over the past 3 days, so that now she can see very little. The eye has been aching. She is otherwise well, but consulted a neurologist a few years ago for 'peculiar sensations', although no precise diagnosis was given.

Introduction

In a patient of this age, with this particular pattern of visual loss and the vague neurological history, this is very likely to be an attack of demyelinating optic neuritis.

History of the presenting problem

There are some key features that might pin down the diagnosis of demyelinating optic neuritis.

- How much of the visual field is affected? In optic neuritis the loss of vision particularly affects the central field, blurring the whole face at a conversational distance, and is larger than that found with retinal (foveal) oedema.

- The pain in optic neuritis may be worse on eye movement, with an unpleasant 'pulling' feeling.

- Spontaneous improvement: one hallmark of optic neuritis is a tendency for visual acuity to get better over the following weeks.

Other optic nerve lesions are less common and usually painless.

Other relevant history

The neurological history is important and full details should be sought: what can the patient remember, what tests were performed and what do the neurologist's notes and letters reveal? It may be that a diagnosis of multiple sclerosis (MS) was considered likely but the patient was not informed at the time of a suspected first event.

Examination

Look for the signs of an optic nerve lesion, expecting to find some or all of the following.

- Reduced visual acuity to a variable degree, although total loss of vision is rare.

- Central scotoma: this is partial to colour or total, and is best mapped with a small coloured target (the conventional red hat-pin in PACES, although any small coloured object will do in routine practice).

- Impaired colour appreciation: compared with the normal eye, colours look 'washed out'.

- Imbalance of the symmetry of pupil response to an alternating bright light: a relative afferent pupillary defect is present.

- Swollen optic nerve head in the acute stage (see Fig. 4), unless the inflammation is 'retrobulbar' in which case its appearance is normal. Optic atrophy follows months later (see Fig. 5).

If features of an optic nerve lesion are not found, and even if the retina appears normal, there is still a possibility of foveal oedema as a cause of central scotoma, in which case a fluorescein angiogram may be helpful.

It would be appropriate to perform a general neurological examination, in particular looking for signs of a cerebellar or spinal cord lesion. These would support the diagnosis of MS in this context.

Investigation and management

Has the patient got MS? Referral back to the neurologist may be appropriate, as may tests such as brain MRI, electrophysiological testing (eg visual-evoked potentials) and lumbar puncture.

Intravenous methylprednisolone is given for severe cases of acute optic neuritis, but mild cases are best treated symptomatically with analgesia if required (see Section 2.5). The eventual level of recovery of visual acuity is difficult to predict and hence a guarded prognosis must be given.

1.2.5 Acute loss of vision in an elderly man

Scenario

A 75-year-old man reports that he suddenly noticed loss of vision in one eye. Recently, he has felt unwell, has lost weight, finds it difficult to get out of bed in the morning and has begun to have headaches.

Introduction

> Consider giant-cell arteritis in any elderly patient with an acute loss of vision that may be caused by acute optic nerve ischaemia.

> ⚠ Cranial arteritis is a medical emergency: visual loss in the affected eye is irreversible and the second eye is at immediate risk.

An elderly patient with acute and painful visual loss has giant-cell arteritis (synonymous with 'temporal' or 'cranial' arteritis) until proved otherwise. Although there may be diagnostic clinical features, many cases hinge on a high index of suspicion in the face of conflicting clinical evidence. In general, the older the patient, the less likely a non-arteritic event. Diagnosis can be confirmed by temporal artery biopsy. Loss of vision, when it occurs in giant-cell arteritis, is pronounced and irretrievable, and the second eye is at immediate risk.

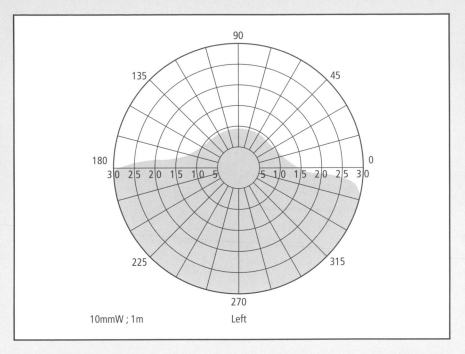

▲**Fig. 14** Inferior altitudinal field defect in giant-cell arteritis with ischaemic optic neuropathy. The field of the right eye was normal. Uniocular altitudinal defects are secondary to an anterior lesion, in either the retina or the optic nerve.

History of the presenting problem

This man has many obvious clues to the diagnosis of giant-cell arteritis, but ask any patient of middle age or older presenting with acute loss of vision about the following.

- Headaches: tend to be lateralised.

- Scalp tenderness: usually noted when brushing the hair.

- Jaw pain: may be the result of claudication.

- Symptoms of polymyalgia rheumatica, including muscular pain (particularly of shoulder girdle), stiffness, general malaise, weight loss and fever.

Examination

If there is established ischaemia of the optic nerve head, there will be signs of an optic nerve lesion (see Section 1.2.4) with the following.

- Vision may be totally lost, without even perception of light.

- The visual field may show a partial pattern of loss, which is often altitudinal, ie affecting the upper or lower part (Fig. 14).

- A relative afferent pupillary defect.

- A pale swollen optic disc visible on ophthalmoscopy (Fig. 15).

Examine the patient specifically for tenderness of the cranial arteries – not only temporal, but also occasionally facial or occipital – with swelling and/or loss of pulsation: these findings are characteristic of, but not necessary for, the diagnosis.

Investigation

> If you suspect cranial arteritis, check erythrocyte sedimentation rate and C-reactive protein (CRP) urgently.

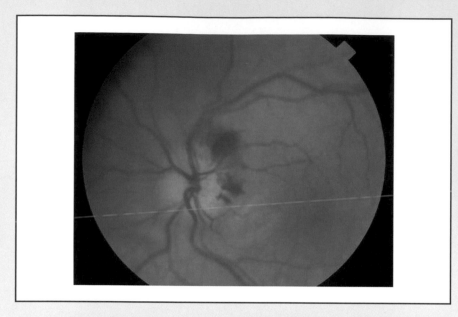

▲**Fig. 15** Optic disc in the acute stage of giant-cell arteritis. The infarcted optic nerve head is pale and swollen with blurred and haemorrhagic margins. Visual loss is usually irreversible.

The pre-steroid CRP is especially important: a normal result virtually excludes the diagnosis of giant-cell arteritis. Although a temporal artery biopsy may be negative, finding a positive result is so important for future strategy that a biopsy should be performed whenever feasible.

Management

🔑 If giant-cell arteritis is a possiblity, give corticosteroids immediately rather than withhold them.

Visual loss in cranial arteritis can progress rapidly, and once present is irretrievable. The second eye could also become affected, and hence steroids should be started immediately on suspicion of the diagnosis. Arterial biopsy can be done within the following 24 hours and then a further decision made about strategy. If both eyes are affected, there is even greater urgency in beginning treatment.

The corticosteroid dose should be tailored to the circumstances.

- If vision is little affected, an initial oral dose of prednisolone 1 mg/kg per day is adequate.

- If both eyes are affected, some clinicians advocate intravenous administration of methylprednisolone, although there is no conclusive evidence of the superiority of this over oral prednisolone.

2.1 Iritis

Aetiology

Most cases of iritis are of unknown aetiology. Some recognised causes are shown in Table 3.

Clinical presentation

The patient has a red aching eye with photophobia, which tends to worsen over hours to a few days. Vision may be blurred, but acuity is not severely affected. The pupil tends to be small and may be irregular because the iris has adhered to the anterior lens, in which case it festoons on dilatation. There may be symptoms or signs to suggest an underlying cause (Table 3), but this would be unusual. Diagnosis is made by slit-lamp examination, which is essential whenever iritis is suspected.

Features of iritis on slit-lamp examination

- 'Flare': leak of protein from inflamed vessels into the anterior chamber makes the fluid in the aqueous look hazy.
- Keratitic precipitates: inflammatory cells in the anterior chamber sometimes deposit on the inner surface of the cornea, forming keratitic precipitates (see Fig. 8). Large precipitates are characteristic of granulomatous iritis such as that caused by sarcoid.

- Hypopyon: if the iritis is severe then inflammatory cells may sediment at the bottom of the anterior chamber, which is characteristic of Behçet's disease or endophthalmitis.

In the absence of systemic symptoms, general examination of the patient is unlikely to give valuable clues.

Investigation

A first uncomplicated attack of unilateral acute iritis does not require investigation. However, investigation should obviously be guided by any clues to an underlying cause (Table 3) in the history. Appropriate investigations might include the following.

- CXR: look in particular for evidence of sarcoidosis.

- Serum C-reactive protein: suggests a systemic inflammatory process if raised.

- Urine dipstick (for haematuria and proteinuria, quantitating proteinuria, if present, by urinary albumin to creatinine ratio) and renal function: for evidence of TINU.

- FBC and liver and bone chemistries: serum calcium may be raised in sarcoidosis.

- Serum angiotensin-converting enzyme: may be raised in sarcoidosis.

- Serology for syphilis in selected cases.

TABLE 3 **CAUSES OF IRITIS**	
Autoimmune	**Drug induced**
Ankylosing spondylitis	Rifabutin
Sarcoidosis	Cidofovir
Behçet's syndrome	
Inflammatory bowel disease	
Juvenile chronic arthritis	
Psoriasis	
Reiter's syndrome	
TINU (Tubulointerstitial nephritis and uveitis)	
Infectious	
Herpes zoster	
Herpes simplex	
Leptospirosis (uncommon)	
Lyme disease	
Syphilis	
Tuberculosis	
Leprosy	

Note
There is a clear association of iritis with human leucocyte antigen (HLA)-B27 positivity. The most likely causes of acute iritis with systemic associations are HLA-B27/spondylitis/sacroiliitis and sarcoidosis.

- Test for HLA-B27 positivity: this does not influence immediate management, but those with HLA-B27 are much more liable to recurrent attacks. 'Birdshot choroidopathy' is a very rare disease in which there is reduced vision as a result of inflammation within the vitreous rather than the aqueous, and this is uniquely correlated with HLA-A29.

Treatment

Iritis responds promptly to topical treatment with steroids and pupil dilators in the vast majority of cases: drops are preferable by day and ointment by night. A typical regimen would include dexamethasone 0.1% every 2 hours for the first 48 hours, then four times daily together with cyclopentolate 1% three times daily until review a week later. The latter prevents the formation of adhesions between iris and lens while the inflammation is active, but will also blur vision, especially for reading.

Prognosis

Iritis settles without sequel provided that treatment is not delayed. Vision is expected to return to normal.

Repeated attacks are more likely if iritis is associated with a persistent systemic disease or if the patient is HLA-B27 positive, when the risk of recurrent iritis is 50%, some 15 times greater than if HLA-B27 negative.

FURTHER READING

Respiratory Medicine, Section 2.8.2 (sarcoidosis) and *Rheumatology and Clinical Immunology*, Section 2.3.4 (spondyloarthropathies and other arthritides).

Nishimoto JY. Iritis: how to recognize and manage a potentially sight-threatening disease. *Postgrad. Med.* 1996; 99: 255–7, 261–2.

2.2 Scleritis

Aetiology

Scleritis is an inflammatory disease of the vessels supplying the sclera that may be associated with rheumatoid arthritis, systemic vasculitis (especially Wegener's granulomatosis) or other autoimmune rheumatic diseases (in about 50% of cases). (See *Rheumatology and Clinical Immunology*, Sections 2.3.3 and 2.5.2.)

Clinical presentation

Scleritis may be anterior or posterior, and anterior scleritis may be nodular, diffuse or necrotising. Posterior scleritis may be associated with anterior disease, but can also occur in isolation unassociated with systemic disease.

Pain is the most common symptom of scleritis, and is typically severe, worse at night and on eye movement, and wakes the patient from sleep. Redness, photophobia and lacrimation are other common symptoms of anterior scleritis, but severe necrotising scleritis in patients with vasculitis associated with polyarticular rheumatoid arthritis may occur without preceding pain or redness. Uncommonly, posterior scleritis may present with ocular pain, reduced visual acuity, proptosis and limitation of extraocular movements, but with a white eye.

When a patient presents with pain in the eye, remember the following.

- Severe eye pain that is worse at night is highly suggestive of scleritis.
- Severe necrotising scleritis associated with rheumatoid arthritis is usually painless.

Physical signs

The sclera is usually red and thickened, with dilatation of episcleral vessels (see Fig. 9). The redness may be localised, as in nodular scleritis, or diffuse. The brick-red colour is best seen in daylight.

In very severe scleritis, the sclera may appear white because it is necrotic as a result of vascular occlusion. This is an important sign that can easily be overlooked and is an indication for urgent treatment with systemic steroids.

Scleral thinning and increased scleral transparency show through the underlying bluish choroid, either after scleritis has healed (see Fig. 10) or in acutely necrotising scleritis (Fig. 16).

General examination of the patient will clearly be directed by the particular history, but should focus especially on the nose (discharge/bleeding and septal perforation), ears (deafness), upper respiratory tract (stridor), lungs (any abnormal signs) and joints (in particular for signs suggestive of rheumatoid arthritis).

Investigation

Any associated systemic disease should be identified by the following.

- Urine dipstick: for haematuria and proteinuria (quantitating proteinuria, if present, by urinary albumin to creatinine ratio) and renal function.

- FBC.

- Inflammatory markers: erythrocyte sedimentation rate and C-reactive protein.

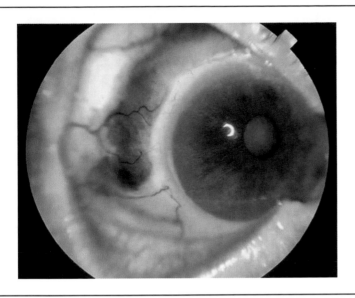

▲ **Fig. 16** Necrotising scleritis in rheumatoid arthritis (scleromalacia perforans) with full-thickness scleral loss. Only thin conjunctiva and episclera cover the choroid.

necessary and the steroid dose cannot be reduced to acceptable maintenance levels; agents used include azathioprine, ciclosporin and methotrexate.

Complications

Frequent complications include keratitis, uveitis, cataract, glaucoma and exudative retinal detachment in posterior scleritis. Rarely, the globe actually perforates.

Prognosis

Of patients with scleritis, 25% lose two or more lines of vision over 3 years, usually as a result of cataract or corneal involvement. Less than 5% of eyes lose useful vision in the longer term.

- Serology for autoimmune rheumatic or vasculitic disorders: rheumatoid factor, antineutrophil cytoplasmic antibody, antinuclear antibody and anti-DNA antibodies.

Ocular ultrasonography is essential for diagnosing posterior scleritis, showing thickening of the posterior eye coat, which may also be evident on CT or MRI of the eye and orbit. Scleral biopsy may be required in the rare event that lymphoma or infection is suspected.

Differential diagnosis

Episcleritis is a mild, non-sight-threatening disease that resolves spontaneously over 6–8 weeks. In contrast to scleritis, pain is not a feature and the redness will usually blanch with phenylephrine drops. Iritis (anterior uveitis) is less painful and the redness is more marked around the cornea. Slit-lamp examination will distinguish these conditions. Rarely, lymphoma may present with scleral inflammation.

Treatment

Severe or necrotising scleritis requires immediate treatment.

NSAIDs, especially flurbiprofen, may be effective for milder cases, but systemic steroids are frequently required to control the disease and immunosuppressive therapy is essential immediately for severe or necrotising disease.

- Flurbiprofen 100 mg three times daily will produce symptomatic improvement within 48 hours if effective.

- For necrotising or severe disease give oral prednisolone 1 mg/kg per day initially, or intravenous pulse methylprednisolone 500–1000 mg. Unresponsive disease may require additional immunosuppressive therapy with cyclophosphamide.

- Steroid-sparing treatment may be required if long-term therapy is

FURTHER READING

Pakrou N, Selva D and Leibovitch I. Wegener's granulomatosis: ophthalmic manifestations and management. *Semin. Arthritis Rheum.* 2006; 35: 284–92.

- - - - - - - - - - - - - - - -

Wirbelauer C. Management of the red eye for the primary care physician. *Am. J. Med.* 2006; 119: 302–6.

2.3 Retinal artery occlusion

Aetiology

Retinal arterial occlusion is caused by acute obstruction of the central retinal artery or its branches as a result of embolism or, less commonly, thrombosis. It occurs most commonly in the fifth or sixth decade. Associated conditions include carotid vascular disease, diabetes, hypertension, valvular heart disease, arrhythmias (especially atrial fibrillation with left atrial thrombus) and, less commonly and especially in younger patients, atrial myxoma, coagulopathies and haemoglobinopathies. Intravenous drug abuse is also an associated factor.

Clinical presentation

Patients present with sudden painless loss of vision. The visual loss may be transient (amaurosis fugax) or sustained, depending on whether arterial blood flow is re-established. Central artery occlusion results in total visual loss and branch occlusion in altitudinal (upper or lower) field loss.

Uncommonly, visual loss may primarily affect the peripheral field with preservation of central vision if the macula is supplied by a cilioretinal artery arising from the short posterior ciliary vessels, a pattern that occurs in 25–30% of the population. Rarely, the converse situation of cilioretinal artery occlusion with sparing of the central retinal artery can occur. Retinal artery occlusion may occasionally result from giant-cell arteritis.

Physical signs

• Visual acuity is usually profoundly reduced, such as to hand movements, or there may even be no perception of light.

• A relative afferent pupillary defect is present.

• Retinal pallor may be sectoral or generalised, the retinal arteries are attenuated, and a 'cherry red spot' may be seen at the macula as a result of the underlying choroidal circulation visible through the fovea (see Fig. 11). Sometimes

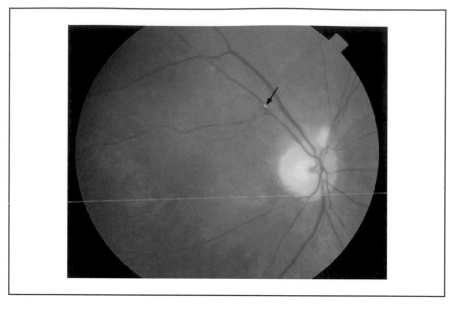

▲ **Fig. 17** Branch retinal artery embolus (Hollenhorst's plaque): a well-defined refractile opacity is seen in the superotemporal branch artery at the first bifurcation (arrow). There is also a cotton-wool spot at the edge of the optic disc at 1 o'clock.

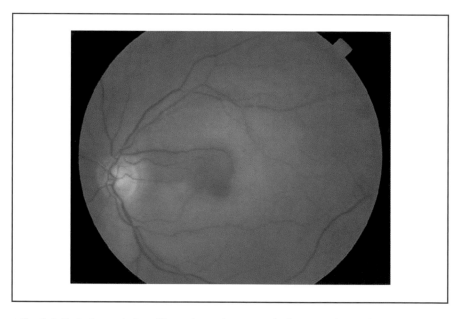

▲ **Fig. 18** Retinal artery occlusion with macular sparing as a result of a patent cilioretinal artery. The central macula/fovea is perfused, but there is surrounding retinal pallor with oedema that causes a 'cherry red patch' rather than a 'cherry red spot'. The visual acuity in this eye recovered to 6/9, but with a permanently restricted peripheral field.

an embolus may be visible within the arterial lumen, a Hollenhorst plaque (Fig. 17), and/or 'cattle-trucking' of the blood column in the arteries may be seen. There are sometimes also appearances indicating patency (Fig. 18)

or occlusion (Fig. 19) of a cilioretinal artery.

A complete cardiovascular examination of the patient is required, looking in particular for arrhythmia (especially atrial

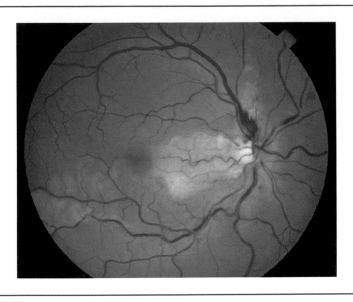

▲**Fig. 19** Cilioretinal artery occlusion. This right eye shows retinal oedema between the optic disc and macula, the opposite of Fig. 18. Visual acuity is poor and there is a large central scotoma that will persist.

fibrillation), hypertension, carotid bruit(s) and cardiac murmurs.

Investigation

- FBC, glucose and renal/liver/bone profile.

- Inflammatory markers: erythrocyte sedimentation rate and C-reactive protein.

- Other tests, eg haemoglobin electrophoresis and coagulation studies, especially in younger patients with no other identifiable risk factors and as directed by clinical suspicion.

- ECG and CXR: look for arrhythmia or evidence of hypertension or valvular heart disease.

- Carotid Doppler studies and echocardiography: important in identifying a remediable source of emboli that may also threaten the brain (see *Cardiology*, Section 3.10 and *Neurology*, Section 3.6).

- Fluorescein angiography: may be of value in atypical situations (Fig. 20).

Differential diagnosis

The clinical features of retinal artery occlusion are difficult to confuse with other causes of acute unilateral visual loss such as retinal vein occlusion, retinal detachment or acute ischaemic optic neuropathy.

Treatment

⚠ Any treatment undertaken more than an hour after the onset of retinal artery occlusion is unlikely to improve visual recovery and it should be emphasised to patients that any visual improvement is a bonus.

No treatment has been shown to be effective in restoring vision and randomised controlled studies are lacking. Most treatments attempt to improve ocular perfusion either by lowering intraocular pressure or by vasodilatation.

Emergency interventions

- Ocular massage: may dislodge an embolus if performed in the very early stages, and is easy to do.

- Paracentesis of the anterior chamber: the removal of aqueous humour with an insulin syringe (after instilling povidone–iodine solution) can dramatically reduce intraocular pressure.

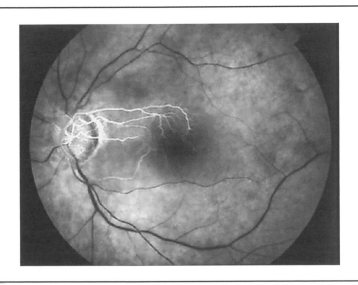

▲**Fig. 20** Fluorescein angiogram corresponding to Fig. 18. Fluorescein dye, which appears white, fills the central cilioretinal circulation in contrast to the non-perfused retinal arteries and veins, which appear black.

Longer-term treatments

- Address any identifiable risk factors: smoking, hypertension, coagulopathy or hyperlipidaemia.

- Anticoagulate: for embolic thrombus from the heart.

- Carotid stenosis: patients shown to have carotid occlusion of >70% should be considered for carotid endarterectomy; consider aspirin therapy for lesser degrees of narrowing.

Complications

Long-term ocular complications after retinal artery occlusion are uncommon, and much fewer than after retinal vein occlusion. Iris neovascularisation may occur, leading to neovascular glaucoma, but retinal neovascularisation is rare. The risk of a similar event in the second eye is very small, unless there is bilateral carotid disease or a cardiac source for emboli.

Prognosis

Of affected eyes, 30% recover visual acuity of 6/60 or better, although 5% have no light perception in the affected eye. Retinal artery occlusion is associated with serious life-threatening conditions that determine the overall mortality.

FURTHER READING

Sharma S and Brown GC. Retinal arterial obstruction. In: Schachat AP, ed. *Retina (Vol. 2 Medical Retina)*, 4th edn. Philadelphia: Elsevier Mosby, 2006: Section 68.

2.4 Retinal vein occlusion

Aetiology

Retinal vein occlusion occurs when the central retinal vein [central retinal vein occlusion (CRVO)] or its branches [branch retinal vein occlusion (BRVO)] become obstructed as a result of thrombosis within the lumen, often preceded by changes within the vessel wall. Hypertension, diabetes, hyperlipidaemia, hyperviscosity syndromes, hypercoagulability and raised intraocular pressure all predispose to this condition. Occlusion usually occurs at the optic disc itself within the central vein, or at an arteriovenous crossing of a branch vein.

Epidemiology

Retinal vein occlusion is the second most common retinal vascular disease after diabetic retinopathy.

Clinical presentation

Presenting symptoms result either from the onset of the occlusion or from the development of complications. Vein occlusions are usually unilateral and, if bilateral, rarely simultaneous.

The commonest presentation is with sudden onset of painless loss of vision. BRVO causes visual loss when the macula is involved, but if the macula is spared the occlusion may be an incidental finding. Painless loss of vision may also arise (uncommonly) from vitreous haemorrhage as a complication of ischaemic CRVO, and in rare instances a red painful eye may result from the late complication of neovascular (rubeotic) glaucoma.

Physical signs

In CRVO, there are widespread flame and blot retinal haemorrhages (see Fig. 12), often with cotton-wool spots (microinfarcts) throughout the retina, in contrast to the sectoral distribution in BRVO (see Fig. 13). A relative afferent pupillary defect is indicative of significant retinal ischaemia, as are numerous cotton-wool spots. BRVO will produce a corresponding visual field defect, but not a relative afferent pupillary defect because much of the retina remains perfused and healthy.

In a few cases the red reflex will be obscured if vitreous haemorrhage is significant (see Fig. 2). Rarely in neovascular glaucoma the cornea is hazy, the conjunctiva red and the eye rock hard.

Patients with retinal vein occlusion are generally those at high risk of atheromatous vascular disease and hence cardiovascular examination is appropriate, looking in particular for hypertension, vascular bruit(s) and peripheral pulses.

Investigation

Should be directed at establishing the aetiology of the venous occlusion: the younger the patient, the greater the chance of finding a cause.

- FBC and coagulation studies.

- Inflammatory markers: erythrocyte sedimentation rate and C-reactive protein.

- Blood glucose, electrolytes, renal/liver/bone profile and lipids.

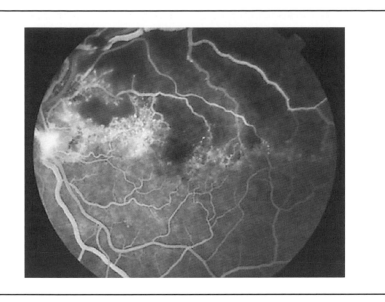

▲ **Fig. 21** Fluorescein angiography in superior BRVO showing darker areas where there is loss of capillary circulation and profound retinal ischaemia.

- Serum immunoglobulins/protein electrophoresis, urinary Bence Jones proteins and (if indicated) plasma viscosity.

Specific ophthalmological investigations include the following.

- Ocular pressure estimation.

- Fluorescein angiography: this may be helpful in cases where there is diagnostic uncertainty but is mainly used to demonstrate the site of occlusion, the degree of retinal ischaemia and determine the risk of complications (Fig. 21).

Differential diagnosis

Characteristic CRVO and BRVO are readily distinguished from most other causes of retinal haemorrhage. Bilateral CRVO is rare and may be mimicked by severe non-proliferative diabetic retinopathy. Waldenström's macroglobulinaemia may produce retinal changes similar to bilateral CRVO. Accelerated hypertensive retinopathy should not be forgotten (see *Cardiology*, Section 2.17.1).

> If you see retinal haemorrhages, always check the BP.

Treatment

> Emergency treatments for retinal vein occlusion, such as haemodilution and anticoagulation, are of no reliable benefit.

In the short term, identifiable risk factors should be treated to reduce the risk of systemic complications and retinal vein occlusion in the other eye. In the long term, laser photocoagulation may be beneficial for macular oedema in some cases of BRVO, but not in CRVO. Panretinal photocoagulation should be performed in ischaemic eyes at risk of neovascularisation.

Complications

Permanent visual impairment from macular damage is more common in CRVO than in BRVO. Uncommonly, retinal and iris neovascularisation may occur secondary to significant retinal ischaemia, leading to vitreous haemorrhage and/or rubeotic glaucoma.

Prognosis

One-quarter of eyes with BRVO recover visual acuity of 6/9 or better without treatment, a sufficient standard for driving. The risk of a similar event in the fellow eye is appreciable but not high.

FURTHER READING

Branch Vein Occlusion Study Group. Argon laser scatter photocoagulation for prevention of neovascularization and vitreous hemorrhage in branch vein occlusion: a randomized clinical trial. *Arch. Ophthalmol.* 1986; 104: 34–41.

Laatikainen L, Kohner EM, Khoury D and Blach RK. Panretinal photocoagulation in central retinal vein occlusion: a randomised controlled clinical study. *Br. J. Ophthalmol.* 1977; 61: 741–53.

Weinstein R and Mahmood M. Case records of Massachusetts General Hospital: weekly clinicopathological exercises. Case 6–2002: a 54-year-old woman with left, then right, central-retinal-vein occlusion. *N. Engl. J. Med.* 2002; 346: 603–10.

2.5 Optic neuritis

Aetiology

Optic neuritis may present in isolation, but ultimately more than 50% of patients who have it will develop clinical evidence of multiple sclerosis (MS) (see *Neurology*, Section 2.5).

Clinical presentation

There is moderate-to-severe loss of central vision of rapid onset, often associated with pain on eye movement. Visual loss may increase during the first week and then slowly recover, although improvement in acuity may be incomplete. Vision may be worse when the patient's body temperature is increased after a bath or exertion (Uhthoff's phenomenon).

Rarely, optic neuritis may be bilateral and associated with a transverse myelitis causing paraparesis or paraplegia (Devic's disease). Occasionally a more chronic onset is suggestive of local inflammatory disease, such as sinusitis or Wegener's granulomatosis associated with posterior scleritis.

Physical signs

Reduced visual acuity, reduced colour perception, central or cecocentral scotoma, relative afferent pupillary defect and a swollen optic disc may be expected (see Fig. 4). Uncommonly, the peripheral retinal veins are sheathed.

If there is clinical suspicion that the patient may have MS, then neurological examination is clearly appropriate, looking in particular for evidence of cerebellar or spinal cord disease.

Investigation

Investigation is usually not necessary at first presentation in a previously healthy patient (unless steroid treatment is planned) because the prognosis for visual recovery is good. MRI may show evidence of demyelination and visual-evoked potentials may show delay and/or reduction in amplitude (see *Neurology*, Section 3.3.2).

Differential diagnosis

- Consider acute anterior ischaemic optic neuropathy in older patients, when the visual field defect is usually altitudinal.

- If bilateral, consider Leber's optic neuropathy, found predominantly in young men, or nutritional or toxic optic neuropathy such as that caused by alcohol, tobacco, ethambutol, quinine or vitamin B_{12} deficiency. In children, consider a postviral phenomenon.

Treatment

If the visual loss or pain is severe, intravenous methylprednisolone should be administered (1 g/day for 3 days) because it will ensure visual function recovers more rapidly and the pain is controlled. Oral steroids should not be used because they are associated with an increased risk of new episodes of optic neuritis, as found by the Optic Neuritis Study Group. Longer term, there is no proven visual benefit from the use of corticosteroids.

Prognosis

Visual recovery after a first episode is normally good or complete; recurrent episodes may be associated with progressive visual impairment that can be profound. Steroid treatment only hastens recovery during acute episodes and does not improve the ultimate visual outcome. The risk of a similar event in the second eye is appreciable but low. The development of MS is associated with increased mortality.

FURTHER READING

Balcer LJ. Clinical practice: optic neuritis. *N. Engl. J. Med.* 2006; 354: 1273–80.

- - - - - - - - - - - - - - - - - - -

Hickman SJ, Dalton CM, Miller DH and Plant GT. Management of acute optic neuritis. *Lancet* 2002; 360: 1953–62.

2.6 Ischaemic optic neuropathy in giant-cell arteritis

Aetiology

Giant-cell arteritis (GCA) is an inflammatory disorder of unknown aetiology affecting small to medium-sized arteries of the head and neck. It is characterised by disruption of the internal elastic lamina, with an inflammatory cell infiltrate of giant cells, lymphocytes and plasma cells (see *Rheumatology and Clinical Immunology*, Section 2.5.1). Visual loss is most commonly caused by involvement of the posterior ciliary arteries, resulting in acute anterior ischaemic optic neuropathy (AION) and in rare cases central retinal artery occlusion.

It is extremely rare in people younger than 60 years, and is twice as common in women. It was first described by Sir Jonathan Hutchinson in 1890, some 2 years after the description of polymyalgia rheumatica by William Bruce, the two syndromes constituting the opposite extremes of a single clinical disorder.

Clinical presentation

Systemic symptoms include scalp tenderness and headache, pain on chewing (jaw claudication), proximal muscle weakness or stiffness, and general malaise.

Visual loss, usually unilateral and severe, occurs in about 5–10% of cases. Altitudinal field loss may be seen (see Fig. 14). Uncommonly, amaurosis fugax may precede more profound central visual loss, and diplopia occurs in about 10% of patients before visual loss. Rarely, occipital blindness may occur as a result of involvement of the vertebrobasilar circulation.

Physical signs

Visual acuity is severely reduced, often to hand movements or light perception, and there is a relative afferent pupillary defect. The optic disc is pale and swollen, and there are often haemorrhages at the disc margin (see Fig. 15).

The temporal arteries may be tender and pulseless, although clinically normal arteries may be pathologically involved. Uncommonly, eye movements may be impaired as a result of involvement of cranial nerves III and VI.

Investigation

- Inflammatory markers: erythrocyte sedimentation rate (ESR) and C-reactive protein (CRP). A normal ESR does not reliably exclude GCA, although a normal CRP effectively does (there is only one documented case report with normal CRP before corticosteroids).

- Temporal artery biopsy or biopsy of another clinically involved artery such as facial or occipital: this should be performed within 48 hours of starting steroids whenever possible to avoid compromising the histology. A positive biopsy is absolute confirmation of the diagnosis, which may prove important in longer-term strategy.

- FBC may show a normochromic/normocytic anaemia.

- A normal CRP (before steroids) effectively excludes GCA.
- A positive biopsy is absolute confirmation of the diagnosis.

Differential diagnosis

The major differential diagnosis is between non-arteritic AION and retinal artery occlusion. It is important to establish the diagnosis because steroid therapy is necessary for GCA, but is inappropriate or even hazardous for non-arteritic AION associated with hypertension or diabetes. In cases of doubt, steroids should be given pending the outcome of investigations.

Treatment

The primary aim of treatment in cases of GCA is to suppress the arteritis and minimise the risk of damage to the fellow eye or other organs.

Immediate

Urgent steroid treatment should be initiated immediately after blood has been taken for ESR and CRP. Oral prednisolone 1 mg/kg per day is appropriate, there being no evidence that intravenous steroids are more effective as long as the initial treatment is supervised.

Short term

The steroid dose is tapered according to the response of clinical features, such as headache, and a fall in ESR and CRP. This can usually be achieved by 10-mg decrements per week to 30 mg, then by 5-mg decrements to 10 mg, followed by a much more cautious reduction in 1-mg steps.

Longer term

The median duration of steroid therapy for GCA is 2 years, so it is important to begin prophylaxis against osteoporosis. It is unusual for GCA to recur after successful treatment, unless the steroids have been withdrawn too quickly. Because the risk of long-term complications is greater from the treatment than from the disease, it is more appropriate for follow-up of patients with GCA to be undertaken by a physician rather than an ophthalmologist. Steroid-induced cataracts may occur in the fellow eye.

Prognosis

Visual recovery is uncommon in the presenting eye, and a few patients lose vision in the second eye even when treatment has been initiated.

FURTHER READING

Hayreh SS. Steroid therapy for visual loss in patients with giant-cell arteritis. *Lancet* 2000; 355: 1572–3.

Hayreh SS, Zimmerman B and Kardon RH. Visual improvement with corticosteroid therapy in giant cell arteritis: report of a large study and review of literature. *Acta Ophthalmol. Scand.* 2002; 80: 355–67.

Liozon E, Herrmann F, Kim L, *et al.* Risk factors for visual loss in giant cell (temporal) arteritis: a prospective study of 174 patients. *Am. J. Med.* 2001; 111: 211–17.

Salvarani C, Cantini F, Boiardi L and Hunder GG. Polymyalgia rheumatica and giant-cell arteritis. *N. Engl. J. Med.* 2002; 347: 261–71.

2.7 Diabetic retinopathy

Aetiology

Retinopathy takes time to develop and is extremely rare before puberty or at presentation in those with type 1 diabetes. However, about 80% of patients have detectable retinopathy after 10 years of type 1 diabetes. In contrast, in type 2 diabetes, where the onset is uncertain, retinopathy is established in up to 25% of patients at the time of diagnosis of the diabetes. Retinopathy is a consequence of chronic hyperglycaemia, and poor diabetic control is now established as contributing to the risk of developing significant retinal changes.

Clinical presentation

Diabetic retinopathy is asymptomatic until sight-threatening complications occur, by which time the disease is in an advanced state. When symptoms do arise, gradual blurring of vision is more common than acute loss, unless there is a vitreous haemorrhage or the patient suddenly becomes aware of the problem and panics. Sight-threatening yet asymptomatic retinopathy must therefore be detected by screening, and maculopathy in type 2 diabetes is the most common cause.

Diabetic retinopathy

- People with type 1 diabetes are more likely to develop proliferative disease than maculopathy; the reverse applies to those with type 2 diabetes.
- In type 2 diabetes, retinopathy may already be established when the diabetes is diagnosed.
- Prevention of retinopathy is far better for the patient than laser treatment when retinopathy is established.

Examination

It is essential to examine the fundus through dilated pupils using at least 1% tropicamide, best combined with 2.5% phenylephrine drops to enable proper assessment of the macula, ie the central area between the major retinal vessels, temporal to the optic disc. Diabetic retinopathy is classified into four types.

Background

Mild-to-moderate non-proliferative retinopathy is characterised by microaneurysms and haemorrhages, sometimes referred to as 'dots and blots' (Fig. 22). Leakage from these can result in retinal oedema and hard exudates, but this is asymptomatic unless the fovea at the centre of the macula is involved (maculopathy).

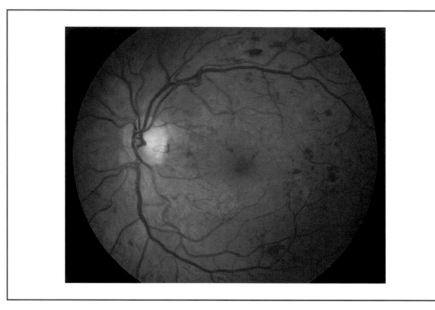

▲ **Fig. 22** Background diabetic retinopathy with dot and blot haemorrhages, although there is no hard exudate.

Maculopathy (exudative or ischaemic)

Clinically significant oedema, hard exudates (Fig. 23) or ischaemia may affect the macula, either alone or in combination. The critical area is within a disc diameter (1.5 mm) of the central fovea. Hard exudates are easily recognised, but retinal oedema and ischaemia are difficult to see by routine ophthalmoscopy

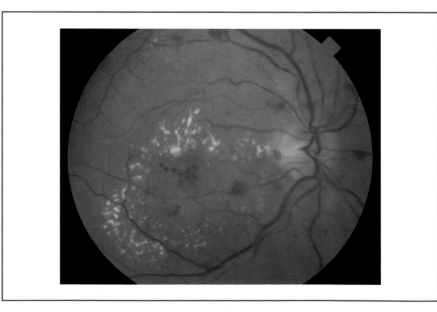

▲ **Fig. 23** Diabetic maculopathy with hard exudates in a circular or circinate pattern at the fovea. In this instance, vision will already be reduced as the fovea is involved.

and are more readily identified by fluorescein angiography. Maculopathy may coexist with preproliferative and proliferative retinopathy.

Preproliferative (ischaemic)

This stage of severe retinopathy, although asymptomatic, indicates retinal ischaemia. The signs include multiple cotton-wool spots, large haemorrhages (more than half a disc in diameter), venous dilatation and irregularity, venous beading (Fig. 24) or loops, and intraretinal microvascular abnormalities.

Proliferative

The hallmark of this stage of retinopathy is the growth of new vessels from the surface of the retina at the disc (Fig. 25) and/or elsewhere along the vascular arcades (Figs 26 and 27). Traction on new vessels may result in preretinal haemorrhage (Fig. 28) and vitreous haemorrhage (see Fig. 2), and contraction may lead to retinal detachment.

Patients with diabetic retinopathy clearly require assessment by clinical examination (and investigation) for other evidence of microvascular or macrovascular disease.

Differential diagnosis

People with diabetes are at increased risk of retinal vein occlusion, which can usually be distinguished from diabetic retinopathy by the greater extent of haemorrhage and asymmetry of findings. Occasionally, diabetic retinopathy may be asymmetrical in the presence of significant carotid stenosis, which appears to 'protect' the ipsilateral eye.

Investigation

Fluorescein angiography can be useful if clinical findings are unclear, or if focal treatment is to be accurately targeted. Ocular ultrasonography can be helpful in detecting whether the retina is detached or if it cannot be visualised because of vitreous haemorrhage or a cataract.

Treatment

Maculopathy is treated by laser coagulation, either focally or as a 'grid', the primary goal being maintenance of vision by sealing leaking areas close to the fovea. Proliferative retinopathy is treated by a more extensive scatter, or panretinal, laser (Fig. 29). Vitreous haemorrhage and advanced retinal fibrosis with detachment may require surgical treatment by vitrectomy and retinal microsurgery.

Patients must stop smoking, and assessment and optimisation of

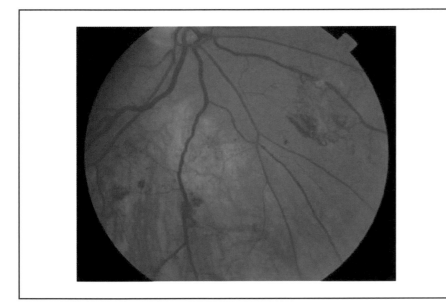

▲ **Fig. 24** Venous beading and proliferative diabetic retinopathy with a fan of new vessels at 2 o'clock.

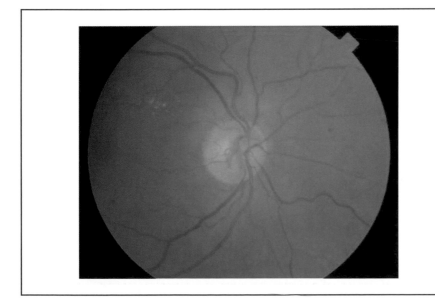

▲ **Fig. 25** New vessels on the optic disc.

183

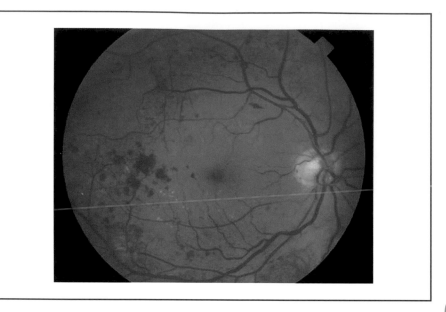

▲ **Fig. 26** New vessels inferotemporal to the macula. Large blot haemorrhages temporal to the fovea are indicative of retinal ischaemia in the watershed area.

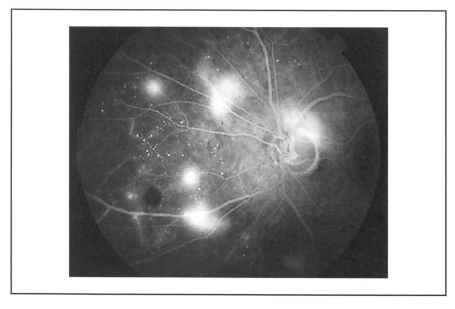

▲ **Fig. 27** Fluorescein angiography of proliferative retinopathy showing profuse focal leakage of fluorescein (white patches) from retinal new vessels.

diabetic and BP control are critically important.

Complications

Irreversible visual loss from untreatable or unresponsive maculopathy or proliferative disease is a common complication. Less frequent is neovascular (rubeotic) glaucoma caused by neovascularisation of the iris and obstruction to the drainage mechanism of the eye.

Prognosis

> Risk of loss of vision depends on the stage of diabetic retinopathy. The approximate percentage of eyes that will lose useful vision irretrievably within 5 years if not treated rises from 3% for those with background retinopathy, through 20% for those with exudative and 30% for those with preproliferative, up to 50% for those with proliferative retinopathy.

In the UK and USA, diabetic retinopathy is still the most common reason for registration as partially sighted or blind in the working age group. In addition to the visual morbidity of diabetic retinopathy, it is also associated with an increased morbidity and mortality from other diabetic complications, including hypertension, ischaemic heart disease, peripheral vascular disease, cerebrovascular disease, peripheral neuropathy and nephropathy.

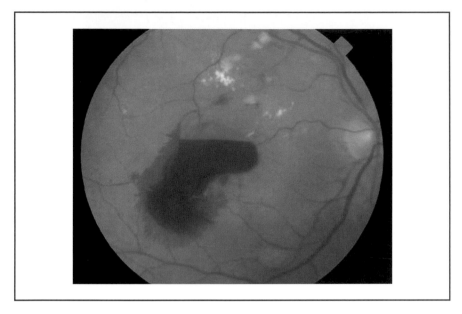

▲ **Fig. 28** Preretinal haemorrhage showing a horizontal fluid level as a result of bleeding from new vessels.

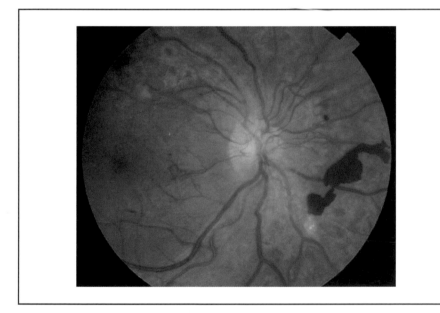

▲ **Fig. 29** Proliferative diabetic retinopathy with focal scars produced by panretinal photocoagulation. Persisting obvious new vessels can be seen on the optic disc.

Prevention

Primary

The most important means of preventing blindness from diabetic retinopathy in both type 1 and type 2 diabetes is good diabetic control, as proven by well-conducted clinical trials in the UK and USA. Other risk factors to be addressed include hypertension, hyperlipidaemia and smoking.

Secondary

The risk of visual loss from diabetic retinopathy can be reduced by undergoing regular eye examination by a trained observer such as an optometrist, physician or GP, or by retinal photography. If sight-threatening retinopathy is identified, treatment by laser photocoagulation will reduce the risk of blindness from maculopathy and proliferative disease by an estimated 60%. Patients with background retinopathy or no retinopathy at all should be examined once a year, those with preproliferative retinopathy more frequently (every 3–6 months).

FURTHER READING

Frank RN. Diabetic retinopathy. *N. Engl. J. Med.* 2004; 350: 48–58.

Towler HMA, Patterson JA and Lightman SL. *Diabetes and the Eye*, 2nd edn. London: BMJ Books, 1998.

Watkins PJ. Retinopathy. *BMJ* 2003; 326: 924–6.

3.1 Fluorescein angiography

Principle
The retinal circulation is normally impervious to fluorescein because of the blood–retinal barrier, similar to the blood–brain barrier. Transit through the retina and choroid can be recorded on film, digitally, by video or by direct observation. Indocyanine green angiography, a very similar technique, gives a better assessment of choroidal disease.

Indications
To enable assessment of the retinal circulation in a variety of diseases, in particular to determine the presence and degree of leakage (see Fig. 27) and ischaemia (see Fig. 21) within the retina.

Contraindications
Contraindications are previous allergy to fluorescein, recent myocardial infarction and pregnancy (relative).

Practical details

Before the procedure
Written informed consent should be obtained and the patient warned that skin and urine will be discoloured for 24 hours. Resuscitation facilities must be available. The pupils should be fully dilated.

The procedure
The dye (3 mL of 20% or 5 mL of 10% sodium fluorescein) is rapidly injected into an antecubital vein with the patient seated at the camera. Venous access must be secure because extravasation is painful. A series of photographs or continuous video is recorded over the initial minute and then periodically over the next 5–10 minutes as the dye enters the eye and is distributed throughout the circulation.

Complications
Complications are transient nausea or vomiting (occurs in 5% of patients), local extravasation and thrombophlebitis, anaphylaxis and circulatory shock. Mortality is less than 1 in 200,000.

3.2 Temporal artery biopsy

Indications
This is used to establish the diagnosis of giant-cell arteritis (cranial or temporal arteritis) in patients presenting with symptoms or signs suggestive of this condition.

Contraindications
There are no contraindications, except known extracranial–intracranial collateral circulation via the superficial temporal artery.

Practical details

1. Written informed consent should be obtained.

2. The procedure should be performed under aseptic conditions in a designated clean area or operating room. The required equipment includes fine-toothed skin forceps, sharp and blunt scissors, skin retractors (cats' paws), scalpel (a D15 scalpel is ideal), suture forceps, absorbable and non-absorbable sutures, and local anaesthetic (a dental syringe is ideal for administration).

3. Identify the frontal branch of the temporal artery where it runs across the forehead, and mark its course with an indelible pen for about 3 cm.

4. Infiltrate the skin with the local anaesthetic in two parallel lines adjacent to, but not directly over, the artery.

5. Remove any overlying hair, cleanse the skin with 5% povidone–iodine solution (or equivalent) and then drape with sterile towels or plastic adhesive drape.

6. Incise the skin with the scalpel along the skin mark.

7. Dissect the subcutaneous tissues to expose the artery for the length of the skin incision. Avoid injury and pathological artefact to the artery by minimising any direct handling.

8. Ligate the ends of the artery and any branches with 5/0 chromic catgut (or similar suture), then excise the artery specimen.

9. Close the skin in two layers and dress the wound.

10. Place the arterial specimen in fixative and send for histopathology.

11. External non-absorbable skin sutures can be removed at 5–6 days.

Complications

Haemorrhage can occur early or late in the procedure, and is the result of either inadequate ligation or secondary infection. The chance of the latter occurring is increased by concomitant steroid therapy. It has been known for a facial nerve to be biopsied in error.

4.1 Self-assessment questions

Question 1

Clinical scenario

A 25-year-old man presents with 6 weeks of malaise, weight loss and fever. He is anxious, with BP 160/100 mmHg. The findings on fundoscopy are shown in Fig. 30.

Question

What is the most likely cause of these appearances?

Answers

A Hypertensive retinopathy
B Cytomegalovirus infection
C Infective endocarditis
D Toxoplasmosis
E Cholesterol embolisation

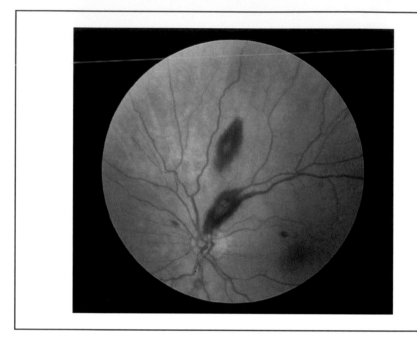

▲ **Fig. 30** Question 1.

Question 2

Clinical scenario

A 50-year-old man is found to have glycosuria. His (random) blood glucose is 13 mmol/L and a diagnosis of type 2 diabetes mellitus has been made. The findings on fundoscopy are shown in Fig. 31.

Question

What is the most likely cause of this appearance?

Answers

A Background diabetic retinopathy
B Proliferative diabetic retinopathy
C Accelerated (malignant) hypertension
D Mucormycosis
E Normal variant of no clinical significance

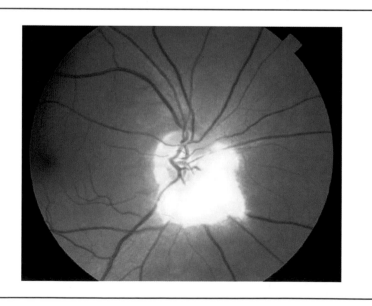

▲ **Fig. 31** Question 2.

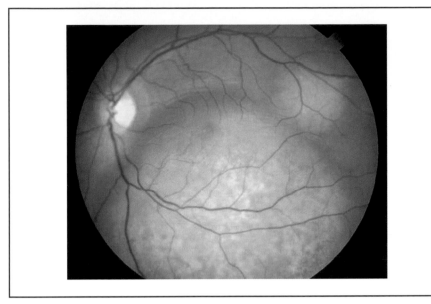

▲**Fig. 32** Question 3.

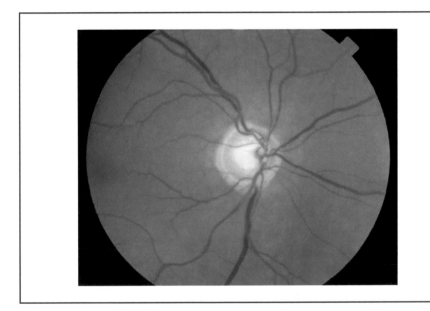

▲**Fig. 33** Question 4.

Question 4

Clinical scenario

A 68-year-old man with type 2 diabetes mellitus and hypertension presents because he is finding it increasingly difficult to read. The appearances on fundoscopy are shown in Fig. 33.

Question

What is the most likely cause of this appearance?

Answers

A Optic atrophy
B Chronic glaucoma
C Papilloedema
D Proliferative diabetic retinopathy
E Background diabetic retinopathy

Question 5

Clinical scenario

A 72-year-old woman with type 2 diabetes mellitus presents with headaches and loss of vision in her left eye. Her BP is 190/110 mmHg and the appearances of the left optic fundus are shown in Fig. 34.

Question

What is the most likely diagnosis?

Answers

A Accelerated (malignant) hypertension
B Papilloedema due to raised intracranial pressure
C Proliferative diabetic retinopathy
D Subarachnoid haemorrhage
E Giant-cell arteritis

Question 3

Clinical scenario

A 45-year-old woman with type 2 diabetes mellitus and a history of breast carcinoma is on long-term tamoxifen treatment. She complains of blurring of vision in her left eye, the fundoscopic appearance of which is shown in Fig. 32.

Question

What is the most likely cause of this appearance?

Answers

A Choroidal metastases
B Background diabetic retinopathy
C Proliferative diabetic retinopathy
D Diabetic maculopathy
E Tamoxifen retinopathy

Question 6

Clinical scenario

A 65-year-old man presents with a red and extremely painful eye. He gives a history of feeling generally under the weather for about 6 months, with generalised joint aches and pains along with 'blocked sinuses' for 6 weeks.

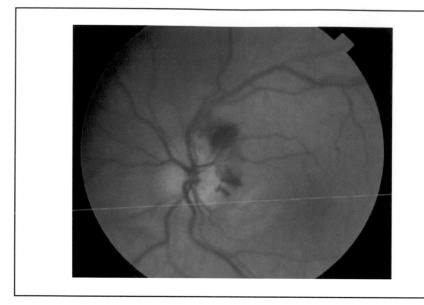

▲ **Fig. 34** Question 5.

Question

What is the most likely diagnosis?

Answers

A Iritis associated with sarcoidosis
B Iritis asociated with Behçet's syndrome
C Episcleritis associated with sinusitis
D Scleritis associated with rheumatoid arthritis
E Scleritis associated with Wegener's granulomatosis

Question 7

Clinical scenario

A 24-year-old woman presents with aching of her left eye and blurring of vision in that eye for 2 days. She is otherwise well. A diagnosis of probable demyelinating optic neuritis is made.

Question

What is the most appropriate treatment?

Answers

A No specific treatment
B Prednisolone 20 mg once daily, adjusted according to clinical response

C Prednisolone 60 mg once daily, adjusted according to clinical response
D Methylprednisolone 1 g iv once daily for 3 days, followed by oral steroids
E Methylprednisolone 1 g iv once daily for 3 days, followed by oral steroids along with cyclophosphamide (oral or iv)

Question 8

Clinical scenario

A 25-year-old man presents because his right eye has become red over the last 4 days. It aches, bright light makes the pain worse and his vision has become slightly blurred. He is otherwise well. A diagnosis of unilateral acute iritis is made.

Question

What is the most appropriate treatment?

Answers

A No specific treatment
B Dexamethasone eye drops
C Cyclopentolate eye drops

D Dexamethasone eye drops and cyclopentolate eye drops
E Prednisolone 40 mg po once daily

Question 9

Clinical scenario

A 38-year-old man has had type 1 diabetes for 20 years. He has neglected his medical care, rarely attending his GP's surgery and not responding to phone calls from the diabetic specialist nurse. He now presents because he has gone blind in one eye due to a vitreous haemorrhage. Examination of the other ('good') eye reveals proliferative diabetic retinopathy.

Question

If the 'good' eye is not treated, what are the chances that he will irreversibly lose vision in it over the next 5 years?

Answers

A 3–5%
B 10–15%
C 20–30%
D 40–60%
E 80–100%

Question 10

Clinical scenario

A 68-year-old woman presents with sudden painless loss of vision in her right eye 4 hours ago. A diagnosis of central retinal artery occlusion is made.

Question

What is the most appropriate treatment?

Answers

A No specific treatment
B Ocular massage
C Intravenous heparin
D Intravenous thrombolysis
E Aspirin 300 mg stat

4.2 Self-assessment answers

Answer to Question 1

C

There are two large dense retinal haemorrhages, each demonstrating a pale centre. These are Roth's spots, which are a classical feature of infective endocarditis. Similar haemorrhages can occasionally be seen in severe anaemia, thrombocytopenia and myeloproliferative disorders.

Answer to Question 2

E

There is a dense white opacity involving the disc margin from 2 to 8 o'clock, which also obscures the inferonasal retinal vessels. This is due to myelinated nerve fibres, which are a normal variant of no clinical significance.

Answer to Question 3

A

The fundus shows two well-defined, rounded and raised lesions typical of choroidal metastases from carcinoma of the breast. Choroidal metastases are more common than is clinically recognised because they often do not affect vision. Tamoxifen can cause fine crystalline deposits at the macula, but these are not present here.

Answer to Question 4

B

The peripheral rim of the optic disc is narrow and pale, and the central cup is wide: these are features ('cupping') of chronic glaucoma.

Answer to Question 5

E

The infarcted optic nerve head is pale and swollen with blurred and haemorrhagic margins in the acute stage of giant-cell arteritis. Papilloedema would not cause significant visual loss.

Answer to Question 6

E

Severe pain indicates that the diagnosis is scleritis and not iritis or episcleritis. Scleritis can occur in rheumatoid arthritis or Wegener's granulomatosis, but the other elements of the history are typical of Wegener's and not rheumatoid arthritis.

Answer to Question 7

A

If visual loss or pain is severe (which they are not in this case), intravenous methylprednisolone (1 g/day for 3 days) should be administered because this will enable visual function to recover more rapidly and the pain will be controlled. However, oral steroids are associated with an increased risk of new episodes of optic neuritis and should not be used.

Answer to Question 8

D

Most cases of iritis respond promptly to topical treatment with steroids (eg dexamethasone 0.1% every 2 hours for the first 48 hours) and pupil dilators (eg cyclopentolate 1% three times daily). The latter prevents the formation of adhesions between iris and lens while the inflammation is active, but will also blur vision.

Answer to Question 9

D

The approximate percentage of diabetic eyes that will lose useful vision irretrievably within 5 years if not treated depends on the stage of retinopathy: background, 3%; maculopathy (exudative or ischaemic), 20%; preproliferative, 30%; proliferative, 50%.

Answer to Question 10

A

No treatment has been shown to be effective in restoring vision. In the very early stages, emergency ocular massage is easy to perform and may succeed in dislodging an embolus.

PSYCHIATRY

Authors:

V Kirchner and MS Lipsedge

Editor:

V Kirchner

Editor-in-Chief:

JD Firth

1.1 History-taking

1.1.1 Eating disorders

Letter of referral to medical outpatient clinic

Dear Doctor,

Re: Ms Alison Jones

Thank you for seeing this 17-year-old schoolgirl whose parents are concerned because she has eaten very little for the past few weeks. She denies that there is any problem at all but her parents tell me that she weighs herself several times a day, exercises compulsively and makes herself sick. She refuses to join her parents for meals. As you can see she is painfully thin. I did not find any obvious physical cause.

Yours sincerely,

Introduction

Control and self-esteem are the issues that patients with eating disorders are usually struggling with. Eating and weight are things they sometimes feel in control of, although a lot of the time even these feel out of control. If they have suffered abuse then these feelings may be even stronger. Anyone telling them to eat and gain weight might be met with considerable hostility and putting undue pressure on them may arouse feelings of abuse. Their beliefs about their weight and appearance will be very strong so they are unlikely to accept the severity of their situation or advice from well-meaning doctors. Approach the situation with empathy and understanding, and concentrate on winning their trust. It may initially be appropriate to address urgent medical complications, not the eating disorder itself. It is important to differentiate between anorexia nervosa and bulimia nervosa, as management is different for each.

International Classification of Diseases (ICD)-10 criteria for anorexia nervosa

- BMI <17.5 or body weight >15% below expected, where BMI = weight (kg)/(height in metres)^2.
- Self-induced weight loss.
- Body image distortion.
- Abnormalities of the hypothalamic–pituitary–gonadal axis.
- If onset is prepubertal, then delayed puberty.

Diagnostic and Statistical Manual of Mental Disorders (DSM)-IV criteria for bulimia nervosa

- Recurrent episodes of binge eating.
- Recurrent inappropriate compensatory behaviour to prevent weight gain.
- The above occurring more than twice weekly for 3 months.

History of the presenting problem

Anorexia nervosa is a clinical diagnosis (see above) and other general medical conditions that may account for the weight loss must be excluded.

Other conditions that may present like anorexia nervosa

- Inflammatory bowel disease.
- Malabsorption: coeliac disease.
- Infection: tuberculosis and HIV.
- Thyrotoxicosis.
- Diabetes.
- Addison's disease.
- Malignant disease.
- Depression.
- Obsessive–compulsive disorder.
- Psychosis.

Focusing on the possible diagnoses of anorexia nervosa and bulimia nervosa, try to establish how much, what and how often she is eating. Explore if she relates to these common behaviours/symptoms:

- intense fear of putting on weight;

- constantly thinking about food;

- hoarding food;

- does not eat with family or in public places;

- binge eating and self-induced vomiting;

- laxative and diuretic abuse;

- ritualistic, excessive and possibly abnormal exercise;

- amenorrhoea.

In most cases the diagnosis is clear and never in substantial doubt, but take care not to rush to conclusions immediately and enquire about bowel habit, abdominal bloating and other symptoms that might indicate malabsorption. Also check for symptoms that might indicate one of the diseases listed in the Key Point box above.

Other relevant history

Ask the patient how old was she when the eating disorder started. What does she believe set it off? How does it affect her life? Has she had previous medical complications? Has she received treatment in the past?

Has she been abused physically, sexually or emotionally? Asking about abuse should only be done when you are alone with her and you perceive that your relationship with her is such that she will not find such a question overwhelmingly intrusive. Exploration and discussion of this issue would not be expected in the context of a PACES scenario, but in clinical practice you would assure confidentiality: you may be the first person she has ever told about this issue.

Collateral history

This will not be available in a PACES scenario, unless given in the letter of referral. However, the patient may feel ashamed of her eating pattern and therefore be unwilling to divulge information. Her parents may be able to provide details, but beware of making the patient feel colluded against.

Plan for investigation and management

Explain the need to exclude general medical causes for her symptoms. Since she may not herself be worried

about her weight loss – in fact she might value it – it might be worth emphasising the amenorrhoea or poor temperature control as these are symptoms she might agree to having investigated. Tell her you will have someone she trusts present during the physical examination, remembering how sensitive she is likely to feel about her body. Establish her height and weight to calculate her BMI.

Investigations are necessary to identify medical complications and exclude other causes for weight loss rather than to aid in making the diagnosis of anorexia or bulimia nervosa. Initial investigations would be blood tests, an ECG and a CXR (Table 1).

General management goals would include:

* treating medical complications;
* restoring a more normal eating pattern;
* providing information;

* referral to psychiatric services or GP so psychotherapy and family counselling can be initiated.

Although psychotherapy is the treatment of choice, there is no agreed 'best' psychological treatment for anorexia nervosa and the outcome is variable.

Arrange a follow-up outpatient appointment to review test results, confirm with the patient that the diagnosis is a primary eating disorder and that specialist follow-up is in place.

Further discussion

Self-starvation is a serious life-threatening problem. The signs of starvation are:

* hypothermia;
* lanugo;
* loss of muscle mass;
* dependent oedema;
* bradycardia;
* hypotension;
* neuropathy.

TABLE 1 ROUTINE INVESTIGATIONS REQUIRED IN PATIENTS PRESENTING WITH PROBABLE ANOREXIA NERVOSA

Investigation	Possible abnormalities
Electrolytes	Hypokalaemia Hypochloraemic alkalosis Renal failure
Calcium	Low
Phosphate	Low
Magnesium	Low
Liver function test	Low proteins Raised liver enzymes
Glucose	Low
FBC	Low white cell count Normochromic or iron-deficient anaemia
Erythrocyte sedimentation rate	Should be normal
Thyroid function test	Low triiodothyronine
ECG	Dysrhythmias T-wave changes, ST depression, lengthened QT interval
CXR	Small heart Osteoporosis

If she is inducing vomiting, tell-tale signs are:

- salivary gland enlargement;
- dental erosion;
- calluses on the fingers/knuckles.

Anorexia nervosa: refusal of treatment

If the patient's situation is life-threatening and she adamantly refuses treatment, she must be assessed by a psychiatrist for treatment under the Mental Health Act 1983 (see Section 2.14).

1.1.2 Medically unexplained symptoms

Letter of referral to medical outpatient clinic

Dear Doctor,

Re: Ms Catherine Davies

Thank you for seeing this 45-year-old solicitor with an 8-month history of feeling exhausted and unable to engage in any activity that requires physical exertion. She has recently been spending up to 15 hours a day in bed and feels miserable because of not being able to do what she could previously. She has been off sick from work for the past 2 months. There is no history of mental illness. I cannot find any abnormality on examination. Her BP is 120/80 mmHg. I have checked her FBC, erythrocyte sedimentation rate, urea and electrolytes, liver and bone function tests and thyroid function tests and they are all normal.

Yours sincerely,

TABLE 2 SOMATOFORM DISORDERS

Disorder	Characteristic features
Undifferentiated somatoform disorder	Unexplained and incapacitating physical complaints, eg fatigue for at least 6 months
Somatisation disorder	Many different symptoms including gastrointestinal, gynaecological and neurological. Pain is common
Conversion disorder	One symptom simulating a disease, eg motor or sensory symptoms and seizures
Hypochondriasis	Preoccupation with having a particular disease
Body dysmorphic disorder	Subjective feelings of a body defect
Pain disorder	Pain syndrome

Introduction

Medically unexplained physical symptoms fall into the category of somatoform disorders (Table 2). In these conditions patients present with physical symptoms that are not explained by any medical condition and are assumed to have an underlying psychosocial cause. Medically unexplained physical symptoms are often dismissed and patients feel they are not being taken seriously despite feeling very ill indeed. These symptoms are difficult to treat and often make doctors feel impotent and frustrated. Although psychological factors are assumed to be important, patients rarely accept a purely psychological explanation. A sensible approach is for physician and psychiatrist to work collaboratively. One physician should investigate possible medical causes and coordinate all investigations and care. An empathic but firm and sensible approach is essential. The involvement of a large number of doctors is likely to do more harm than good.

History of the presenting problem

A full medical and functional history is required, with any leads followed appropriately, but it is very likely that nothing convincing will emerge

in the medical enquiry. Look for predisposing, precipitating and perpetuating factors. These may be biological, psychological or social, for example a high-achieving person who is not reaching self-imposed targets at work.

Ask the patient the following.

- When did the symptoms start?
- When did her mood change?
- What was the first symptom?
- What is her explanation?
- In what sequence did symptoms develop?
- What was going on in her personal, family and work life just prior to the onset?
- Is she taking any medication that might have troublesome side effects?
- Does she have a history of mental illness, eg mood or eating disorders?
- Does she have alcohol or other substance misuse problems?

When asking about past history, factors such as invalidism within the family may provide a model of illness behaviour. Periods of extended absence from school or work may indicate a predisposition to using physical symptoms to deal with psychological distress or social pressures. Enquire about the coexistence of other medically unexplained syndromes or idiosyncratic beliefs about her health, eg irritable bowel syndrome, fibromyalgia or beliefs about food allergies.

> Remember to ask about travel to foreign countries to exclude unusual infections.

Plan for investigation and management

Explain to the patient that a full and thorough physical examination must be performed. Also explain that repeated examinations are not helpful unless new circumstances warrant it. Reassure the patient that any abnormal physical findings will be followed up.

Tell the patient that a well thought-out battery of investigations will be carried out as the next step (see below). This will reassure her, and also other doctors involved in her care, that possible physical causes are being taken seriously. However, if physical examination and investigations are negative, then in this patient a likely diagnosis is chronic fatigue syndrome, the criteria for which are listed below.

> **Diagnostic criteria for chronic fatigue syndrome**
>
> Clinically evaluated, medically unexplained fatigue of at least 6 months' duration that is:
>
> • of new onset;
> • not a result of ongoing exertion;
> • not substantially alleviated by rest;
> • a substantial reduction in previous levels of activity.

> Along with the occurrence of four or more of the following symptoms:
>
> • subjective memory impairment;
> • tender lymph nodes;
> • muscle pain;
> • joint pain;
> • headache;
> • unrefreshing sleep;
> • postexertional malaise.

To successfully manage chronic fatigue symptoms it is essential to establish a collaborative relationship with the patient and use a comprehensive treatment approach, addressing physical disabilities and using psychological strategies. Establishing whether the illness-related behaviour has some secondary gain is helpful in understanding and resolving the situation (eg is there an intolerable situation at work?).

The following are management strategies that have been investigated.

• Graded exercise programmes and cognitive-behaviour therapy are the only two treatments shown to be of definite benefit.

• Antidepressants have limited effectiveness.

• Immunotherapy, dietary supplements and NADH are of no benefit.

• Prolonged rest is ineffective and tends to be harmful.

Review the patient in the outpatient clinic on a regular basis, eg at 6-weekly intervals. It is important to ensure reliable communication with the other clinicians involved (GP and cognitive-behaviour therapist). The reason for regular review is to provide reassurance and pre-empt her making numerous urgent appointments.

Further discussion

What routine tests would be reasonable to request in this case?

Routine tests should include the following.

• Urine dipstick for protein and sugar.

• FBC and white cell differential.

• Erythrocyte sedimentation rate and C-reactive protein.

• Urea, creatinine and electrolytes.

• Bone function tests (including calcium).

• Liver function tests.

• Glucose.

• Creatine phosphokinase.

• Thyroid function tests.

• Autoantibodies profile, eg antinuclear factor and antiendomysial antibody.

• Coeliac disease test.

• CXR.

• ECG.

Other investigations will be guided by findings from history and examination or by abnormalities detected on the routine tests listed above. It is important, but sometimes extremely difficult, to avoid a situation where every interaction with the patient leads to a new symptom, which then triggers a new battery of tests. The mature physician, having taken details of the new history and repeated the physical examination if relevant, will say 'I have followed what you have been saying, but I don't think that there's anything new to worry us here [assuming that there isn't]. I don't think any more tests are needed'.

1.2 Communication skills and ethics

1.2.1 Panic attack and hyperventilation

Scenario

Role: you are a junior doctor working in the Emergency Department

A 21-year-old university student is brought to the Emergency Department by her tutor with difficulty in breathing. She is very worried about her final examinations that start the next day because she has not completed her revision programme. In addition to the breathing difficulty she complains of palpitations, shakiness, sweating and pins and needles in her hands and around her mouth. She is distressed and tearful. Other than hyperventilation, a physical examination and investigations including CXR and ECG are normal. You conclude that her symptoms are due to an anxiety state with hyperventilation.

Your task: to explain the psychological nature of her problems and suggest how matters might be helped.

Key issues to explore

- What are her fears and her own explanation of what is happening to her at present?
- Can she see the link between psychological distress and her physiological response?

Key points to establish

- Introduce yourself appropriately.

- Demonstrate good listening skills and an empathic approach.
- Explain the reassuring results of both the physical examination and the investigations.
- Emphasise the link between her anxiety and her physical symptoms, and explain the physiology of hyperventilation in terms she would understand: 'When you get anxious and worried your heart rate and breathing naturally speed up, and this has effects on the body. It can make you feel light-headed and dizzy, and this can make you feel more anxious which makes things worse, a sort of vicious cycle.'
- Reassure her that this is anxiety and not a more severe mental illness, and that it is understandable in her current stressful situation.
- Reassure her that her condition is not life-threatening.
- Suggest simple strategies to manage the anxiety: 'We need to find a way of getting out of the vicious cycle. Sitting down and concentrating on taking slow breaths may help. Sometimes breathing into a paper bag can help to slow the breathing down. Deliberately trying to think of something calm and pleasant is also useful.'

Appropriate responses to likely questions

Patient: am I going to die?

Doctor: no. What are you worried you may die from?

Patient: I think I am going to have a heart attack or stop breathing altogether.

Doctor: I have done a physical examination and carried out tests

including an ECG, which shows how your heart is functioning. All of the results are normal, including the ECG which shows that your heart is fine. The chest X-ray shows there is nothing wrong with your lungs. Panic and hyperventilation are common symptoms and are never fatal.

Patient: is it going to get worse?

Doctor: what do you mean by 'get worse'?

Patient: will it come back?

Doctor: you might have more attacks like this one, but now that you know what is going on and understand the link between frightening thoughts and physical symptoms, you will feel less out of control if it does come back.

Patient: will these attacks get longer?

Doctor: no, I don't think that's likely: as you have seen today, the distressing feelings settled down quite quickly. The more you use the methods we discussed to deal with them, the more likely you are to control them and prevent them.

Patient: what if these attacks do not go away?

Doctor: I think that they will – they almost always do. But if they didn't, we would then arrange for you to see a specialist. There are highly effective psychological treatments, for example a treatment called cognitive-behaviour therapy.

Patient: are there any medicines that might help me?

Doctor: yes, sometimes we use antidepressant drugs that have been shown to be helpful in treating this condition, even in patients who do not have depression.

Patient: should I sit my exam tomorrow?

Doctor: what are your concerns about sitting your exam?

Patient: *that I will have another attack.*

Doctor: I think it would be a good idea for you to do it, because we know that one of the things that reinforces anxiety is avoiding the problem, whatever it is. As you are feeling now do you feel able to sit the exam?

Patient: *no, I do not think I have done enough revision.*

Doctor: that's a thing you'll have to discuss with your tutor, but many people doing an exam feel that they haven't done as much revision as they should have done.

1.2.2 Deliberate self-harm

Scenario
Role: you are a junior doctor in the Emergency Department. Mrs Freda Smith, a 64-year-old widow, was brought to hospital after taking an overdose of her antihypertensives. She has a history of depression. Over the years she has become estranged from her children and increasingly isolated. She is not in contact with psychiatric services. You have assessed her mental state and found all the features of a depressive illness. She told you she had been planning this overdose for a long time and had been collecting the tablets to carry this out. She still wishes she was dead and is disappointed that she was found by her neighbour who called the ambulance. You have assessed her physical health and no further medical treatment is required for the overdose. She

is anxious to go home and is reluctant to see a psychiatrist.

Your task: explain to Mrs Smith that she needs to speak to a psychiatrist and she would benefit from help from the mental health service.

Key issues to explore

• Address her concerns about seeing a psychiatrist.

• Explain that depression is a treatable illness.

Key points to establish

• Approach her empathically and above all avoid giving the impression that you are criticising or condemning her for the suicide attempt.

• Reassure her that you expect her to recover physically from the overdose.

• Establish why she does not want to see a psychiatrist.

• Explain that she is depressed and that this is a treatable condition.

• Prepare her psychologically for admission to a psychiatric ward.

Appropriate responses to likely questions

Patient: *I am not mad so why do I need to see a psychiatrist?*

Doctor: what do you mean when you say 'mad'?

Patient: *that you think I do not know what I am doing.*

Doctor: I don't think that. I think that you were feeling very miserable and you took the overdose to end those feelings of hopelessness.

Patient: *I don't see how a psychiatrist could help me with that.*

Doctor: you told me that you have been feeling miserable and lonely. The overdose shows us how desperate you have been feeling. What you have is depression, which is an illness that can be treated. Psychiatrists specialise in this.

Patient: *what sort of treatments are there?*

Doctor: the commonly used treatments are a combination of talking therapies and antidepressant medication. Have you come across these treatments before?

Patient: *I have heard about antidepressants. I have heard they are addictive.*

Doctor: antidepressants have been used for many years and doctors have a lot of experience with them. They are effective in treating depression and they are not addictive in the sense that they don't make people feel as though they want to take more and more of them. A few people can feel out of sorts if they stop taking them suddenly, but this only lasts a few days and we prevent it by gradually reducing the dose before stopping.

Patient: *will I be locked up if I see a psychiatrist?*

Doctor: I strongly feel that you need treatment and hospital might be the best place for you to get that treatment, even if that is not want you want. Once you feel better you may feel differently about being in hospital.

Patient: *how long would they keep me in hospital?*

Doctor: treatments for depression take a few weeks to start working, so it is likely that you would be in hospital for a few weeks.

Patient: *if I try to leave, will you stop me?*

Doctor: I very much hope that you won't just walk out. I think that you are depressed and that we can help this. I very much hope that you will agree to talk to someone from the psychiatry team so that we can find out what they think would be best for you. At the end of the day, I will insist that you see a psychiatrist even if that means stopping you from leaving.

1.2.3 Medically unexplained symptoms

Scenario

Role: you are a junior doctor in a medical outpatient clinic.

You have been following up a 34-year-old woman in the medical outpatient clinic. She presented with a 12-month history of fatigue. On examination there were no abnormal physical findings. You have done a battery of laboratory investigations and they have all been negative. There is no evidence of an underlying depressive illness.

She had suffered a brief flu-like illness about a week before the onset of her fatigue. She returned to work before she had fully recovered because she did not want to let her colleagues down. As things turned out, she was not able to cope with her job as a trader in an international bank and was sent on sick leave. She is an articulate woman who is a perfectionist and sets herself high standards. She is convinced that the virus has damaged her immune system and is still making her ill. She spends most of the day either in bed or resting on a couch. Any attempt to do tasks that are physically

demanding, for example climbing up the stairs, causes breathlessness, rapid heart beat and weakness of her legs. She attributes this to an ongoing disturbance of her immune system. She has spent a lot of time and money pursuing complementary therapies, including high doses of vitamins and trace elements. You have made a diagnosis of chronic fatigue syndrome (see Section 1.1.2).

Your task: to explain her illness to her and introduce a treatment approach of graded exercise.

Key issues to explore

- Explore her explanatory model for her illness and offer an alternative.

- Introduce the idea of graded exercise and explain its rationale.

- Introduce the idea of cognitive-behaviour therapy.

- Encourage problem-solving that will enable her to get back to work.

Key points to establish

- Summarise the position both in terms of her history and investigations.

- Acknowledge the distressing nature of her symptoms and disabilities.

- Acknowledge her own explanatory model, ie her conviction that all her symptoms are caused by a damaged immune system.

- Reassure her that there is no laboratory evidence of any ongoing disturbance to her immune system.

- Offer her an alternative explanatory model, acknowledging

that the original viral illness was the initial cause but that she has since developed secondary symptoms due to a lack of exercise.

Appropriate responses to likely questions

Patient: if my immune system is back to normal, why do I feel so exhausted?

Doctor: for the past year you have been spending most of your time in bed or on the sofa. We have a nervous system in the body called the autonomic nervous system. This regulates things like your blood pressure and heart rate. When this system is underused through lack of exercise it becomes inefficient and uncoordinated: your system has been underused for a long time now so you are bound to feel fatigued for some time after any exertion, no matter how minor.

Patient: why does any physical effort make me feel much worse?

Doctor: when you don't exercise your muscles, they become very weak, the opposite to what happens when you train in the gym. Your heart also becomes unfit, so any exertion will cause it to beat rapidly. The same goes for your breathing. So over the past year the combination of your muscles, heart and lungs becoming weaker and out of condition is now causing you to feel exhausted all the time.

Patient: if there is nothing wrong with my central nervous system, why can't I concentrate better?

Doctor: you are used to being in an environment at work were your brain is challenged continuously. Since being at home you have been out of this environment and mostly preoccupied with dealing with the exhaustion. Like anything else, your brain needs stimulation and exercise. You will find that your concentration will gradually improve as you stimulate your brain. We can talk about how to do this.

Patient: I am receiving income protection benefit and the insurers and my employers are pressurising me to return to work, but I cannot possibly do that at the moment. What should I do?

Doctor: at what point do you see yourself returning to work?

Patient: I would need to be completely recovered to cope with my job.

Doctor: perhaps that is looking at things in an 'all or nothing' way. You may want to consider ways that you can gradually get back to work. If your employers and insurers see that you are making progress and have a plan in place, they will be more sympathetic.

Patient: what if they don't respond favourably?

Doctor: I hope they will, but if they do not then the Disability Discrimination Act ensures that people can return to work in a graded and flexible fashion, thereby protecting you from undue pressure.

Patient: in the self-help group that I subscribe to, they say that there are bound to be underlying problems with my immune system and it may take me another year or two to recover.

Doctor: we know from research that the longer you remain inactive the harder it is to recover. People who make an early start to a graded exercise programme combined with cognitive-behaviour therapy begin to recover more quickly.

1.3 Acute scenarios

1.3.1 Acute confusional state

Scenario
A middle-aged man has an acute confusional state after coronary artery bypass graft surgery. His mental state had appeared normal on admission, but 48 hours after the operation he has pulled out his intravenous line, refuses to allow the nurses anywhere near him and is cowering in a corner of the ward. He is clearly terrified and suspicious, and accuses the staff of trying to kill him.

Introduction

What is the most likely cause of this disruptive behaviour?

The most likely cause is an acute confusional state (delirium), but occasionally patients might develop a brief psychosis or a severe affective (mood) disorder after major surgery.

In general what are the cardinal feature of an acute confusional state?

- Clouding of consciousness, which may fluctuate.

- Disorientation in time, place and person.

- Impaired grasp of the situation and diminished attention.

- Reversal of the sleep–wakefulness cycle.

- The confusion worsens at night, but with a lucid interval in the morning.

What are the common causes of an acute confusional state?

After coronary artery surgery, delirium following a lucid interval is probably due to metabolic disturbance, medication, sleep deprivation or alcohol withdrawal. The common causes of delirium are shown in Table 3.

History of the presenting problem

What would you like to know about how this developed?

You know the patient was mentally well prior to the surgery. Think of

TABLE 3 COMMON CAUSES OF A POSTOPERATIVE ACUTE CONFUSIONAL STATE

Common causes	Conditions
Systemic	Infection (eg pneumonia, septicaemia, urinary tract infection) Respiratory or cardiac failure Electrolyte imbalance Metabolic disorder, eg hypoglycaemia, renal or hepatic failure Severe hypotension due to reduced cardiac output secondary to myocardial infarction, pulmonary embolus or arrhythmia Severe anaemia
Intracranial	Cerebrovascular accident Postictal state
Drug-induced	Steroids, theophylline or beta-blockers Drug intoxication (eg with analgesics) Withdrawal of alcohol or benzodiazepines
Other	Pain Urinary retention

what may have happened during the surgery, for example were there problems with the anaesthetic or with the surgery that might have affected cerebral perfusion or caused a cerebrovascular event. People are commonly confused and disorientated as they recover from a general anaesthetic. Did this man gain lucidity within the expected time-frame? What medication was he given in the last 48 hours? Analgesics are a common cause of confusion. Also look for drug errors. Consider the fluids he was given: he may be dehydrated or have an electrolyte imbalance. He may also be hypotensive. Other postoperative complications such as bleeding or infection may cause confusion.

What would you like to know from the nursing staff?

The nursing staff are likely to be the main source of information in a case such as this, although any relatives present may give a useful history and for a variety of reasons may be keen to do so. Ask the nurses if the patient has had vomiting and/or diarrhoea. In addition enquire about early warning signs of impending delirium, for example:

- daytime drowsiness;

- if there was a lucid interval in the morning, which might have given a misleading impression of normality during the morning ward round.

Other relevant history

What collateral information would you like to have?

Try to establish the underlying cause of the delirium by looking for information in the notes and/or asking relatives.

- Estimate the patient's usual daily alcohol intake.

- Check whether there has been increasing absent-mindedness and progressive impairment of memory over the preceding 6–12 months or so, indicating dementia with superimposed delirium.

- Has there been a recent head injury? Unlikely in this context, but you need to consider the possibility of subdural haematoma.

- Is there a history of a previous psychiatric disorder that might point towards a relapse of schizophrenia or a manic-depressive disorder precipitated by the psychological stress of the operation?

- Is there a history of seizures? Rarely a presentation such as this can be due to a prolonged ictal state.

- Do not forget to ask about unusual conditions that may catch you out, eg have they recently returned from a tropical area? (In which case consider malaria.)

Examination

When you examine the mental state, what features should you look for in order to establish the diagnosis of delirium?

How may the person's appearance be different?

The patient generally appears more frightened than hostile, although he may act aggressively in self-defence against an imaginary enemy. In some cases the patient will appear apathetic and withdrawn rather than agitated.

What behaviour would you expect?

The patient is commonly restless and may pluck at the bedclothes. The patient may attempt to escape

from the ward. In contrast to this picture of 'noisy' delirium, patients may be withdrawn and underactive, and it might only be on close questioning that the clinician learns that they are disorientated and unable to grasp what is going on around them.

What changes in speech and thinking may occur?

The patient's speech may be incoherent. There may be fleeting and sketchy ideas of persecution or ideas of reference (eg the ward television is showing a police drama which the patient interprets to mean that he is about to be arrested). Delusional themes might include the patient being convinced that he is being held in prison, or that staff are trying to poison him.

How may mood be affected?

Mood is often changeable and can fluctuate from intense fear and agitation to milder forms of anxiety, depression and irritability.

> In delirium there is clouding of consciousness. This helps to distinguish delirium from the agitation of severe depression or the excitement of mania, in which consiousness is unimpaired.

What perceptual disturbances are possible?

There may be illusions and hallucinations. The latter are mainly visual but can also be auditory and tactile. A telephone wire may be perceived as a snake, while the ringing of a telephone might sound like a fire alarm.

How would you know cognitive function is impaired?

There is disorientation in both time and place, and misidentification of members of staff or members of his own family. The patient is likely to appear dazed and unclear about his surroundings: he has difficulty in grasping what is happening around him, his attention to what is going on is greatly reduced and he tends to drift off. His attention span is also decreased (unable to correctly repeat seven digits listed to him).

How may you test this further?

In this particular patient testing may be difficult, but in a less disturbed and somewhat more cooperative patient you could ask him or her to recite the days of the week and then the months of the year in reverse order. Another test of attention and concentration is to serially subtract 7 from 100 or 3 from 20. Other general tests of cognitive function that are commonly used are the Abbreviated Mental Test and the Mini-Mental State Examination. When interpreting the patient's performance on these tests, you need to take into account educational attainment, fluency in the language of the examination and any impairment of sight or hearing.

Does the person with delirium have insight into their condition?

This fluctuates with the patient's level of consciousness. After the episode the patient will have little recollection of what he thought, how he behaved and how he was treated.

> 🔑 In assessing a patient with an acute confusional state you should always try to perform a full physical examination (after sedation if necessary), looking for evidence of any of the conditions listed in Table 3. This may be very difficult to do: your notes in the medical record must detail your findings or, if relevant, explain the circumstances that prevented thorough examination.

TABLE 4 INVESTIGATIONS TO DETERMINE THE CAUSE OF AN ACUTE CONFUSIONAL STATE

Investigation	Comment
ECG	Has he had an infarct or developed an arrhythmia?
Glucose (fingerprick test plus laboratory)	Hypoglycaemia is common after surgery
Electrolytes and calcium	Hyponatraemia is common postoperatively
Renal and liver function	Acute renal failure is common postoperatively
FBC and erythrocyte sedimentation rate	Look for anaemia or evidence of infection
Culture of urine, blood and sputum	
Pulse oximetry and arterial blood gases	
CXR	
CT head scan	If focal neurological signs are present and/or no other obvious explanation for confusion
Other tests as determined by clinical findings or results from initial investigations	

Investigations

These should be performed (after sedation if necessary) to establish the presence of any of the conditions listed in Table 3. In the absence of obvious clinical clues, which would direct investigations, the tests shown in Table 4 would be appropriate.

Management

The patient with delirium is often unable to cooperate with nursing and medical care. He might refuse medication and investigations. He may become dehydrated or sustain an injury when falling or fighting.

The priorities are as follows.

- Establish and treat the cause of the delirium, eg electrolyte imbalance, dehydration, infection or anaemia.

- Review all current medication and withdraw any that can be stopped.

- Keep the patient in touch with his surroundings: a window increases awareness of the contrast between day and night.

- 24-hour nursing care is indicated, preferably with a single nurse on

each shift rather than a succession of nurses 'dropping in'.

What sedatives/tranquillisers may be useful?

For severe agitation, haloperidol in a dose of 5–10 mg (po or im; 0.5–1 mg in the elderly) is a useful major tranquilliser. In cases of delirium tremens, administer chlordiazepoxide 30 mg four times a day (reducing doses and less in the elderly) to relieve the agitation and prevent withdrawal fits (see Section 1.3.4). Give parenteral vitamin B and C to prevent Wernicke–Korsakoff syndrome.

> 🔑 Delirium is an urgent situation and the staff have a clear duty of care. If the patient clearly lacks the capacity to give meaningful consent or refuses potentially life-saving investigation and treatment, then emergency measures are covered by common law. If more than emergency interventions are required because the problems persist, then it would be advisable to call in the duty psychiatrist to discuss the use of the Mental Health Act or Mental Capacity Act.

1.3.2 Panic attack and hyperventilation

Scenario

A 35-year-old office manager presents to the Emergency Department complaining of intense discomfort in his chest. This had developed as he was driving to work. Over the previous few weeks, since his firm had been taken over by a larger company, he had felt tense, sweaty, shaky and light-headed just before meetings and had been increasingly aware of his heart beating rapidly. New management have imposed stringent targets but he has lost half of his administrative and secretarial staff. He has been reluctant to take any time off work because the firm is downsizing and he fears redundancy.

Introduction

In a case such as this it is important to remember the following.

- What is the most important consideration when confronted with symptoms like panic that might have an underlying medical rather than a psychological cause?

- Although this is likely to be a primary anxiety disorder, there may be an underlying physical cause, such as substance misuse.

What general medical conditions could lead to this presentation?

- Thyrotoxicosis: there may be a history of heat intolerance and weight loss. Look for goitre, eye signs, tremor and tachycardia. Check thyroid function.

TABLE 5 *INTERNATIONAL CLASSIFICATION OF DISEASES (ICD)-10 CLASSIFICATION OF THE NEUROTIC AND STRESS-RELATED DISORDERS*

Disorders	Further information
Panic disorder	See Section 2.7.2
Generalised anxiety disorder	See Section 2.7.1
Adjustment disorders	See Section 2.6
Mixed anxiety and depressive disorder	
Acute stress reaction	See Section 2.9.1
Obsessive–compulsive disorder	See Section 2.8
Post-traumatic stress disorder	See Section 2.9.2
Phobic disorder	See Section 2.7.3

- Hypoglycaemia: there may be a history of diabetes or alcohol intoxication. Check blood sugar.

- Paroxysmal supraventricular tachycardia: check ECG.

- Phaeochromocytoma: very unlikely indeed, but this rare condition can present with episodic sweating, headache, tremor and fluctating high BP.

What substance misuse problems may present with symptoms of panic?

- Alcohol withdrawal: symptoms may include restlessness, overactivity, disorientation, inability to register new information, fearfulness, sweating, tremulousness, visual hallucinations and illusions (sensory distortions). Look for evidence of chronic liver disease and check liver function tests, especially γ-glutamyl transpeptidase, and also mean corpuscular volume.

- Drug intoxication: some of the symptoms are similar to alcohol withdrawal, ie restlessness, overactivity, disorientation and inability to register new information. In addition the patient may be preoccupied with bizarre psychological

experiences and have rapid fluctuations of mood.

- Drug withdrawal: look for evidence of drug use, eg injection sites, track marks and abscesses.

Having excluded an underlying organic cause, consider the different types of anxiety disorder listed in Table 5.

History of the presenting problem

What symptoms is he getting?

He might be having both physical and psychological symptoms. For example, he may have been feeling tense and apprehensive, and in addition having chest pain and a headache like a 'tight band' around his skull. See the list of possible symptoms in Table 6.

What are the characteristics of a panic attack?

Typically these are episodes of extreme anxiety with abrupt onset and fairly short duration. They occur out of the blue, but as the condition develops they may be linked to specific situations, thoughts or physical symptoms, eg a rapid heart beat. Hyperventilation and palpitations commonly occur along with shakiness and sweating.

TABLE 6 SYMPTOMS AND SIGNS OF AN ANXIETY STATE

Symptoms and signs	Features
Psychological symptoms	Irritability Intolerance of noise Poor concentration and memory Fearfulness Apprehensiveness Restlessness Continuous worrying thoughts
Physical symptoms	Dry mouth Difficulty in swallowing Shakiness Diarrhoea Urinary frequency Paraesthesiae, especially in fingers and around mouth Dizziness Hot flushes
Physical signs	Tense Sweating Shaky Pale Restless Hyperventilation

What information would be useful to understand psychosocial triggers for the anxiety?

There may be stressful personal situations that precipitate the initial anxiety. For example, this man felt overwhelmed by his workload, and this was exacerbated by a fear of losing his job. Other factors may come into play, eg excessive reliance on coffee with the caffeine worsening the symptoms of anxiety, or the use of alcohol to treat the anxiety symptoms causing a vicious circle (Fig. 1).

In anxiety the enhanced awareness of physiological sensations combined with increased autonomic arousal can induce fear of a catastrophic medical event. For example, this man who is having anxiety-related chest pain may believe he is going to die from a heart attack.

Other relevant history

There may be a personal or family history of an anxiety-based disorder or mood disturbance, especially at times of stress and adverse life events. Also ask about any separations and insecurity during childhood.

Examination

The primary reason for a physical examination is to exclude any underlying physical problems.

In this case, although you suspect a primary anxiety disorder, it is important to perform a thorough cardiac and respiratory examination, since the main complaint is of chest pain. Myocardial infarction makes people anxious – indeed many think that they are going to die – and it is a mistake to jump to the diagnosis of anxiety-related chest pain too readily. Carry out a careful examination for evidence of any organic causes of anxiety.

Investigations

Since the presenting feature was chest pain, an ECG is vital. In a 35-year-old man with no previous cardiac history the ECG is likely to be normal. The only finding on examination was hyperventilation so pulse oximetry should be performed, and most would think it appropriate to check arterial blood gases, with a normal Po_2 and a low Pco_2 being the expected result.

Thyroid function, routine biochemistry and haematology tests should be done. Further medical tests may be indicated, but if the clinical diagnosis seems clearly to be that of an anxiety disorder then it is not helpful to embark on an extensive range of investigations as these might actually reinforce the anxiety.

Management

What explanation and reassurance would you give?

It is important to elicit the patient's own 'explanatory model', eg his conviction that he is about to have a heart attack may lead to frequent checking and recording his own pulse rate, which in turn makes him feel more anxious. Give him some understanding of the link between his symptoms and his faulty physiological assumptions.

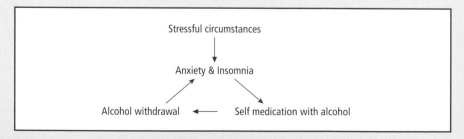

▲ **Fig. 1** An example of how anxiety and alcohol use can develop a vicious circle with each exacerbating the other.

What physical interventions can be used to help a person presenting during a panic attack?

Take the patient to a quiet room (if possible) and reassure him, explaining how anxiety induces the physiological effects of excessive adrenaline release. If he is hyperventilating and if quiet discussion and encouragement do not slow his respiratory rate, then breathing in and out of a paper bag to raise plasma P_{CO_2} can be helpful. This should not be performed in the middle of an open area, where the patient might think he was being made to look a fool. Consider oral benzodiazepines eg lorazepam 2–4 mg or diazepam 5–10 mg.

What is the longer term treatment of panic disorder?

Cognitive-behaviour therapy is the treatment of choice. Sometimes selective serotonin reuptake inhibitor antidepressants may be helpful.

Would you prescribe benzodiazepine anxiolytics?

These should be avoided if possible as tolerance quickly develops and there is a high risk of dependence.

1.3.3 Deliberate self-harm

Scenario

A 30-year-old unemployed woman is brought into the Emergency Department after taking an unknown quantity of paracetamol and vodka 90 minutes earlier. She is alert and tearful. She is able to tell the triage nurse that she was feeing desperate because her partner had left her and she had just been evicted for rent arrears. Some years ago she took an overdose and cut her wrists after one of her children was taken into care.

Introduction

Why is deliberate self-harm important?

Firstly, because it is common. Deliberate self-harm (DSH) leads to about 100,000 hospital admissions in England and Wales every year and its incidence is increasing. Secondly, an episode of DSH indicates a greatly increased risk of suicide.

> During the 10-year period following any episode of DSH the risk of suicide is increased to 30-fold higher than that expected in the general population, with the first 6 months being the period of greatest risk. Take note of the following:
>
> - 1% of patients kill themselves in the year after an episode of DSH;
> - one-fifth to one-quarter of patients who die by suicide have presented to a general hospital following episodes of DSH in the year before their death.

Who is at greatest risk of suicide?

The highest suicide rate occurs in people aged over 75, but the rate among young men has increased greatly over the past 20 years. Men tend to use violent means such as hanging; women are more likely to kill themselves by self-poisoning with drugs. Most people who commit suicide have a psychiatric disorder such as:

- depression (15% lifetime risk of suicide);
- schizophrenia (10% lifetime risk);
- alcohol addiction (3–4% lifetime risk).

What personal or social circumstances increase the risk of suicide?

- Divorce.
- Loss of job, long-term unemployment and retirement.
- Social isolation.
- Recent bereavement.
- Chronic painful or terminal illness.
- History of mood disorder, alcoholism or attempted suicide.
- Death of a parent in childhood.

History of the presenting problem

What questions should you ask the patient about her preparation for the overdose?

- Had she planned the overdose for some time or did she take it on impulse?
- Had she hoarded the pills?
- Had she taken precautions to make sure that she was alone and undisturbed?
- Did she leave a suicide note?
- Had she given away her most treasured possessions?
- Had she arranged for the children to be sent away or had her pet dog or cat put down?
- Did she plan more than one means of killing herself, eg overdose plus jumping out of a window or in front of a lorry, using a firearm or hanging?

> ⚠ • Patients are not experts in pharmacology. When evaluating risk do not assume that a small overdose of a relatively safe drug necessarily implies minimal lethal intent.
> • Patients do not have a sophisticated knowledge of the therapeutic index of medicines and they might think that a few temazepam tablets are as dangerous as a handful of digoxin pills.

What recent depressive symptoms should you enquire about?

Symptoms that suggest severe depression include:

- hopelessness, helplessness, despair, anhedonia and morbid guilt;

- command hallucinations and depressive delusions;

- severe insomnia;

- self-neglect;

- agitation;

- panic attacks.

Other relevant history

What else do you ned to know in order to asses the short-term risk of a further suicide attempt?

Assess the patient's state of mind before, during and since the episode. Does she regret that she has survived the overdose? Establish whether she has a psychiatric disorder that puts her at risk of suicide. Chronic, painful, disabling or life-threatening illnesses also increase the risk. This patient has a history of self-harm, which makes her more vulnerable to future suicide attempts, as would a family history of suicide. She has also recently separated from her partner and lost her home; recent events of this type are risk factors. Explore the quality of her social support network, eg does she have access to a supportive relative or friend who she can turn to? Having a confidante is protective.

What other source of information would be extremely helpful?

Because suicidal people are often reluctant to reveal information, speaking to someone else who knows her well may tell you more about the suicide attempt and her personal circumstances. This would also help you to assess whether she

has an impulsive or aggressive personality, which is important because these traits are known to be additional risk factors.

> **Difficulties in the assessment of suicide risk**
>
> - The degree of suicide intent can fluctuate.
> - Even gravely suicidal patients can deliberately conceal their intentions.
> - Patients may appear misleadingly calm after having made a firm but undisclosed plan to kill themselves.

Management

What broad principles do you need to address in your management plan?

The immediate priority in any patient presenting with DSH is dealing with the physical consequences of the self-harm. In this patient that would be managing paracetamol poisoning by establishing blood levels, monitoring liver function and and possibly administering acetylcysteine. Also check blood for the presence of other drugs that may have been taken.

The second priority is to prevent further episodes of self-harm. It is good practice to request an opinion from the psychiatric duty team to determine whether admission or discharge with follow-up are appropriate.

> ⚠ • Patients who discharge themselves from the Emergency Department before psychosocial screening have three times the rate of repetition of DSH.
> • Failure to resolve precipitating circumstances and failure to establish a rapport with the medical staff are two things that should alert you that this person is still at high risk.

What should you do if the patient insists on leaving prematurely or refuses life-saving treatment?

Firstly, evaluate her capacity to make an informed decision. Explain the risks to the patient of not receiving treatment. Is she able to retain the information and understand it? Is she able to weigh it up in the balance when making her decision? Is she able to communicate her decision to you?

After this, record your assessment of her capacity. If she lacks capacity, she can receive life-saving treatment under common law. It is good practice to enlist the support of family or friends to persuade her. If she is at high risk of suicide, she should be admitted either voluntarily or under the Mental Health Act 1983 (see Section 2.14).

1.3.4 The alcoholic in hospital

Scenario

A 54-year-old man is admitted to hospital in a neglected state. He appears anxious, agitated, shaky and sweaty. He reports that he stopped drinking alcohol 2 days previously.

History of the presenting problem

What should you ask the patient about his drinking to determine the severity?

The important aspects to try to establish are as follows.

- When was his last drink?

- What is he drinking?

- What is the strength?

- How much? How many units per week (see Table 7)?

TABLE **7** UNITS OF ALCOHOL IN COMMON BEVERAGES, WHERE **1** UNIT OF ALCOHOL CONTAINS **8** G OF ETHANOL

Type of drink	Units of alcohol
Pint of lager	2
Pint of extra-strong lager	5
150-mL glass of wine	1
One shot of spirits (25 mL)	1

- How often?

- When in the day?

- Does he relate drinking to any particular pattern or situation?

- Does he drink alone or with people?

How would you establish alcohol dependence?

The *Diagnostic and Statistical Manual of Mental Disorders* (DSM)-IV criteria for alcohol dependence are:

- inability to reduce alcohol consumed;

- repeated efforts to control drinking;

- amnesic periods;

- drinking increasing amounts;

- ongoing drinking despite detrimental consequences;

- withdrawal symptoms.

What are withdrawal symptoms

The DSM-IV criteria for alcohol withdrawal symptoms are:

- sweating;

- tremor;

- agitation and anxiety;

- tachycardia;

- raised BP;

- nausea and vomiting;

- insomnia;

- hallucinations (tactile, visual and auditory);

- grand mal seizures.

What recommendations have been made regarding a safe level of alcohol consumption?

The Royal College of Physicians (1995) recommended that the maximum total units per week for safe use are 21 in men and 14 in women. The Department of Health (1995) recommended that women consistently consuming 2–3 units daily and men 3–4 units daily will not accrue any significant health risk. Haemorrhagic stroke, cancer, accidents and hypertension are all associated with alcohol consumption above recommended levels.

Other relevant history

What associated medical conditions would you look for?

- Oesophagitis.

- Gastritis.

- Gastric ulcer.

- Alcoholic hepatitis and cirrhosis.

- Oesophageal varices.

- Pancreatitis.

- Cardiomyopathy.

- Thiamine deficiency (Wernicke–Korsakoff syndrome).

- Neuropathy.

- Head injuries (subdural haematoma).

- Cerebellar atrophy.

What psychiatric conditions may coexist?

One-third of people with alcohol dependence also have another mental illness, most commonly a mood disorder, an anxiety disorder or an antisocial personality disorder. Suicide is also commonly associated with alcohol.

- A grasp of his current social circumstances and supports will help this man feel understood as a person and will give you an insight into why he continues to drink.
- A blaming, moralistic attitude focusing exclusively on alcohol abuse will result in a frustrating, ineffective, therapeutic relationship.

In longer-term management, what issues are helpful to better understand the patient?

The age he started drinking and why may reveal continuing psychological reasons for drinking. Problem drinking may have started later. Previous withdrawal symptoms and their outcome may help to predict what happens now. Also, examining the outcome of previous alcohol treatment programmes and why they failed may help him to overcome obstacles to abstinence. Discuss precipitants of previous relapses. A family history of alcohol abuse may indicate a genetic propensity and/or exposure to a heavy drinking microculture where alcohol is routinely used as an inappropriate coping device. Explore with the patient the negative social effects of heavy drinking such as drinking and driving offences, losing jobs or partners, in addition to the medical consequences.

Examination

Look for signs of:

- withdrawal (see above);

- infection (especially pneumonia);

- malnutrition;

- possible medical complications of chronic alcohol abuse (see above);

- confusion, ie being disorientated, having impaired attention and registration, etc.

If he is confused, conditions to consider include the following.

- Hypoglycaemia.

- Delirium tremens, which can occur within 72 hours of the last drink.

- Wernicke's encephalopathy.

- Postictal state: however, before attributing seizures to alcohol withdrawal, exclude other causes such as hypoglycaemia, hyponatraemia, hypomagnesaemia and any other central nervous system pathology, eg subdural haematoma.

- In cases of delirium exclude the possibility of infection, hepatic failure or any other general medical condition.

- Head injury.

Wernicke's encephalopathy classically presents with:

- ocular abnormalities (horizontal and vertical nystagmus, weakness/paralysis of lateral rectus muscles and weakness/paralysis of conjugate gaze);
- ataxia;
- confusion;
- peripheral neuropathy;
- malnutrition.

Wernicke's encephalopathy is due to thiamine deficiency. If missed and not treated with parenteral thiamine, it will result in death or permanent neurological and cognitive damage.

Management

The important aspects are as follows.

- Benzodiazepines: treat withdrawal symptoms with a 7–10 day course of diazepam or chlordiazepoxide, usually orally. Occasionally intravenous treatment is required for seizures. Never use intramuscular injection because of erratic absorption. Initially titrate the oral dose until symptoms are controlled, then taper the dose until stopping.

- Nurse the patient in a well-lit, quiet environment.

- Give thiamine supplementation (parenterally if Wernicke's encephalopathy is suspected).

- Monitor for and prevent hypoglycaemia.

- Rehydration.

- A high-calorie, high-carbohydrate diet.

- Avoid antipsychotics because they lower the seizure threshold.

- Refer the patient to alcohol services for follow-up, support, advice, cognitive-behaviour therapy; and also to a psychiatrist if comorbid mental illness is present.

1.3.5 Drug abuser in hospital

Scenario

A 29-year-old woman has been admitted to a surgical ward for drainage of an abscess on her forearm. She uses heroin intravenously and says that she is about to go into opioid withdrawal. Your opinion is sought.

History of the presenting problem

What would you ask about her substance misuse?

Important points to elucidate are as follows.

- What substances is she using? (This list may be extensive.)

- Since when?

- By what method?

- How much?

Heroin can be smoked, injected or snorted, and may be used in conjunction with other opioids. Ask her to describe any withdrawal symptoms she may be experiencing or has experienced in the past. Has she developed tolerance? Does she have any plans to kick her habit?

What are the symptoms of opioid withdrawal?

The *Diagnostic and Statistical Manual of Mental Disorders* (DSM)-IV symptoms of opioid withdrawal are:

- dysphoric mood;

- nausea or vomiting;

- muscle aches;

- lacrimation or rhinorrhoea;

- pupillary dilation, piloerection or sweating;

- diarrhoea;

- yawning;

- fever;

- insomnia.

What features indicate drug dependence?

- Tolerance.

- Withdrawal symptoms on cessation.

- Greater use than initially intended.

- Time spent on drugs at the expense of other daily activities.

- Unsuccessful attempts to cut down.

- Continued use despite physical and psychological complications.

What social issues do you need to explore?

Ask the patient about her current social circumstances and social supports. What was happening in her life at the time her drug abuse started? Does she have children or might she be pregnant? Does she have a safe place to live? How does she fund her drug habit? Understanding these issues will help establish a therapeutic alliance as well as giving you a more holistic view of her problems.

> Poly-substance abuse is common among heroin users, but does not necessarily mean dependence on all the substances. Withdrawal symptoms from one substance may be altered by the presence of others.

What medical complications of drug abuse is it important to look for?

Chronic liver disease and its complications, endocarditis and HIV are the most common serious conditions seen with intravenous drug use.

Examination

People with drug-dependence problems may present in a demanding and overwhelming manner, but do not let this deter you from establishing objective evidence of drug use. Look for needle track marks, discoid scars from subcutaneous injection, burn marks on fingers and neglected self-care.

Look for the signs of opioid withdrawal (see above), and also for hypertension, tachycardia and temperature dysregulation.

Investigations

Urine test kits are now available in most emergency departments that will tell you within 10 minutes whether any drug or its metabolites are present in a urine sample. They usually just indicate the presence or absence of a drug, not the amount.

In this woman with an obvious septic focus it will be appropriate to check FBC, glucose, electrolytes, renal and liver function tests, clotting and blood cultures, and also to swab the abscess. These tests, including swabs of any areas that might be infected on clinical grounds, should be performed routinely on any drug users admitted to hospital since they are at risk of malnutrition and infections.

Further tests may be required if there are specific indications, eg echocardiography if there is a suspicion of endocarditis. It will also be appropriate to discuss with the patient whether she would like to be tested for hepatitis B and C, HIV and syphilis.

Management

In addition to drainage of the abscess, appropriate antimicrobial therapy and treatment of any other medical problems, the problem to be tackled is how opioid withdrawal should be prevented or treated.

How should opioid withdrawal be prevented or treated?

Always get advice from substance misuse specialists. If you have determined that the patient is dependent on opioids and is in withdrawal, then she will need methadone substitution to relieve her symptoms. If she is pregnant this is mandatory as opioid withdrawal is associated with spontaneous abortion and fetal death. Initially prescribe 10 mg methadone bd and monitor 4-hourly for withdrawal symptoms. Increase by 5–10 mg increments if withdrawal symptoms occur, up to a maximum of 20 mg bd in the first 24 hours. Observe for signs of opioid infection. Determine how much methadone is required over a 24-hour period and then that dose can be given as a single or divided dose. Beware of overdosing as this could result in respiratory arrest. Remember that she may be getting opioids from an alternative source while she is in hospital, so look for

TABLE 8 EQUIVALENT OPIOID DOSES

Drug	Dose	Methadone equivalent
Street heroin	Purity varies, hence impossible to make an accurate estimate	Purity varies, hence impossible to make an accurate estimate
Pharmaceutical heroin	10-mg tablet or ampoule	20 mg
Morphine	10-mg ampoule	10 mg
Dihydrocodeine (DF 118)	30-mg tablet	3 mg
Buprenorphine hydrochloride	200-μg tablet	5 mg
	300-μg ampoule	8 mg
Codeine phosphate	15-mg tablet	1 mg
J. Collis Browne 100 mL	10-mg extract of opium	10 mg

signs of intoxication and ensure that naloxone is available in case this occurs.

> ⚠ Methadone can cause fatal respiratory depression at a dose of 30 mg, or even lower if combined with other opioids, alcohol or benzodiazepines. Remember:
>
> - *never* give a methadone dose equivalent to what patients report they are using (Table 8);
> - *never* prescribe methadone to occasional opioid users.

Are there other drugs that can be used to relieve withdrawal symptoms?

Clonidine and lofexidine are centrally acting agents used to dampen down sympathetic tone, thereby reducing the severity of withdrawal symptoms. Try to avoid the use of benzodiazepines as these are frequently also abused.

When and where should opioid withdrawal be embarked upon?

An acute admission unit is not a suitable setting to embark on an opioid withdrawal programme. Aim to stabilise the dose of methadone the patient is receiving and then refer to a drug rehabilitation unit if withdrawal is deemed appropriate. Withdrawal should take 10–14 days.

Thinking ahead, what else would you want to do for this patient?

This may be the only contact she has with medical services, so try to provide her with some information about safer drugs use (harm minimisation), the availability of services and the dangers of HIV and hepatitis. Refer her to a psychiatrist if comorbidity is suspected or her behaviour is very challenging. Encourage attendance at a drug rehabilitation unit.

Strategies used here include motivational interviewing, cognitive-behaviour therapy, methadone maintenance or withdrawal programmes, inpatient treatment programmes, drug substitution and assistance with social problems. Naltrexone may be used to prevent relapse.

1.3.6 The frightening patient

> **Scenario**
>
> A tall and physically intimidating man is brought to the Emergency Department by the police. He appears dishevelled, is shouting abuse and lashing out at anyone who approaches him.

Introduction

What practical safety measures would you take when approaching a person who might be violent?

If you are concerned that a patient might be violent, observe the following precautions.

- Do not take any risks.

- Never see the patient alone.

- Call back-up, eg hospital security and/or police.

- Remove your tie, scarf or necklace.

- Make sure that you and other staff always have easy access to an exit door.

- Remove other patients from the area.

- Remove potential weapons from the area.

- Do not let hospital security and/or police leave until you feel the situation is safe.

- Check for concealed weapons.

What factors are known to be associated with violent behaviour?

- Men.

- Individuals under 30 years.

- Access to weapons.

- Drug and alcohol abuse.

> 🔑 When dealing with aggressive people in hospital, the first distinction you need to make is between people who are aggressive as a result of medical or mental illness (or from distress) and those who are habitually violent.
>
> The approach and management will be different in each case and the more information you can gather about the person, the better you will be equipped to make good decisions in a calm and rational manner. However, common themes include the following.
>
> - Medical or mental illness: some people react in an angry and blaming way to the feelings of uncertainty and loss of control that may accompany an illness. People with mental illness might be aggressive because they are very frightened by their symptoms. Understanding and reassurance go a long way to resolve these situations, while being rigidly authoritarian will just escalate matters.
> - Habitually violent or armed people need to be dealt with by the police service.

History of the presenting problem

Recognising that information from the patient may be sparse and that you may have to rely on collateral information from family, friends, the police and medical notes, ask the following questions.

- What is he normally like?

- When did this behaviour start?

- Did anything precipitate it?

- What was he doing when he was found by the police?

- Has he threatened or injured anyone?

- Has he destroyed property?

- Has he used drugs or alcohol?

- What has he been saying?

- Has he been making sense?

Having established information about the incident that led to the patient's arrest, what further information about him do you need to determine the underlying cause of his violent behaviour?

- Has he got any medical conditions, eg epilepsy or diabetes?

- Is he normally on medication and is he compliant?

- Has he received treatment for a mental illness?

- Does he have a history of aggressive behaviour?

- Does he have a history of drug and alcohol abuse?

- Has he been arrested or convicted in the past?

What mental disorders may present with violence?
If the violence is thought to be a result of mental illness, then consider the following:

- delirium/acute confusional state (see Section 1.3.1);

- mood disorders (see Section 2.12);

- psychotic disorders (see Sections 2.3 and 2.13).

Examination
The patient's general appearance may give clues to an underlying condition. What he is saying may indicate that he is confused or deluded. If he is behaving bizarrely or appearing to respond to hallucinations, then this may

suggest the presence of delirium or psychosis.

It is imperative to try to get his cooperation to do a physical examination, or as much of one as he can tolerate, in order to look for an underlying physical condition. However, if this is not possible you should record precisely why in the medical notes. Write down exactly what is said by the patient, including expletives!

Investigations
It may not be possible to perform any investigations before sedation is administered. If you are able to get the patient to cooperate, then only do what is absolutely necessary as excessive demands may irritate him. The following should certainly be considered.

- Check for drug abuse: urine drug screen (see Section 1.3.5).

- Check for alcohol abuse: breathalyser test or saliva alcohol test.

- Check for delirium: always check fingerprick blood glucose, and perform those tests listed in Section 1.3.1 that are indicated and possible. If the tests cannot be done, then your notes should explain precisely why, eg 'Patient would not allow venepuncture (told me to "xxxx off")'.

Management

How should you behave towards this man to calm him down?
Remember first and foremost not to risk your safety or that of other patients and hospital staff.

- Keep a calm, reassuring appearance.

- Be pleasant, clear and firm.

- Do not bargain with, argue with or threaten him.

- Minimise confrontational direct eye contact.

- Maintain a safe distance: do not invade his body space.

- Offer food and drink (cooled tea, not hot!).

- Reassure the patient and let him know that you appreciate how frightened or angry he must be and say that you would like to help.

- Praise any attempts at self-control, no matter how minor.

- Try to establish a rapport.

What about physical restraint?
Physical restraint should not be used and may be construed as assault. The police or staff trained in control and restraint may restrain him if necessary, but beware of positional asphyxia if a patient's movement or breathing is in any way restricted. Particularly hazardous is restraining the patient lying face down and applying pressure downwards on his back as this impairs breathing. If physical restraint is unavoidable, his vital signs must be continuously monitored.

What sedation can you use?
Always offer oral sedation first, but often intramuscular sedation is necessary. Start with lorazepam 1–4 mg po or im. If this is not effective, then add haloperidol in an initial dose of 2.5 mg po or im, rising to 5 mg or 10 mg if necessary.

What are the legal aspects of giving sedation against his will?
In extreme situations, sedation can be administered compulsorily as an emergency treatment under common law to contain the situation. The patient should immediately be assessed for treatment and admission under

the Mental Health Act 1983 (see Section 2.14).

What factors can reduce aggression in emergency and outpatient departments?

- Do not keep agitated patients waiting.

- Encourage patients to air their grievances.

- Keep patients informed about what you are doing.

- Staff in high-risk areas should receive training in control and restraint.

- Better security measures, eg video surveillance and security staff.

- The design and layout of clinics should be relaxing and pleasant, but with security in mind.

⚠ Caution must be taken if antipsychotics are required in patients with heart disease.

2.1 Dissociative disorders

Psychopathology

There is a temporary but drastic modification of an individual's character or sense of personal identity, usually to avoid emotional distress, but also occurring at times of extreme emotion, eg religious experiences.

Epidemiology

The exact prevalence is unknown. Dissociative disorders are more common in women and adolescents/young adults. They may occur in epidemics, especially in children. Dissociative amnesia is the most common, whereas fugue is rare. Dissociative identity disorder is less frequently diagnosed in the UK than in the USA. In the UK the symptoms are often felt to fit better with borderline personality disorder. As a symptom depersonalisation is very common, but as a recurrent persistent problem it is rare.

Clinical presentation

Dissociative disorders present in different ways and the features of recognisable syndromes are described in Table 9.

Differential diagnosis

Conditions that may present with dissociative symptoms include:

- schizophrenia;
- temporal lobe epilepsy;
- depression;
- head injury;
- delirium;
- dementia;
- drugs;
- acute stress disorder.

Treatment

Treatment needs to be tailored to the individual and the following are guiding principles.

- Treat any underlying medical and psychiatric illnesses that may be the primary problem.
- Identify and address stressors.
- Use psychological interventions to help the person process and integrate stressful feelings.

Prognosis

Dissociative amnesia and fugue usually remit as abruptly as they started and recovery is usually complete with few relapses. Dissociative identity disorder is often associated with borderline personality disorder and usually has a chronic course, seldom with complete resolution of symptoms.

FURTHER READING

Frankel FH. Dissociation: the clinical realities. *Am. J. Psychiatry* 1996; 153 (7 Suppl.): 64–70.

Gelder M, Harrison P and Cowen P, eds. *Shorter Oxford Textbook of Psychiatry*, 5th edn. Oxford: Oxford University Press, 2006: 212–16.

Sadock BJ and Sadock VA. *Kaplan & Sadock Synopsis of Psychiatry*, 9th edn. Philadelphia: Lippincott Williams and Wilkins, 2003: 676–91.

TABLE 9 TYPES OF DISSOCIATIVE DISORDER	
Type	**Characteristics**
Amnesia	Sudden inability to recall periods of past life or own identity
Fugue	Travel away from usual surroundings, amnesia for past identity and sometimes may even assume new identity
Identity disorder	Presence of two or more distinct identities/personality states
Depersonalisation	Mental processes or body are perceived as unreal, remote or automatised: individual is in a 'dream-like state'

2.2 Dementia

Psychopathophysiology

Dementia is characterised by:

- memory impairment;
- impairment in several other cognitive domains;
- a decline from previous levels of functioning;

- mood and behaviour changes;

- no impairment of consciousness.

Epidemiology

In community residents, 5% of those aged over 65 years and 20% of those aged over 80 years have dementia, comprising:

- 50% due to Alzheimer's disease;

- 10–20% due to dementia with Lewy bodies;

- 10–20% due to vascular dementia.

Huntington's disease affects women and men equally, and is usually diagnosed in the late thirties and forties. Prion diseases, eg Creutzfeldt–Jakob disease (including the new variant type), are rare and age of onset depends on the age at exposure to the prions and the incubation period. HIV and head injury affect a younger population. Minor cognitive problems due to HIV are common and AIDS dementia complex is the AIDS-defining illness in about 4.5% of cases.

Clinical presentation

The typical clinical presentations of the different types of dementia are shown in Table 10.

Executive dysfunction

Problems with planning, organisation, sequencing and abstraction, all of which are functions of the frontal lobe.

Differential diagnosis

Exclude reversible cause of cognitive dysfunction:

- 'pseudo-dementia' due to depression;

- delirium;

- alcohol;

TABLE 10 CLINICAL PRESENTATION OF DEMENTIA

Types of dementia	Clinical presentation
Alzheimer's disease	Gradual onset and decline. Features include forgetfulness, lack of spontaneity, disorientation, depressed mood, deterioration in self-care, dysphasia, apraxia, agnosia and executive dysfunction
Vascular dementia	Presence of vascular disease elsewhere. Course is typically fluctuating with stepwise progression. Is similar to Alzheimer's disease and differentiation is difficult, although the presence of strokes or localising signs are highly suggestive
Lewy body dementia	Fluctuating cognition, visual hallucinations, parkinsonism, sensitivity to antipsychotic drugs, falls/transient loss of consciousness/syncope, delusions
Frontal lobe dementia	Personality changes, executive dysfunction, deterioration in social skills, emotional blunting, disinhibition, language problems
HIV	Forgetfulness, slowness, poor concentration, problem-solving difficulty, apathy, neurological abnormalities
Head injury	Depends on the location and extent of brain injury. Features include memory impairment, attention problems, irritability, lability and apathy
Huntington's disease	Depression, irritability, anxiety, paranoia, choreoathetosis, memory impairment and problems with executive functioning (single autosomal dominant gene on chromosome 4)
Prion diseases	Fatigue, anxiety, poor concentration, involuntary movements, periodic abnormal electroencephalogram activity, progressive cognitive impairment

- hypothyroidism;

- syphilis;

- vitamin B_{12} deficiency;

- normal-pressure hydrocephalus;

- subdural haematoma.

Treatment

Consider the following.

- Social support.

- Behavioural problems managed through behavioural and environmental modifications. Rarely a short course of low-dose antipsychotic drugs (eg amisulpride) may be used as an adjunctive, but only when psychotic symptoms are present. Also antidepressants can be used to treat low mood and regulate sleep.

- Cholinesterase inhibitors in Alzheimer's disease, eg donepezil, rivastigmine and galantamine.

- Memantine (reversible N-methyl-D-asparate antagonist).

Complications

Be aware that the complications of dementia are not only medical but also social and behavioural problems, including:

- distress of care-givers;

- social isolation;

- self-neglect;

- risk of personal injury, eg accidents, falls and wandering;

- vulnerability to exploitation;

- aggression and other behavioural problems.

Prognosis

Alzheimer's disease has a variable course, but death usually occurs within 5–8 years of onset. Except for dementia due to head injury, all dementias are progressive, but in some their progression can be halted temporarily (eg HIV and Alzheimer's disease) or permanently (eg hypothyroidism and syphilis).

> Head injury predisposes to normal-pressure hydrocephalus, characterised by:
> - enlarged ventricles;
> - progressive dementia;
> - urinary incontinence;
> - gait disturbance.

Prevention
Consider the following:

- genetic counselling (Huntington's);

- cardiovascular disease prevention and treatment;

- intellectual stimulation.

Factors found to reduce risk in research (although not used clinically):

- antioxidants, eg vitamin E and selegiline;

- hormone-replacement therapy in Alzheimer's disease;

- NSAIDs in Alzheimer's disease.

Important information for patients
People with dementia should be encouraged to plan early for the eventual cessation of driving. Also financial planning needs to be done.

FURTHER READING

American Psychiatric Association. *Diagnostic and Statistical Manual of Mental Disorders: DSM-IV*, 4th edn. Washington, DC: American Psychiatric Association, 2000: 135–80.

Gelder M, Harrison P and Cowen P, eds. *Shorter Oxford Textbook of Psychiatry*, 5th edn. Oxford: Oxford University Press, 2006: 321–58.

Jones RW. Dementia. *Scott. Med. J.* 1997; 42: 151–3.

Khouzam HR, Donnelly NJ and Ibrahim NF. Psychiatric morbidity in HIV patients. *Can. J. Psychiatry* 1998; 43: 51–6.

Patterson CJ, Gauthier S, Bergman H, *et al.* The recognition, assessment and management of dementing disorders: conclusions from the Canadian consensus conference on dementia. *Can. Med. Assoc. J.* 1999; 160 (12 Suppl.): S1–S15.

2.3 Schizophrenia and antipsychotic drugs

2.3.1 Schizophrenia

Aetiology/psychopathology
Schizophrenia is currently believed to be a neurodevelopmental disorder. There is strong evidence of genetic risk, eg identical twins have a 48% chance of concordance. Structural changes seen in MRI studies include decreased volume of areas such as the parahippocampus, thalamus, superior temporal gyri and frontal lobes. Older neurotransmitter theories focused on defects in the dopamine system, but newer theories include defects in glutaminergic neurotransmission involving hippocampal N-methyl-D-aspartate receptors.

Epidemiology

- Prevalence: 0.5–1.5% of the general population.

- Incidence: 0.5–5 per 10,000 per year.

- Median age at onset: early to mid twenties for men, and late twenties for women.

Clinical presentation
An important aspect of schizophrenia is its devastating effect on an individual's interpersonal relationships, work, self-care and other goal-directed behaviours. The diagnosis of schizophrenia requires the presence of two or more of the symptoms listed in Table 11 for at least 1 month, and the total duration of the illness, including prodromal and residual symptoms, should be 6 months or longer. Take care to exclude mood disorders, substance abuse and general medical conditions.

TABLE 11 CORE SYMPTOMS OF SCHIZOPHRENIA

Symptoms	Characteristics
Delusions	False, unshakeable beliefs held with extraordinary conviction that are not amenable to logic, and out of keeping with the patient's social, cultural and educational background
Hallucinations	A perception experienced in the absence of an external stimulus to the sense organ involved, most commonly auditory
Disorganised speech	Loss of normal structure of thinking
Negative symptoms	Blunted affect, apathy, poverty of speech, attentional impairment, poor motivation
Disorganised behaviour	Excitement, stupor and mutism

Differential diagnosis

Other disorders presenting with schizophrenia-like symptoms include the following.

- Schizophreniform disorder: symptoms present for 1–6 months.

- Schizoaffective disorder: concurrent mania or severe depression.

- Delusional disorder: encapsulated delusions with minimal hallucinations.

- Brief psychotic disorder: duration less than 1 month.

- Shared psychotic disorder (*folie à deux*): a person without psychosis taking on the pyschotic symptoms of someone close.

- Due to general medical condition, eg high-dose steroids.

- Substance induced, eg amphetamine intoxication.

Treatment

This is a complex illness that needs a comprehensive treatment approach. Always obtain collateral information. Physical examination and special investigations are needed to exclude concurrent medical problems. A useful approach to treatment is to use the 'biological, psychological and social' guidelines shown in Table 12.

High expressed emotion, ie criticism, hostility and over-involvement of parents or care-givers towards people with schizophrenia is a significant risk factor for relapse.

Complications

! **Suicide**
Of patients with schizophrenia, 10% die by suicide and up to 50% attempt suicide.

Prognosis

Prognosis is variable and difficult to predict for any individual. Estimates are as follows:

- 10–15% have a good prognosis;

- 10–15% have a chronic, unremitting course;

- the remainder vary from occasional to frequent relapses.

Predictors of a poor outcome include the following:

- male sex;

- obstetric complications;

- abnormal premorbid personality;

- low IQ;

- single;

- early age at onset;

- insidious onset;

- substance abuse;

- family history of schizophrenia;

- absence of obvious precipitant.

2.3.2 Antipsychotics

General principles

About 70% of patients with schizophrenia respond to standard antipsychotic drugs, and a further 10% respond to atypical antipsychotics. Antipsychotics also significantly reduce relapse rates.

The main mechanism of action of antipsychotics is via blockade of dopamine receptors. The atypicals also act by blocking serotonin receptors in the striatal system and the frontal cortex, hence there are fewer extrapyramidal side effects and greater efficacy for negative symptoms.

Antipsychotics can be divided into low-potency, high-potency and atypical drugs (Table 13).

Indications

The main indication is for psychosis, and use in any other condition (Table 14) must be carefully considered because these drugs have severe side effects that can be permanent, most notably tardive dyskinesia.

! Use antipsychotics judiciously because of the risk of tardive dyskinesia.

TABLE 12 BIOLOGICAL, PSYCHOLOGICAL AND SOCIAL APPROACH FOR THE TREATMENT OF SCHIZOPHRENIA

Approach	Treatment
Biological	Antipsychotic medication
Psychological	Cognitive therapy Crisis management Social skills training
Social	Family therapy Vocational rehabilitation Psycho-education, eg recognising early signs of relapse

TABLE 13 SUBGROUPS OF ANTIPSYCHOTICS

Subgroup	Examples	Discussion
Low-potency drugs	Chlorpromazine	Generally associated with more anticholinergic, antihistaminergic and α-adrenergic blocking side effects. Therefore more epileptogenic and cardiotoxic (prolonged QT interval)
High-potency drugs	Haloperidol, trifluoperazine	Associated with greater extrapyramidal side effects
Atypical drugs	Clozapine, risperidone, olanzapine, quetiapine, amisulpride, aripiprazole	Far fewer side effects (except clozapine) Agranulocytosis is a serious problem with clozapine Weight gain and sedation can be problematic Can lead to metabolic syndrome, ie hypertension, diabetes and hyperlipidaemia

TABLE 14 OTHER CONDITIONS IN WHICH ANTIPSYCHOTICS ARE USED

Condition	Example of antipsychotic
Severe anxiety	Low doses used
Severe impulsivity	Low doses used
Tourette's syndrome	Haloperidol
Nausea	Prochlorperazine
Chronic hiccoughs	Chlorpromazine
Infant opioid withdrawal	Chlorpromazine
Emergency sedation	Haloperidol

TABLE 15 SIDE EFFECTS OF ANTIPSYCHOTICS

Side effect	Characteristic
Extrapyramidal symptoms	Stiffness, tremor, hypersalivation, acute dystonia, akathisia, tardive dyskinesia, tardive dystonia
Anticholinergic symptoms	Blurred vision, constipation, urinary retention, dry mouth, confusion, agitation, seizures
Antihistaminic symptoms	Sedation
α-Adrenergic blockade	Orthostatic hypotension
Leucopenia	Agranulocytosis can occur with all antipsychotics, but has a high incidence with clozapine
Increased prolactin secretion	Amenorrhoea, galactorrhoea, sexual dysfunction
Metabolic syndrome	Weight gain, hypertension, diabetes, hyperlipidaemia
Obstructive jaundice	Phenothiazines
Allergic dermatitis and photosensitivity	
Neuroleptic malignant syndrome	Muscle rigidity, hyperthermia, fluctuating level of consciousness and autonomic dysfunction, leucocytosis, elevated creatine phosphokinase

Antipsychotics

When using these drugs, remember:

- always use the lowest dose possible;
- start with a low dose and slowly titrate up until therapeutic effect is achieved;
- always be aware of side effects;
- do not use more than one antipsychotic at a time.

Contraindications

- Drowsiness, confusion, coma due to central nervous system depressants.
- Bone-marrow suppression.
- Phaeochromocytoma.
- If at all possible avoid use in patients who are pregnant or breast-feeding.

Complications

Side effects

Side effects to antipsychotics are common, and they can be severe and even life-threatening. These are listed and briefly described in Table 15.

Most important adverse effects of antipsychotics

- Agranulocytosis.
- Neuroleptic malignant syndrome.
- Acute dystonia.
- Tardive dyskinesia.
- Akathisia.

FURTHER READING

American Psychiatric Association. *Diagnostic and Statistical Manual of Mental Disorders: DSM-IV*, 4th edn. Washington, DC: American Psychiatric Association, 2000: 297–344.

Kane JM. Management strategies for the treatment of schizophrenia. *J. Clin. Psychiatry* 1999; 60 (Suppl. 12): 13–17.

McGrath J and Emmerson WB. Treatment of schizophrenia. *BMJ* 1999; 319: 1045–8.

Sadock BJ and Sadock VA. *Kaplan & Sadock Synopsis of Psychiatry*, 9th edn. Philadelphia: Lippincott Williams and Wilkins, 2003: 1104–12.

Schultz SK and Andreasen NC. Schizophrenia. *Lancet* 1999; 353: 1425–30.

2.4 Personality disorder

Psychopathology
Personality disorder (PD) is defined in the *Diagnostic and Statistical Manual of Mental Disorders* (DSM)-IV as an enduring pattern of inner experience and behaviour that:

- deviates markedly from the expectations of the individual's culture;

- is pervasive and inflexible;

- has an onset in adolescence or early adulthood;

- is stable over time;

- leads to distress or impairment in interpersonal and social functioning.

PD is often accompanied by a history of being abused or having behavioural disturbances during childhood. There are different types of PD (Table 16).

Epidemiology
Prevalence ranges between 2 and 13% in the general population. There are gender differences:

- antisocial PD is diagnosed more frequently in men;

- histrionic, borderline and dependent PDs are diagnosed more frequently in women.

Clinical presentation
The diagnosis needs a longitudinal view of a person's lifelong behaviour patterns. Difficult and odd behaviour in reaction to a stressful situation can easily be confused with a PD.

Factors that must always be assessed in PD

- Deliberate self-harm.
- Aggression.
- Violence.
- Impulsivity.
- Suicide.

Comorbid mental illness is frequently present, eg depression, drug dependence, alcohol dependence and anxiety disorders.

Treatment
Psychotherapy remains the mainstay of treatment. The success rate of patients recovering sufficiently to no longer meet the diagnostic criteria for PD can be as high as 52%. Types of psychotherapy used include:

- psychodynamic therapy;

- cognitive-behaviour therapy;

- interpersonal therapy;

- dialectic therapy;

- group therapy.

Certain PDs tend to be resistant to treatment, eg antisocial PD.

Drug treatments are only occasionally effective in reducing problematic behaviours and should be prescribed in a specialist setting only. The following have been found to have some limited efficacy:

- antipsychotics and selective serotonin reuptake inhibitors at low doses for impulsive, deliberate self-harm behaviour;

- carbamazepine for aggressive behaviour.

Drug treatments can be effective when they are used to treat a comorbid illness, eg treat depression and problem behaviours may abate.

Prognosis
The course of PD is variable, but as a general rule it ameliorates with age and may even remit.

FURTHER READING

American Psychiatric Association. *Diagnostic and Statistical Manual of Mental Disorders: DSM-IV*, 4th edn. Washington, DC: American Psychiatric Association, 2000: 685–730.

TABLE 16 CLASSIFICATION OF PERSONALITY DISORDERS

Cluster	Types	Characteristics
A	Paranoid, schizoid and schizotypal	Often appear odd or eccentric
B	Antisocial, borderline, histrionic and narcissistic	Often appear dramatic, emotional and erratic
C	Avoidant, dependent and obsessive–compulsive	Often appear anxious or fearful

Dhossche DM and Shevitz SA. Assessment and importance of personality disorders in medical patients: an update. *South. Med. J.* 1999; 92: 546–56.

– – – – – – – – – – – – – – – – –

Marlowe M and Sugarman P. Disorders of personality. *BMJ* 1997; 315: 176–9.

– – – – – – – – – – – – – – – – –

Perry JC, Banon E and Ianni F. Effectiveness of psychotherapy for personality disorders. *Am. J. Psychiatry* 1999; 156: 1312–21.

2.5 Psychiatric presentation of physical disease

Epidemiology

Psychiatric symptoms are common in general medical conditions, for example:

- on general medical wards, 15–25% of patients experience delirium;

- 30–50% of patients with epilepsy have a psychiatric difficulty at some time.

Clinical presentation

When medical conditions have psychiatric symptoms as part of their presentation, it is necessary to decide whether the psychiatric symptoms are:

- a result of the medical illness;

- part of a separate mental disorder;

- a psychological reaction to having an illness (see Section 2.6).

Symptoms should be elicited that identify serious mental illness or distress, and which need to be addressed urgently. These symptoms include:

- hopelessness;
- thoughts of suicide;
- guilt;
- loss of interest;
- severe insomnia;
- psychosis.

Common mental disorders that may be the result of an underlying medical condition or medication are as follows:

- delirium;

- dementia;

- amnesia;

- mood disorders;

- anxiety disorders;

- sleep disorder;

- sexual dysfunction.

Medical conditions that commonly present with symptoms and signs of mental disorder include:

- epilepsy;

- degenerative disorders, eg Parkinson's, Huntington's and Wilson's diseases;

- brain tumours;

- head trauma;

- demyelinating disorders;

- infectious disease, eg syphilis, encephalitis, meningitis, Creutzfeldt–Jakob disease and HIV (AIDS);

- autoimmune disorders, eg systemic lupus erythematosus;

- endocrine disorders, eg thyroid, pituitary and adrenal disease;

- metabolic disorders, eg hepatic, uraemic, hypoglycaemic encephalopathies and porphyria;

- nutritional disorders, eg thiamine and niacin deficiencies;

- toxins, eg organophosphates and heavy metals.

Other comorbid problems that may complicate the picture

- Alcohol and drug abuse.
- Personality disorders.
- Factitious disorders and malingering.

Treatment

A general principle is to address medical problems as far as possible before attempting to treat any psychiatric symptoms or suspected mental disorders, because these may resolve. However, circumstances may be such that recovery from the medical condition is dependent on the person's mental health and his or her ability to cooperate, in which case the psychiatric symptoms should be treated early. For example, a person with diabetes may find that motivation to remain compliant with treatment is poor because of concurrent depression.

Psychiatric treatments in physical illness

Treatments are the same as would be used in patients who do not have concurrent physical illness, but be aware of drug interactions and adverse effects, eg anticholinergic effects of tricyclic antidepressants.

Treatment strategies to help alleviate psychiatric symptoms include the following.

- Use an empathic, reassuring approach.

- Ensure the patient's physical needs are met, eg hydration and nutrition.

- Provide information about illness, investigations, treatments and their likely effects to help allay any fears and anxieties.

- The nursing environment should be well lit, quiet and tranquil.

- Invite the patient's family or other people who are familiar to visit.

- Hypnotics and anxiolytics should only be used if the patient is not responding to the above treatment strategies.

If there is concern that the patient is severely depressed or psychotic, a psychiatric opinion should be sought immediately. Furthermore, a psychiatric assessment may be helpful in identifying the psychological processes that are affecting recovery and compliance.

TABLE 17 POSSIBLE INTERACTIONS BETWEEN THE MIND AND PHYSICAL ILLNESS	
Relationship with physical illness	**Clinical example**
Coincidental	A person with schizophrenia contracts pneumonia
Causal	Physical illness causing psychiatric disorder, eg hypothyroidism causing depression
Reactive	Anxiety and depression are the commonest reactions to threatening or progressive illness
Iatrogenic	Treatment of physical illness causes a psychiatric disorder, eg L-dopa causing delirium
Reciprocal	Failure to mobilise after a stroke causing or caused by depression
Compliance	Poor compliance, eg in the depressed diabetic or in the patient with memory impairment
Somatisation	Psychiatric illness presents as a physical one
Denial	A psychological defence mechanism by which frightening news, eg a diagnosis of cancer, is excluded from conscious awareness and the patient behaves as if unaware of the distressing facts

FURTHER READING

Gelder M, Harrison P and Cowen P, eds. *Shorter Oxford Textbook of Psychiatry*, 5th edn. Oxford: Oxford University Press, 2006: 165–8.

– – – – – – – – – – – – – – – – –

Sadock BJ and Sadock VA. *Kaplan & Sadock Synopsis of Psychiatry*, 9th edn. Philadelphia: Lippincott Williams and Wilkins, 2003: 350–70.

2.6 Psychological reactions to physical illness (adjustment disorders)

Aetiology/psychopathology
When considering the possibility of a psychiatric disorder in a physically ill person, think of the possible interactions between mind, body and behaviour (Table 17).

The commonest reactions to physical illness and disability are adjustment disorders. These are generally seen in primary care, but 5–20% of psychiatric outpatients may present with this clinical picture. The stressor is usually much less intense and severe than in cases of post-traumatic stress disorder. The onset should be within 1 month or so of the stressful event. Predisposing factors include personality disorder or immature personality or a succession of major life events.

Epidemiology
Males and females are equally affected.

Clinical presentation

- Usually presentation is with severe subjective distress and emotional disturbance (this is based on the clinician's own subjective judgement).

- Impairment of social functioning and performance.

- Onset is within 1 month of a significant life change, leading to continued unpleasant circumstances.

Symptoms include:

- depressed mood;

- tearfulness and/or hopelessness;

- nervousness;

- anxiety;

- disproportionate worrying;

- inability to cope or plan ahead;

- disability in performance of daily routine.

The symptoms are not sufficiently severe to justify a more specific diagnosis such as major depression. The usual duration is a maximum of 6 months. Symptoms can last longer in a chronic disabling medical condition.

Diagnosing depression in physical illness

Approximately 30% of patients with cancer develop depression, a generalised anxiety disorder or an adjustment disorder within the first 2 years of diagnosis, but only a small proportion of this morbidity is recognised and treated.

Depression in physical illness

Be aware of the following:

- dismissing depression as an understandable reaction to severe illness;
- biological symptoms are unreliable, therefore use the Hospital Anxiety and Depression (HAD) Scale;
- depressive cognitions, eg 'I deserve to be ill' or 'I am not worth treating'; also a loss of interest in other people;
- suicidal ideas;
- tearfulness (especially in men);
- indecisiveness;
- any past history of depression.

The diagnosis of depression in patients with physical illness can be complicated by the presence of:

- fatigue;
- loss of appetite and sex drive;
- insomnia.

These symptoms can also be the typical biological symptoms of depression. Therefore, it is helpful to use the HAD Scale that excludes somatic symptoms and concentrates on the psychological symptoms of depression and anxiety (Fig. 2). This self-rating scale has only 14 items and is easy to complete and to score. It was designed specifically for use in non-psychiatric hospital departments. A score of 11 or more on either the anxiety or the depression subscale indicates 'caseness' (the range on each subscale is 0–21).

Treatment

- Encourage discussion and ventilation of feelings to help overcome denial and avoidance.

- Teach a problem-solving technique.

Problem-solving technique

Problem-solving is a straightforward counselling technique with the following components:

- listing the problems;

- selecting one specific problem to focus on;

- listing alternative courses of action;

- evaluating each action plan;

- selecting and implementing the most promising course of action;

- evaluating results of the trial;

- repeating the process until positive results are obtained.

This technique is applied collaboratively with the patient, who takes responsibility for the process, thereby enhancing their sense of autonomy and control.

Complications

- Decreased compliance with medical treatment.

- Increased length of hospital stay.

- Impaired performance at work.

- Disruption of social relationships.

- Increased risk of suicide attempts and suicide.

FURTHER READING

Hawton K, Salkovskis PM, Kirk J and Clark DM. *Cognitive Behaviour Therapy for Psychiatric Problems: a Practical Guide.* Oxford: Oxford University Press, 1989.

House A, Mayou R and Mallinson C, eds. *Psychiatric Aspects of Physical Disease.* London: Royal College of Physicians and Royal College of Psychiatrists, 1995.

Murray Parkes C and Markus A, eds. *Coping With Loss: Helping Patients and Their Families.* London: BMJ Publishing Group, 1998.

Van Der Molen B. *Communication and Cancer: How to Give and Receive Information.* London: The Cancer Resource Centre, 1999.

Zigmond AS and Snaith RP. The Hospital Anxiety And Depression Scale. *Acta Psychiatr. Scand.* 1983; 67: 361–70.

2.7 Anxiety disorders

Anxiety is familiar to everyone as an adaptive response to external threat. Normal fear and apprehension are accompanied by increased activity of the sympathetic nervous system in preparation for 'fight or flight'. Anxiety becomes pathological when it is excessive, prolonged or recurrent, and also focused on bodily sensations (Table 18).

TABLE 18 COMPARISON OF NORMAL AND MORBID (PATHOLOGICAL) ANXIETY

Feature	Normal anxiety	Morbid (pathological) anxiety
Reaction to a threat	Proportionate	Excessive
Duration	Brief	Prolonged
Focus of attention	Towards the external world	Morbid preoccupation with a physiological response, eg rapid heart beat means imminent heart attack

This questionnaire will help you to let us know how you are. Read each item and underline the response which comes closest to how you have felt in the last few days. Don't take too long over your replies, your Immediate reaction will probably be more accurate than a long thought-out response.

I feel tense or 'wound up'

Most of the time

A lot of the time

From time to time, occasionally

Not at all

I still enjoy the things I used to enjoy

Definitely as much

Not quite as much

Only a little

Hardly at all

I get a sort of frightened feeling as if something awful is about to happen

Very definitely and quite badly

Yes, but not badly

A little, but it doesn't worry me

Not at all

I can laugh and see the funny side of things

As much as I always could

Not quite so much now

Definitely not as much now

Not at all

Worrying thoughts go through my mind

A great deal of the time

A lot of the time

From time to time but not often

Only occasionally

I feel cheerful

Not at all

Not often

Sometimes

Most of the time

I can sit at ease and feel relaxed

Definitely

Usually

Not often

Not at all

I feel as if I am slowed down

Nearly all the time

Very often

Sometimes

Not at all

I get a sort of frightened feeling like 'butterflies' in my stomach

Not at all

Occasionally

Quite often

Very often

I have lost interest in my appearance

Definitely

I don't take as much care as I should

I may not take quite as much care

I take just as much care as ever

I feel restless as if I have to be on the move

Very much indeed

Quite a lot

Not very much

Not at all

I look forward with enjoyment to things

As much as ever I did

Rather less than I used to

Definitely less than I used to

Hardly at all

I get sudden feelings of panic

Very often indeed

Quite often

Not very often

Not at all

I can enjoy a good book or radio or TV programme

Often

Sometimes

Not often

Very seldom

▲ **Fig. 2** Hospital Anxiety and Depression Scale. Four options follow each statement: the best response (least anxious or depressed) scores 0; the worst response (most anxious or depressed) scores 3.

TABLE 19 DISTINCTION BETWEEN GENERALISED ANXIETY DISORDER (GAD), PANIC DISORDER AND PHOBIAS

Diagnosis	Characteristics of morbid anxiety
GAD	Continuous, pervasive and persistent ('free floating')
Panic disorder	Episodic with intense unpredictable panic attacks lasting up to 30 minutes. Can occur in any situation
Phobias	Situation specific

Morbid anxiety can be:

- generalised (generalised anxiety disorder) (see below);

- episodic (panic disorder) (see Section 2.7.2);

- situational (phobias) (see Section 2.7.3).

The distinction between these is shown in Table 19. See also Section 1.2.1.

2.7.1 Generalised anxiety disorder

Aetiology/psychopathology

A genetic contribution to generalised anxiety disorder (GAD) has not yet been established.

Biology of anxiety

- Release of noradrenaline, eg by yohimbine, increases anxiety.

- γ-Aminobutyric acid inhibits anxiety.

There may be an underlying anxious personality disorder (see Section 2.4) with long-standing persistent and pervasive feelings of tension, apprehension and inferiority, along with an intense fear of disapproval and rejection.

The precipitating event is generally a threat to the person's security in a relationship or at work, or being given the diagnosis of a serious physical illness. Thus, 'danger events' (ie the expectation of loss or deprivation) precede anxiety, whereas depression tends to be preceded by actual loss. Anxiety reactions are more likely to occur where there is lack of social support due to separation, divorce or bereavement. Some physical disorders and drugs may mimic GAD (Table 20).

Epidemiology

- The 6-month prevalence is 2.5–6.5%. The Office for Population Censuses and Surveys National Survey of Psychiatric Morbidity found that in the week before they were interviewed nearly 3% of the population had a GAD and over 7% had a mixed anxiety–depression.

- More common in females. This might be due to conflict between work and the responsibilities of child care.

- Rates of neurotic disorders such as anxiety are much commoner in those with lower socioeconomic status.

- Onset is commonest in late adolescence and early adulthood.

Clinical presentation

Anxiety states are characterised by a combination of psychological and somatic symptoms.

Psychological symptoms

- Inappropriate and excessive sense of apprehensiveness and dread that impairs everyday functioning.

- Excessive fear of loss, illness, death, accidents, losing control and going insane.

- Irritability, restlessness, worrying, poor concentration and insomnia.

- Thoughts of impending personal catastrophe.

TABLE 20 MEDICAL DISORDERS AND DRUGS THAT MAY CAUSE ANXIETY

Medical disorders	Hyperthyroidism Hypoglycaemia Cardiac dysrhythmia Phaeochromocytoma Respiratory dysfunction
Prescribed drugs	Selective serotonin reuptake inhibitors Sympathomimetics
Recreational drugs	Caffeine Amphetamine Cocaine LSD
Drug withdrawal	Alcohol Benzodiazepines Opiates

TABLE 21 SOMATIC SYMPTOMS OF ANXIETY

Somatic symptom	Signs
Autonomic arousal	Palpitations
	Muscle tremor
	Sweating
	Epigastric discomfort
Muscle tension	Constricting headaches
	Backache
Hyperventilation	Paraesthesiae
	Headache
	Dizziness
	Faintness

Somatic symptoms

These arise from autonomic arousal, muscle tension and hyperventilation (Table 21). Hyperventilation causes a low $P\text{co}_2$ and alkalosis.

GAD can affect various systems of the body.

- Cardiac: tachycardia and palpitations.

- Pulmonary: hyperventilation, tightness in chest and breathlessness.

- Gastrointestinal: dry mouth, difficulty in swallowing, 'butterflies in the stomach', nausea and frequent bowel motions.

- Urinary: frequency.

- Neurological: headache, light-headedness, paraesthesiae around mouth and in hands, tremor and muscle aches.

- Autonomic: sweating, shakiness, feeling too hot or cold, and erectile impotence.

Treatment

- Be circumspect with benzodiazepines. Beta-blockers might help to reduce tremor. A sedative antidepressant, eg trazodone, reduces insomnia.

- Cognitive-behaviour therapy is the safest and most effective treatment.

Complications

- Anxiety disorders are associated with increased mortality due to suicide as well as alcohol and smoking-related disorders.

- Dependence on benzodiazepines, hypnotics and alcohol.

Prognosis

Good prognostic indicators

- A stable premorbid personality.

- Development of acute symptoms in response to transitory stress.

Poor prognostic indicators

- Chronic or severe symptoms.

- Agitation, depersonalisation or conversion symptoms.

- Suicidal preoccupations.

- Persistent social/occupational factors.

- Inadequate social support.

Patients with an anxiety disorder:

- might have a concurrent depressive illness;
- might later develop a depressive illness;
- might present with somatic rather than psychological symptoms;
- might have an underlying medical disorder (see Table 20).

2.7.2 Panic disorder

Aetiology/psychopathology

Panic disorder consists of recurrent bouts of intense and rapidly escalating anxiety associated with the unrealistic anticipation of imminent personal catastrophe. The condition is probably caused by the interaction between biochemical and psychological events, perhaps from a biochemical abnormality associated with poorly regulated autonomic responses. Patients with panic disorder are more likely than normal subjects to experience panic attacks when given yohimbine (an α-adrenergic antagonist) or sodium lactate infusions.

Panic disorder is five times commoner in first-degree relatives than in the general population.

Psychological factors

Patients with panic disorder are more likely than those with generalised anxiety disorder (GAD) to make alarming deductions from the physical symptoms of anxiety. According to this cognitive hypothesis, there is a vicious circle of fear (Fig. 3) that intensifies the autonomic response so that the patient interprets an increase in heart rate as a sign of an imminent heart attack, which in turn heightens anxiety and further accelerates heart rate.

Epidemiology

There is a lifetime prevalence of 1.5%, with onset usually before the age of 40. There is a female to male ratio of 2:1.

Clinical presentation

The patient experiences repeated unexpected bouts of severe anxiety that can occur in any situation and which are not restricted to certain places. The physical and

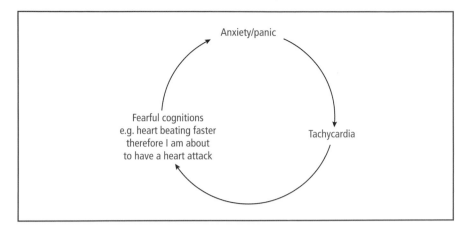

▲ **Fig. 3** The vicious circle of emotion, autonomic response and negative thoughts.

psychological symptoms of panic disorder are similar to those of GAD, but are episodic and more intense. There is an overwhelming fear of loss of control and of imminent death, generally from a heart attack. As the disorder progresses, fear and avoidance of specific situations develops, generally of places such as supermarket checkout queues and public transport where the patient fears becoming trapped and unable to obtain emergency medical assistance. As the patient becomes increasingly house-bound, the disorder might be more appropriately labelled 'panic disorder with agoraphobia'.

Differential diagnosis

Panic attacks can occur in the course of GAD, agoraphobia, depression and alcohol withdrawal. The diagnosis of panic disorder depends on the characteristics and severity of the panic attacks, and on whether their onset precedes one of these other conditions.

Treatment

- Provide reassurance and explanation by describing the interaction between fear and overactivity of the sympathetic nervous system.

- Give the patient a simple diagram of the vicious circle that develops

when fear caused by the physical symptoms of anxiety intensifies thoughts of imminent catastrophe (see Fig. 3).

- Benzodiazepines are to be avoided in the longer-term treatment of panic disorder because of the risk of dependence.

- Antidepressants have anti-panic effects.

- Cognitive-behaviour therapy: this is as effective as antidepressants and has a lower relapse rate.

Antidepressents used include the following.

- Imipramine: low starting dose of 10 mg daily (a higher initial dose can actually exacerbate anxiety and insomnia). The dose is gradually increased over a period of weeks to about 150 mg daily. Be aware of cardiovascular and anticholinergic side effects as well as α-adrenoceptor blockade and the risk of seizures. Note that about one-third of patients with panic disorder relapse when imipramine is withdrawn.

- Selective serotonin reuptake inhibitors: be aware of rebound anxiety when the antidepressant is withdrawn as well as common gastrointestinal and sexual side effects.

Complications

- Major depressive disorder occurs in at least half of those who have panic disorder.

- Agoraphobia is a common complication.

- Some patients become dependent on alcohol as a form of self-medication.

- Benzodiazepine dependence is not uncommon.

Prognosis

The course tends to fluctuate. Even with treatment 20–30% of patients with panic disorder are symptomatic at 6-year follow-up.

FURTHER READING

Allgulander C. Suicide and mortality patterns in anxiety neurosis and depressive neurosis. *Arch. Gen. Psychiatry* 1994; 51: 702–12.

Clark DM and Fairburn CG. *Science and Practice of Cognitive Behaviour Therapy.* Oxford: Oxford University Press, 1997.

Finlay-Jones R. Anxiety. In: Brown GW and Harris TO, eds. *Life Events and Illness.* London: Unwin Hyman, 1989: 95–112.

Melzer H, Gill B and Petticrew M. *The Prevalence of Psychiatric Morbidity Among Adults Aged 16–64 Living in Private Households in Great Britain.* OPCS Surveys of Psychiatric Morbidity in Great Britain, Report no. 1. London: Office of Population Censuses and Surveys, 1995.

Rickels K and Schweizer E. The clinical presentation of generalized anxiety in primary-care settings: practical concepts of classification and management. *J. Clin. Psychiatry* 1997; 58 (Suppl. 11): 4–10.

Snaith RP. *Clinical Neurosis*, 2nd edn. Oxford: Oxford University Press, 1991.

2.7.3 Phobic anxiety disorders

Aetiology
The cardinal features of phobias are fear and avoidance. The fear is disproportionate to the circumstances and the patient recognises this. Despite this insight, the phobic patient feels intensely anxious at the very thought of a particular situation.

Phobias are classified as:

- specific (simple);
- blood/injection/injury;
- agoraphobia;
- social phobia.

Specific (simple) phobias
Simple phobias can sometimes be traced to a single traumatic incident, such as being stuck in a lift or underground train, being attacked by a vicious dog or having been involved in a road traffic accident. Specific phobias might sound trivial but they can severely impair performance at work and in social life (eg due to inability to travel by plane). Specific phobias include familiar fears of:

- spiders;
- snakes;
- heights;
- flying;
- thunder.

Blood/injection/injury phobia
Blood/injection/injury phobia can occur after a traumatic medical incident, and is the most important phobia in the hospital setting. Triggers include the sight of blood, injury or medical apparatus, especially syringes and needles. There might also be excessive fear of contamination. A phobia of diseases such as AIDS might lead to total

avoidance of physical contact with other people, repeated medical consultations or multiple requests for HIV testing. These phobias can lead to:

- delay in seeking medical help;
- refusal to have blood tests;
- reluctance to submit to any invasive medical procedure.

Blood/injection/injury phobia is associated with an unusual physiological response. Whereas other specific phobias are associated with an acceleration of the heart rate on exposure to the focus of fear and avoidance, those suffering from blood/injection/injury phobia have a strong vasovagal response with deceleration of heart rate and a fall in BP, which could lead to syncope.

Agoraphobia
Agoraphobia sometimes follows the occurrence of one or two isolated panic attacks in a public, crowded or confined space. Fear of further episodes subsequently discourages the patient from leaving home. This avoidance behaviour prevents habituation and perpetuates the condition. The phobia is reinforced by the conviction that further potentially harmful panic attacks

will occur if the patient ventures out again.

Social phobias
Social phobias tend to occur in shy and unconfident people, and might be precipitated by an embarrassing incident. Thus, a sensitive person whose credit card is rejected due to a computer error might subsequently be afraid to sign cheques in public because of a fear that an anxious tremor will be noticed.

Epidemiology
The epidemiology of various phobias is shown in Table 22.

Clinical presentation
The phobic patient experiences both the psychological and the somatic symptoms of morbid anxiety in specific circumstances. Even the anticipation of those situations provokes anxiety and this leads to avoidance. Patients may postpone seeking treatment until there is a change in their domestic or occupational circumstances which forces them to seek help. For example, the social phobic may be given the responsibility of making a public presentation; an agoraphobic may lose a relative who used to do

TABLE 22 EPIDEMIOLOGY OF PHOBIAS

	Age of onset, general	Male/female ratio	Other features	Prevalence in population (%)
Specific phobias	From childhood	F > M	Might follow traumatic event, eg being trapped in a lift	10
Blood/injury/injection phobia	From childhood	F > M	Vasovagal reaction and a positive family history	Not known
Agoraphobia	Age 20–40	F > M	Often associated with panic attacks	3
Social phobia	Mid-teens	F = M		2.5

his or her shopping; whilst a blood/injection/injury phobic might develop severe anaemia and need to have laboratory tests.

Agoraphobia

Agoraphobics fear and avoid any situation from which escape might be difficult or embarrassing. Agoraphobic people are afraid of:

- leaving home;
- going into crowded places (eg supermarkets);
- collapsing, having a convulsion or fainting;
- going mad;
- being incontinent in a public place;
- having a heart attack without access to immediate help.

Social phobia

Social phobia is the fear and avoidance of social situations (eg restaurants, parties, public speaking and committee meetings). In social phobia the fear is that others will regard the person as socially clumsy or will notice his or her anxiety-induced tremulousness or sweating.

Differential diagnosis

A delusional disorder (see Section 2.13) has to be excluded in both social phobias and agoraphobia.

- Social phobic people retain insight and recognise that the fear that other people will observe and judge them critically is excessive and disproportionate. They are aware that their discomfort derives from their own self-consciousness. In contrast, paranoid persons suspect that other people regard them with unjustified hatred and malevolence.

- Both agoraphobic and paranoid people will be afraid to venture out of their homes, but agoraphobics are house-bound because they fear their own anxiety and panic, while the paranoid person locates danger in other people's actions and intentions.

Patients with dysmorphophobia (body dysmorphic disorder) might also eschew social events and public places.

Treatment

Cognitive-behaviour therapy is the treatment of choice.

Complications

Dependence on alcohol and benzodiazepines.

Prognosis

Without treatment phobias tend to follow a chronic course.

FURTHER READING

Clark DM and Fairburn CG. *Science and Practice of Cognitive Behaviour Therapy.* Oxford: Oxford University Press, 1997.

Hawton K, Salkovskis PM, Kirk J and Clark DM. *Cognitive Behaviour Therapy for Psychiatric Problems: a Practical Guide.* Oxford: Oxford University Press, 1989.

Liebowitz MR. Update on the diagnosis and treatment of social anxiety disorder. *J. Clin. Psychiatry* 1999; 60 (Suppl. 18): 22–6.

Marks IM. *Fears, Phobias and Rituals: Panic, Anxiety and Their Disorders.* New York: Oxford University Press, 1987.

Stravynski A and Greenberg D. The treatment of social phobia: a critical assessment. *Acta Psychiatr. Scand.* 1998; 98: 171–81.

2.8 Obsessive–compulsive disorder

Aetiology/psychopathology

There is a possible genetic contribution to obsessive–compulsive disorder. A significant proportion of sufferers have a previous personality characterised by extreme punctuality, orderliness and cleanliness. Obsessive–compulsive disorder can be accompanied by soft neurological signs. Obsessional symptoms can also occur in a number of organic disorders including Huntington's chorea and Tourette's syndrome. Obsessive–compulsive disorder can follow head injury and encephalitis. Studies of cerebral metabolic function show an association between obsessive–compulsive symptoms and striatal and orbitofrontal activity.

Epidemiology

The prevalence is 1.3% of the general population. Men and women are equally affected.

Clinical presentation

- Obsessions: unwanted, distressing and intrusive thoughts, images or impulses which the patient recognises as coming from his or her own mind. They are involuntary and the sufferer tries to suppress them, but this resistance only heightens their frequency and intensity. Both the obsessions themselves and the attempts to resist them cause severe anxiety.

- Compulsions: stereotyped actions which are carried out to neutralise either the anxiety caused by obsessional urges and images or their imaginary disastrous consequences.

	Obsessive–compulsive disorder	Phobia	Paranoid delusions
TABLE 23 DIFFERENTIAL DIAGNOSIS OF OBSESSIVE–COMPULSIVE DISORDER			
Focus of fear	Fear of consequences of obsessions or of failure to carry out compulsive rituals	Fear and avoidance of specific situations which induce marked anxiety	Fear of danger to self from imaginary enemies
Insight	Retained (the patient partly recognises that fears are irrational and absurd)	Retained (the patient is aware that fear is disproportionate to objective danger)	Absent (the patient is absolutely convinced that the danger is real and does not try to suppress unusual thoughts)

The clinical features of obsessions are:

- recurrent;
- unbidden;
- unwelcome;
- distressing;
- resisted;
- cannot be got rid of;
- accompanied by anxiety;
- lead to 'cancelling out' rituals.

Compulsive rituals include repetitive washing of hands, cleaning and checking, which provide temporary relief from the anxiety caused by the obsession itself or its feared consequences, eg that a blasphemous thought might cause a beloved relative to develop a malignant disease. Compulsive rituals are often performed a specific number of times. Many patients have obsessional doubts (*folie de doute*) which make them feel uncertain about whether they have actually carried out their rituals, so they then feel compelled to repeat this activity.

The content of obsessions is often obscene, sadistic or blasphemous. The patient might have recurrent ruminations about danger, disaster, disease or contamination. Obsessions and compulsions can occur in the course of a depressive illness and might remit on recovery from the depression.

Differential diagnosis

The main differential diagnoses to be considered are phobias and paranoid delusions: see the specific characteristics in Table 23.

> Of patients with major depression 30% have obsessional symptoms, while 30% of patients with obsessive–compulsive disorder also suffer from major depression.

Treatment

This consists of either behaviour therapy and/or pharmacotherapy.

Behaviour therapy

This treatment consists of exposure to the environmental triggers that provoke compulsive rituals (eg contact with dirt), combined with prevention from carrying out the ritual activity such as compulsive hand washing (prolonged exposure and response prevention). This treatment produces long-lasting improvement in up to two-thirds of patients. Behaviour therapy can be supplemented by cognitive therapy which teaches the patient to challenge the content of the obsessions.

Medication

Serotonergic antidepressants such as clomipramine and fluoxetine reduce obsessive–compulsive symptoms, especially where there is concurrent clinical depression. The prognosis is more favourable if obsessive–compulsive disorder is secondary to depression.

Complications

Severe depression.

Prognosis

The course tends to be chronic.

FURTHER READING

Marks IM. *Fears, Phobias and Rituals: Panic, Anxiety and Their Disorders*. New York: Oxford University Press, 1987.

Marks IM, Lelliot P, Basoglu M, *et al*. Clomipramine, self-exposure and therapist-aided exposure for obsessive–compulsive rituals. *Br. J. Psychiatry* 1988; 52: 522–34.

Piccinelli M, Pini S, Bellantuono C and Wilkinson G. Efficacy of drug treatment in obsessive–compulsive disorder: a meta-analytic review. *Br. J. Psychiatry* 1995; 166: 424–43.

Pigott TA and Seay SM. A review of the efficacy of selective serotonin reuptake inhibitors in obsessive–compulsive disorder. *J. Clin. Psychiatry* 1999; 60: 101–6.

Salkovskis PM. Understanding and treating obsessive–compulsive disorder. *Behav. Res. Ther.* 1999; 37 (Suppl. 1): S29–S52.

2.9 Acute stress reactions and post-traumatic stress disorder

These conditions are produced by exceptionally stressful and life-threatening events.

- Acute stress reactions tend to develop rapidly and are short-lived.

- Post-traumatic stress disorder (PTSD) runs a more protracted course.

Adjustment disorders (Section 2.6) are provoked by major adverse life events which are less intense and immediately traumatic than those which cause acute stress reactions and PTSD. The characteristics of acute stress disorders, PTSD and adjustment disorder are shown in Table 24.

2.9.1 Acute stress reaction

Aetiology/psychopathology
By definition the necessary and immediate causative factor for this condition is an exceptionally stressful life event. Some individuals might be more prone to developing this disorder than others, and the reaction is more likely to occur in the elderly or if the person is physically exhausted. A previous history of psychiatric disorder also increases vulnerability.

Epidemiology
The prevalence of acute stress reactions depends on the severity of the trauma that instigates them and the degree of exposure to it. Thus, the incidence of acute stress reactions among the survivors of an industrial explosion and fire at a Norwegian paint factory was directly proportionate to the individual's proximity to the centre of the explosion and conflagration. On the other hand, one-fifth of police officers who had to handle bodies after an aeroplane crash developed a severe stress reaction although there was no direct personal threat.

Clinical presentation and prognosis
This is a short-lived but severe disorder caused by an overwhelming, psychologically traumatic experience. The condition generally subsides within hours or days. Examples of such exceptional stressors include rape, assault, a life-threatening accident, a transport disaster, a domestic fire or multiple bereavements.

The symptoms of an acute stress reaction develop rapidly and tend to vary in character and fluctuate in intensity during the first few hours after exposure to the precipitating event (Table 25). The condition tends to resolve within a matter of days but some survivors will go on to develop PTSD (see Section 2.9.2). Some victims might withdraw into a dissociative stupor (see Section 2.1) or run away from the scene in a state of fugue.

Treatment

- If there is persistent denial that the event has occurred, the survivor should be cautiously prompted to recall the facts.

- A very short course of a benzodiazepine tranquilliser and/or hypnotic is indicated for severe agitation or insomnia.

2.9.2 Post-traumatic stress disorder

Aetiology/psychopathology
The individual is involved in or witnesses an event that is an extreme threat to themselves or others, such as:

- a large-scale disaster (eg Hillsborough Football Stadium in 1989, the Kings Cross Station fire, the Paddington rail crash or the July 7th bombings);

- a personal trauma such a rape, torture or assault.

The psychological impact of the traumatic event is known to be more severe when the stressor is 'man-made' rather than an act of God such as a natural disaster.

	Trigger	**Onset**	**Duration**	**Clinical features**
Acute stress disorder	Exposure to sudden and unexpected danger, eg an assault	Immediate	Brief: days	Anxiety Panics Autonomic arousal Denial Numbing
Post-traumatic stress disorder	Extreme event, eg natural disaster, transport disaster, torture, rape	Immediate or delayed	Prolonged: months/years	Hypervigilance Avoidance Increased arousal, intrusions and memories of that life event
Adjustment disorder	Major adverse life event, such as being informed of life-threatening illness, eg AIDS or cancer	Gradual	Prolonged: weeks/months	Anxiety Depression

TABLE 24 THREE TYPES OF REACTION TO STRESSFUL EXPERIENCES

TABLE 25 CLINICAL PRESENTATION OF ACUTE STRESS DISORDER	
Symptoms	**Clinical presentation**
Psychological	Feeling numb and detached, or dazed and disorientated
	Disbelief that the precipitating event has occurred
	Agitation and overactivity
	Fear, dejection, irritability and anger
	Hypervigilance and enhanced startle response
	'Action replays' of the incident in intrusive memories and dreams
	Withdrawal and avoidance of reminders of the incident
	Irrational guilt about surviving or failing to help others
	Poor concentration
	Loss of interest
Physical	Sweating
	Shakiness
	Rapid heart beat
	Fatigue
	Insomnia
	Nightmares
	Loss of appetite
	Nausea and diarrhoea

Vulnerability factors include a previous history or family history of psychiatric disorder. Children and the elderly have an increased risk of developing PTSD. In some cases physical injury might also increase the risk, but in other victims (eg civilians exposed to bomb outrages in Northern Ireland) survivor guilt was more frequently encountered in those who were physically unscathed.

Epidemiology

The incidence of PTSD is proportionate to the intensity of the psychological trauma. For example, 70% of rape victims are found to have PTSD at 9-month follow-up. In general about 25% of individuals exposed to exceptionally traumatic events develop full-blown PTSD, but the frequency can vary. Thus, about 16% of London Underground train drivers who witnessed a train striking a person on the track developed PTSD, while careful psychological preparation of the police officers who handled the bodies of the Piper Alpha oil rig victims prevented the occurrence of any post-traumatic illness.

Clinical presentation

PTSD is a protracted psychological and behavioural reaction to an exceptionally threatening or catastrophic event that immediately induces intense fear, horror and/or helplessness.

The onset can be delayed for some years and it might only emerge when the victim is exposed to a new extreme stressor.

The symptoms of PTSD are:

- recurrent, distressing and intrusive images of the event;

- dreams and nightmares which do not necessarily depict the incident;

- avoidance of reminders of the trauma;

- detachment and numbness;

- hyperarousal, anxiety, insomnia, poor concentration, enhanced startle response and irritability.

The patient may also experience:

- survivor guilt, defined as the irrational sense that one's life was purchased at the cost of another's;

- phobic avoidance of any situation that resembles the original traumatic event;

- depression;

- generalised anxiety disorder;

- substance misuse.

Some patients become aggressive while others (surprisingly) behave recklessly.

Treatment

- Psychological: direct exposure therapy, anxiety management training and cognitive therapy all improve PTSD by 20–80%.

- Pharmacological: both serotonergic tricyclic antidepressants (eg clomipramine) and selective serotonin reuptake inhibitor antidepressants may help to suppress flashbacks and nightmares as well as reducing the frequency of panic attacks, in addition to their specific antidepressant effect.

Prognosis

This has not yet been clearly established. About one-quarter of rescuers involved in an oil rig disaster were found to have PTSD almost 12 months after the event. There was still a high rate of PTSD in severely abused former prisoners of war 50 years after their release. Prevalence rates for PTSD can range from about 30% among Australian fire fighters to over 80% among Cambodian refugees.

Prevention

- Remind survivors that it is perfectly normal to react emotionally to an abnormal event.

- Gently encourage survivors to talk about the traumatic event rather than sweep it under the carpet. Go at their own pace and without intrusive pressure.

- Advise them to avoid using alcohol to suppress symptoms, because it can delay resolution.

- Encourage them to keep up their usual routine activities.

There have been no large-scale, controlled and prospective studies of the efficacy of early crisis intervention.

FURTHER READING

Alexander DA. Stress among police body handlers: a long term follow up. *Br. J. Psychiatry* 1993; 163: 806–8.

Black D, Newman M, Harris-Hendriks J and Mezey G, eds. *Psychological Trauma: a Developmental Approach.* London: Royal College of Psychiatrists, 1997.

Carlson EB and Rosser-Hogan R. Trauma experiences, posttraumatic stress, dissociation and depression in Cambodian refugees. *Am. J. Psychiatry* 1991; 148: 1548–61.

Farmer R, Tranah T, O'Donnell I and Catalan J. Railway suicide: the psychological effects on drivers. *Psychol. Med.* 1992; 22: 407–14.

Green BL. Psychosocial research in traumatic stress: an update. *J. Trauma Stress* 1994; 7: 341–62.

Joseph S, Williams R and Yule W. *Understanding Post-traumatic Stress: a Psychosocial Perspective on PTSD and Treatment.* Chichester: John Wiley & Sons, 1997.

McFarlane AC. The longitudinal course of posttraumatic morbidity: the range of outcomes and their predictors. *J. Nerv. Ment. Dis.* 1988; 176: 30–9.

O'Brien LS. *Traumatic Events and Mental Health.* Cambridge: Cambridge University Press, 1998.

Weisaeth L. A study of behavioural responses to an industrial disaster. *Acta Psychiatr. Scand. Suppl.* 1989; 355: 13–24.

2.10 Puerperal disorders

Psychiatric disorders associated with childbirth include:

- maternity blues;

- depressive disorder;

- puerperal psychosis.

2.10.1 Maternity blues

Aetiology/psychopathology

Biological factors include the following:

- more common in first pregnancy;

- more common in those with history of premenstrual tension;

- not related to complications at delivery;

- modestly associated with marked postnatal fall in progesterone levels.

Epidemiology
Occurs in 50–70% of women, mainly on the third to fourth day after delivery.

Clinical presentation
The midwives or partner might report:

- lability of mood;

- tearfulness;

- irritability.

There tends to be a rapid and spontaneous resolution to these problems.

Treatment
Provide support and reassurance.

2.10.2 Postnatal depressive disorder

Aetiology/psychopathology
Predisposing factors include:

- previous depressions;

- recent adverse life events;

- marital conflict;

- lack of social support;

- younger age;

- poor relationship with own mother.

Epidemiology
Occurs in 10–15% of women.

Clinical presentation
It usually starts about 2 weeks after childbirth, but can start at any point up to 3 months after delivery. The clinical picture is as in non-psychotic depression.

Treatment

- Psychosocial interventions.

- Antidepressants for severe or persistent symptoms (see below).

- Counselling and mother and baby groups to reduce isolation.

Prognosis

Outcome of postnatal depression

Untreated postnatal depression can last for up to 2 years with damage to:

- relationships;
- emotional and cognitive development of the baby;
- any other children.

Risk of further episode is 1 in 6.

2.10.3 Puerperal psychosis

Aetiology/psychopathology

- Genetic: if there is a strong family history of an affective disorder.

- Environmental: social stress is not implicated (unlike postnatal depression).

- Hormonal: postpartum fall in oestrogen causes supersensitivity of dopamine receptors.

Epidemiology

The frequency is 1 in 500 births. Risk factors include:

- past history or family history of mood disorder;
- primipara;
- older age;
- giving birth by Caesarean section.

Clinical presentation

Usually an affective (especially manic) disorder, but 20% of cases are schizophrenia-like. Onset tends to be abrupt and in the first 2 weeks post partum.

Management of puerperal psychosis

- Antenatal identification of high-risk mothers.
- Move those identified to a specialist mother and baby unit with nurses trained in both mental health and baby care.
- Attempt to preserve mother–child bonding.
- Conventional treatment of depression, mania or schizophrenia, including electroconvulsive therapy if necessary.
- Breast-feeding (see below).
- Assessment of mother–baby interaction before discharge.
- Monitor the mother carefully during subsequent childbearing.

Risks of puerperal psychosis

- Suicide.
- Neglect of child (and of other children).
- Harm to the baby if the mother holds delusional ideas about the child, and of infanticide followed by suicide.

Prognosis

The prognosis is good for immediate recovery but there is a risk of recurrence in 30–50% of patients if they have subsequent deliveries and 50% of patients develop non-puerperal depression.

Perinatal psychiatric drug treatments

Lithium

Avoid lithium in pregnancy and after delivery if possible because:

- in the first trimester it can cause atrialisation of the right ventricle;
- the renal clearance of lithium falls abruptly after delivery, which causes a dangerous rise in serum lithium;
- lithium is secreted in breast milk and if the infant becomes dehydrated, toxic lithium levels develop rapidly.

Carbamazepine and valproate

- Avoid in pregnancy if possible.

Antidepressants

- Amitriptyline or imipramine are used because more data about possible teratogenic effects are available.
- Tricyclics in the third trimester may cause neonatal withdrawal effects, eg irritability and seizures.

Other psychotropic drugs and breast-feeding

When giving a mother psychotropic drugs remember the following.

- All psychotropic drugs are secreted in breast milk, therefore use the lowest effective dose.
- Time feeds to avoid peak levels of drugs.
- Avoid use of more than one psychotropic drug.
- Monitor for development, sedation and irritability in the baby.
- Check the baby's hepatic and renal function.

- Use sertraline or tricyclic antidepressants (amitriptyline or imipramine because more data are available about their effects).
- Use chlorpromazine, trifluoperazine or olanzapine for the same reason.

Pseudocyesis

Pseudocyesis is a rare condition in which the patient erroneously believes that she is pregnant. She has amenorrhoea and abdominal distension. The conviction that she is pregnant is so strong that the patient prepares for the delivery by buying a cradle and baby clothes, etc. In addition to amenorrhoea and abdominal enlargement, there may be swelling and tenderness of the breasts, together with morning sickness and sometimes pica. The majority of patients claim to feel fetal movements.

The psychological basis obviously includes an intense desire for children. Hyperprolactinaemia can mimic pseudocyesis since it causes amenorrhoea, galactorrhoea and abdominal enlargement due to obesity or water retention.

FURTHER READING

Altshuler LL, Hendrick V and Cohen LS. Course of mood and anxiety disorders during pregnancy and the postpartum period. *J. Clin. Psychiatry* 1998; 59 (Suppl. 2): 29–33.

Brockington IF. *Motherhood and Mental Health*. Oxford: Oxford University Press, 1998.

Pritchard DB and Harris B. Aspects of perinatal psychiatric illness. *Br. J. Psychiatry* 1996; 169: 555–62.

Taylor D, Paton C and Kerwin R, eds. *The Maudsley Prescribing Guidelines 2005–2006*, 8th edn. London: Informa Healthcare, 2005.

Yoshida K, Smith B and Kumar R. Psychotropic drugs in mothers' milk: a comprehensive review of assay methods, pharmacokinetics and of safety of breast-feeding. *J Psychopharmacol.* 1999; 13: 64–80.

2.11 Depression

Aetiology/psychopathology

Impaired neurotransmission in depression has been explained by the catecholamine and indoleamine hypotheses, ie low mood is associated with reduced synaptic noradrenaline (NA) or 5-hydroxytryptamine (5HT or serotonin). Reserpine, a monoamine-depleting drug, can cause depression. Conversely, tricyclic and monoamine oxidase (MAO) inhibitor antidepressants increase the synaptic availability of NA and 5HT in the synaptic cleft. However, there is a delay between the antidepressant-induced rise in synaptic NA and 5HT in an individual and any improvement in mood. Furthermore, depressed patients do not have decreased levels of NA, 5HT or the metabolites of either in their blood, urine or cerebrospinal fluid. There is an excess of 5HT reuptake receptors in the frontal cortex of people who have committed suicide.

Some common exogenous causes of depression are shown in Table 26.

Vulnerability factors in women include:

- being responsible for the care of three or more young children;
- lack of a confiding relationship;
- lack of a job outside the home;
- separation from their own mother before the age of 11.

These vulnerability factors sensitise the individual to major adverse life events that are characterised by loss or threat of loss, eg redundancy or physical illness.

Other aetiological factors include the following.

- Genetic: identical twins reared apart show 60% more concordance than dizygotic twins.

- Brain physiology: decrease in rapid eye movement latency.

- Endocrine: loss of cortisol circadian rhythm, ie overactivity of hypothalamic–pituary–adrenocortical system. This might be primary or secondary.

- Psychological: learned helplessness, based on the model of harnessed dogs subjected to recurrent aversive stimuli who become apathetic and fail to escape when restraints are removed.

See also Section 2.10.2.

Epidemiology

Of the general population, 5% will experience an episode of moderate to severe depression. Prevalence is 2–3% of men and up to 9% of women. It is commoner in lower socioeconomic groups because of chronic adversity.

Clinical presentation

The commonly seen mood disorders are depression or bipolar disorder. Depression is much commoner than bipolar disorder.

- Bipolar disorder: there are episodes of persistent lowering of mood interspersed with bouts of sustained elation and overactivity.
- Depression: there are only downward mood swings.

Common

A mixture of psychological and biological symptoms present most days for at least 2 weeks (Table 27). Patients may be agitated or retarded (Table 28).

Uncommon

Psychotic depression Depression can be of psychotic intensity with delusional convictions of disease, putrefaction, poverty, contaminating others or causing evil. There may also be hallucinations, especially accusing or derogatory voices.

Seasonal affective disorder
There is a female to male ratio of 6:1. Onset is in the mid-twenties. Depression tends to occur in the winter months and is often accompanied by oversleeping and overeating. It can be treated with antidepressants and phototherapy, which artificially lengthens the day and optimises biological rhythms.

TABLE 26 COMMON EXOGENOUS CAUSES OF DEPRESSION

Psychosocial factors (mainly loss)	Medical conditions	Drugs
Bereavement	Cerebrovascular accident	Reserpine
Unemployment	Carcinoma of pancreas and bronchus	Beta-blockers
Divorce/separation	Hypothyroidism	Calcium antagonists
Mutilating surgery	Cushing's disease	Oral contraceptives
Disability	Systemic lupus erythematosus	Corticosteroids
	Parkinson's disease	Alcohol
	Multiple sclerosis	Cocaine withdrawal
		Amphetamine withdrawal

TABLE 27 CLINICAL PRESENTATION OF MAJOR DEPRESSION.

Symptoms	Clinical presentation
Psychological	Persistent lowering of mood, often worse in the mornings Slowing of thought and speech Pessimism, self-criticism, guilt and worthlessness Helplessness and hopelessness Poor concentration and memory Loss of a sense of enjoyment (anhedonia) Loss of interest Thoughts of death and/or suicide Suicide attempts
Biological	Insomnia with early-morning wakening (occasionally hypersomnia) Diminished appetite with weight loss (occasionally increased appetite) Loss of sex drive Lack of drive, energy and motivation

TABLE 28 SIGNS OF PSYCHOMOTOR AGITATION AND RETARDATION

Condition	Signs
Psychomotor agitation	Pacing and hand wringing Repetitive and futile activity Quest for reassurance
Psychomotor retardation	Avoidance of company Self-neglect Mutism Slowed movements

Recurrent brief depressions

Bouts of brief (2–5 days) but intense depression occurring every month or so but not related to menstruation.

Anxiety and depression often coexist.

Treatment

Treatment should be both psychological and pharmacological.

- Psychological: cognitive behaviour therapy.

- Pharmacological: antidepressants. Add antipsychotic drug for delusions and/or hallucinations. Electroconvulsive therapy in very severe cases.

Excersise caution when using antidepressants in bipolar affective disorder: there is a risk of inducing mania.

Antidepressants

These tend to be more effective in severe depression and where biological symptoms are prominent.

- Tricyclics, eg lofepramine (less cardiotoxic) and amitriptyline.

- Selective serotonin reuptake inhibitors (SSRIs), eg fluoxetine.

- Combination reuptake inhibitors, eg mirtazapine, venlafaxine.

- MAO inhibitors: these inhibit the reuptake of NA and 5HT, thereby increasing the amount of available neurotransmitter at the synapse.

Management of severe depression

- Assess the patient for suicide risk (see Sections 1.2.2 and 1.3.3). If the risk is high, then admission to a psychiatric unit is indicated, if necessary under the enforcement of the Mental Health Act (see Section 2.14).
- Social isolation, severe self-neglect and failure to eat or drink also require hospital admission.
- Mobilisation of support from carers and mental health professionals is required, especially community psychiatric nurses.

MAO inhibitors

These carry a risk of tyramine response ('cheese reaction'), which causes a dangerous rise in BP. They are also incompatible with opioids, especially pethidine and with sympathominetics.

Tricyclics The side effects of these include:

- anticholinergic, eg dry mouth, blurred vision, constipation, ileus, precipitation of glaucoma, urinary retention and delirium in the elderly;

- α-adrenergic, eg postural hypotension;

- cardiac dysrhythmias;

- lowering the seizure threshold;

- cardiotoxicity in overdose;

- weight gain;

- sexual dysfunction.

Selective serotonin reuptake inhibitors These have fewer cardiovascular effects than tricyclics and are less sedative. They also have no anticholinergic side effects, but can cause gastrointestinal problems, agitation, insomnia and headache.

Tricyclics and SSRIs are probably of equal efficacy. In depression of psychotic intensity, an antipsychotic should be added to the antidepressant.

Electroconvulsive therapy This is the treatment of choice in:

- severe depression;
- refusal to eat or drink;
- grave suicide risk;
- failure of other treatment methods.

Electroconvulsive therapy

Contraindications include raised intracranial pressure, a recent myocardial infarction or cerebrovascular accident, or a recent ventricular dysrhythmia.

Electroconvulsive therapy is applied under general anaesthesia with muscle relaxants. The usual course is six to eight applications, with two applications per week. Major risk factors are those of the general anaesthetic. Side effects include:

- headache;
- transient and persistent memory problems;
- seizures between treatments;
- delirium in the elderly;
- cardiovascular complications.

Prognosis
Most episodes of depression remit within 6 months, although 15% of sufferers experience chronic symptoms. There is a high risk of recurrence if recovery from a particular episode is incomplete. The risk of recurrence increases with age. Mortality due to suicide is 15%.

Prevention

- Cognitive behaviour therapy reduces the risk of further episodes.
- Also consider the continuation of treatment with antidepressants and mood stabilisers (see Section 2.12).

FURTHER READING

Brown GW and Harris T. *Social Origins of Depression: a Study of Psychiatric Disorder in Women.* London: Tavistock, 1978.

Wijeratne C, Halliday GS and Lyndon RW. The present status of electroconvulsive therapy: a systematic review. *Med. J. Aust.* 1999; 171: 250–4.

Williams JMG. Depression. In: Clark DM and Fairburn CG, eds. *Science and Practice of Cognitive Behaviour Therapy.* Oxford: Oxford University Press, 1996: 259–85.

Wolpert L. *Malignant Sadness: the Anatomy of Depression*, 3rd edn. London: Faber, 2006.

2.12 Bipolar affective disorder

This consists of recurrent episodes of mania and depression. Episodes of elevated mood are called mania if they are severe and have psychotic features (delusions and hallucinations). Less severe cases are labelled hypomania. Minimum duration of symptoms is 4 days.

Aetiology/psychopathology
There is a concordance rate of about 75% in monozygotic twins and about 54% in dizygotic twins. A cyclothymic personality is a predisposing factor, ie someone who is prone to spontaneous, subclinical mood fluctuations.

Mania might be secondary to the following:

- antidepressant treatment;
- head injury;
- stroke;
- amphetamine or cocaine use;
- exogenous steroids.

Epidemiology
The lifetime risk of mania is 0.6–1%. The mean age of onset is 30. The incidence is the same in men and women. The age of onset of bipolar disorder is earlier than in depressive disorder.

Clinical presentation
Mania is characterised by the following:

- sustained elevation of mood or irritability;
- abundant energy;
- disinhibition;
- reckless behaviour with extravagant spending, fast driving and promiscuity;
- pressure of speech;
- increased self-esteem;
- grandiose and self-important ideas;
- sometimes a sense of special mission;
- acceleration of thinking and flight of ideas;
- reduced need for sleep;
- poor concentration;
- distractibility;
- lack of insight;
- sometimes delusions of grandeur;
- auditory hallucinations in the second person (ie talking to the patient).

Mixed affective states (ie concurrent depression and manic symptoms) can occur in at least 16% of bipolar patients, usually while the mood is shifting between poles.

For mania, admission to hospital (which is compulsory if necessary) is usually indicated to prevent personal and social damage due to frenetic and reckless behaviour. Hypomania might be contained at home provided the patient can be supervised and is prepared to take regular medication.

McElroy SL, Keck PE and Strakowski SM. Mania, psychosis, and antipsychotics. *J. Clin. Psychiatry* 1999; 57 (Suppl. 3): 14–26.

Taylor D, Paton C and Kerwin R, eds. *The Maudsley Prescribing Guidelines 2005–2006*, 8th edn. London: Informa Healthcare, 2005.

Tohen M and Grundy S. Management of acute mania. *J. Clin. Psychiatry* 1999; 60 (Suppl. 5): 31–4.

Schizoaffective disorder

This diagnostic category is used for manic or depressive symptoms and schizophrenic symptoms occurring concurrently or within a few days of each other.

Rapid-cycling bipolar affective disorder

This is uncommon. There are more than four episodes of severe depression or mania in a year. It is more common in women and in those taking antidepressants.

Differential diagnosis

Differential diagnosis of hypomania and mania in bipolar disorder is as follows.

- Drug-induced overactivity and euphoria: amphetamines, cocaine and Ecstasy.

- Organic states: hypothyroidism (surprisingly), HIV, general paralysis of the insane and multiple sclerosis.

Treatment

- Atypical antipsychotics, eg olanzapine, risperidone and quetiapine.

- Valproate, lithium and carbamazepine.

- Rarely (and paradoxically) electroconvulsive therapy.

- Benzodiazepines may be useful to control agitation in the short term.

⚠ Watch for severe depressive down-swing with risk of suicide.

Prophylaxis

Lithium is indicated after two severe episodes within 2 years. Check renal and thyroid function, and an ECG because of the risk of cardiac dysrhythmias in older patients. Monitor serum lithium, aiming for a level of 0.6–1.0 mmol/L. Watch for hypothyroidism (treat with L-thyroxine) and nephrogenic diabetes insipidus.

Complications

- Risk of death from suicide in a depressive phase.

- Risk of death from exhaustion after weeks of untreated mania.

- Manic stupor.

Prognosis

Untreated episodes might last between 3 and 6 months. Over 50% of sufferers will have further episodes if the disorder begins before the age of 30.

FURTHER READING

el-Mallakh RS. Bipolar illness. *South. Med. J.* 1997; 90: 775–9.

Goodwin FK and Jamison KR. *Manic–Depressive Illness*. Oxford: Oxford University Press, 1990.

2.13 Delusional disorder

Epidemiology

Delusional disorder is less common than schizophrenia. It can occur at any age, but onset is most frequent between 34 and 45 years of age. Prevalence is 0.03% in the general population.

Clinical presentation

Patients usually do not perceive themselves as having a mental illness and so generally do not present themselves for treatment. Their delusions frequently have internal logic and are systematised. They may have olfactory and tactile hallucinations that provide confirmatory evidence to support their beliefs, but hallucinations are generally not prominent. Apart from the delusions and their ramifications, the patient's functioning is not markedly impaired. However, the condition should be taken seriously as patients may be at risk of impulsivity, suicide and homicide. The different subtypes of delusional disorder are shown in Table 29.

TABLE 29 DIFFERENT SUBTYPES OF DELUSIONAL DISORDER

Subtype	Typical preoccupation
Somatic type	Undiagnosed disease
Persecutory type	Conspiracy
Grandiose type	Missionary zeal
Jealous type	Morbid jealousy (Othello syndrome)
Erotomanic type	Impossible love relationship (de Clerambault's syndrome)

Risk factors for delusional disorder

- Social isolation.
- Stress of immigration/exile.
- Family history.
- Personality disorder.

Morbid jealousy carries a significant risk of violence, and concurrent alcohol abuse increases this risk.

Differential diagnosis

The following conditions present with either delusional thinking or preoccupations that can be confused with delusional thinking:

- schizophrenia and other psychotic disorders (see Section 2.3);

- mood disorders;

- dementia (see Section 2.2);

- somatoform disorders (see Section 1.1.2);

- obsessive–compulsive disorder (see Section 2.8);

- neurological disorders, eg after head injury;

- substance abuse (see Section 1.3.5).

Treatment

Reassurance, compassion and support. Cognitive behaviour therapy may ameliorate delusional thinking. Antipsychotic medication and selective serotonin reuptake inhibitors have been shown to be of some value. Hospitalise the patient if there are concerns about aggression, suicide, homicide or extreme impulsivity.

Prognosis

Often a chronic lifelong problem; 33–50% of cases go into remission.

FURTHER READING

American Psychiatric Association. *Diagnostic and Statistical Manual of Mental Disorders: DSM-IV*, 4th edn. Washington, DC: American Psychiatric Association, 2000: 323–9.

Manschreck TC. Delusional disorder: the recognition and management of paranoia. *J. Clin. Psychiatry* 1996; 57 (Suppl. 3): 32–8.

2.14 The Mental Health Act 1983

The Mental Health Act deals with the compulsory detention and treatment of people suffering from mental disorders who are considered to be:

- a danger to themselves and/or;

- a danger to others and/or;

- at risk of deterioration.

The term 'mental disorder' includes all the psychiatric disorders described in this module, with two important exceptions.

- Substance abuse or acute intoxication with drugs and/or alcohol. Note that psychiatric disorders arising out of substance misuse, such as alcoholic hallucinosis or drug-induced psychosis, are covered by the Act.

- Individuals whose personality disorder is regarded as untreatable. Note that although a particular patient's personality disorder might be deemed untreatable, patients with comorbidity, such as a person with an antisocial personality disorder who also has a major depressive disorder and a high risk of suicide, would be covered by the Act.

Physicians only need to be familiar with a limited number of Sections ('Sections' referring to main paragraph numbers of the Act). Clinicians may encounter psychiatric emergency situations in a wide range of settings:

- accident and emergency departments (see Sections 1.2.2 and 1.3.6);

- medical and surgical intensive-care and high-dependency units (see Section 1.1);

- general medical and surgical wards;

- obstetric wards (see Section 2.10.3).

Accident and emergency departments

This is probably the commonest setting for psychiatric emergencies and the most frequent situation is the gravely suicidal patient who declines to be admitted for observation and treatment.

Action should include the following.

- Ensure that a member of staff stays with the patient at all times.

- Call the duty psychiatrist.

- If the suicidal patient attempts to abscond before or during psychiatric assessment, staff have a duty under common law to restrain and detain the patient.

If the duty psychiatrist (who has to be formally approved by the Department of Health as having special experience in the diagnosis and treatment of mental disorders) concludes that the patient requires compulsory admission for observation and/or treatment, he or she will inform the duty approved social worker who will arrange for a second medical assessment to be carried out.

Ideally this second medical assessment would be carried out by the patient's own GP. However, since many patients attending the accident and emergency department

in these circumstances are not actually registered with a GP or might have one who is unavailable, the approved social worker will summon a second psychiatrist (who must be from a different hospital to prevent 'collusion').

If all three agree that compulsory admission is indeed necessary, then they will complete Section 2 or Section 3 documentation.

- Section 2 authorises admission for observation (and any necessary treatment) for up to 28 days.

- Section 3 authorises admission for treatment for up to 6 months.

Patients have the right to appeal against both Sections.

Medical and surgical wards

If the patient is already being nursed on a medical, surgical or obstetric ward, or in an intensive-care or high-dependency unit, and develops a mental illness *de novo* or has an exacerbation or relapse of a pre-

existing disorder, then the physician or surgeon can authorise the patient's compulsory detention for up to 72 hours under Section 5(2) of the Mental Health Act. The Section form can be obtained from the nearest inpatient psychiatric unit.

During those 72 hours the medical or surgical team must request a formal assessment by:

- a consultant psychiatrist;

- the patient's own GP;

- an approved social worker.

Again, if the GP is not available, the patient's own surgeon or physician is authorised to complete the Section.

It is important to note that a patient with a mental illness may be detained under the Mental Health Act on the grounds of risk of deterioration of their mental health alone, ie the patient does not necessarily have to present an active danger to themselves and/or others.

3.1 Self-assessment questions

Question 1

Clinical scenario

A middle-aged man is brought to a London Emergency Department by the British Transport Police. He was found sleeping at a mainline station. He says he cannot remember his name, address or job, or anything about his family. He does not know how he came to be at the station. He speaks coherently with a strong Glaswegian accent. He is fully alert and orientated, and there is no sign of self-neglect or depression.

Question

Which one of the following diagnoses is the most likely?

Answers

A Obsessive–compulsive disorder
B Dissociative fugue
C Phobic anxiety state
D Mania
E Hypomania

Question 2

Clinical scenario

An 86-year-old man, who has lived alone since his wife's death one year previously, is found wandering in the street in the middle of the night after falling down a step. His limbs are stiff. He is bewildered and frightened, and shows signs of self-neglect. He is disorientated and his speech is very hesitant. He describes visual hallucinations that started 6 months previously.

Question

Which one of the following conditions needs to be considered?

Answers

A Dementia with Lewy bodies
B Depressive pseudo-dementia
C Mania
D Obsessive–compulsive disorder
E Dissociative fugue

Question 3

Clinical scenario

A 50-year-old woman has accidentally caused a number of small fires in her home because she forgets to switch off the oven. Her family report that she has been increasingly forgetful. She has been incontinent of urine and her balance is poor. She had a severe head injury 9 months ago. Her symptoms started 6 months ago. Clinical examination of her central nervous system is unremarkable, but her CT head scan shows markedly enlarged ventricles.

Question

Which one of the following is the most likely diagnosis?

Answers

A Normal-pressure hydrocephalus
B Vascular dementia
C Prion disease
D Huntington's disease
E Dementia with Lewy bodies

Question 4

Clinical scenario

A 20-year-old university history student is not allowed to continue with his course because of poor attendance. For several months his written work has been characterised by bizarre, detailed and complex theories about the influence of intergalactic aliens on political events. He has smoked up to eight 'joints' of cannabis a day since he was 16. At interview his speech is slow and hesitant, and he constantly reverts to the theme of being controlled by trans-planetary visitors, who communicate with him and influence his feelings and actions.

Question

Which two of the following diagnoses are the most likely?

Answers

A Dissociative disorder
B Obsessive–compulsive disorder
C Dementia
D Phobia
E Antisocial personality disorder
F Depression
G Schizophrenia
H Post-traumatic stress disorder
I Cannabis-induced psychosis
J Malingering

Question 5

Clinical scenario

A young woman with a diagnosis of schizophrenia asks you about the potential side effects of antipsychotic drugs.

Question

Which two of the following are *not* recognised side effects?

Answers

A Repetitive mouth and tongue movements

B Frequent menstruation
C Weight loss
D Increased risk of sunburn
E Reduced white blood cells and tendency to infection
F Sedation
G Lactation
H Loss of sex drive
I Sudden stiff neck and/or tongue
J Severe restlessness

Question 6

Clinical scenario

You are asked to see a 28-year-old woman in the Emergency Department. She has swallowed half a dozen zopiclone tablets in front of her boyfriend. She is drowsy, but can communicate. On taking the history you learn that she was abused as a child and she has taken many overdoses. She also reports fleeting paranoid ideas and visual hallucinations. She has never been able to settle for long with one partner or at any job. While examining her you find numerous scars on her wrists. You conclude that she has a personality disorder.

Question

Which one of the following is the most likely personality disorder?

Answers

A Antisocial
B Schizoid
C Obsessive–compulsive
D Dependent
E Borderline

Question 7

Clinical scenario

You are looking after an inpatient with carcinoma of the pancreas. He is in pain and has lost weight. He appears miserable and preoccupied, and he barely talks to the other patients or staff.

Question

Which one of the following symptoms is *not* helpful in deciding whether he has a severe depressive illness that requires treatment with an antidepressant?

Answers

A Pessimism
B Self-blame
C Loss of interest
D Thoughts of suicide
E Difficulty sleeping

Question 8

Clinical scenario

A 40-year-old woman was referred to medical outpatients with breathlessness on exertion and palpitations. Her GP has observed that she was very pale. She has suspected anaemia, but has refused to have any blood tests. You think she may have a blood/injection/injury phobia.

Question

Which one of the following would confirm your diagnosis?

Answers

A Hallucinations of corpses
B Paranoia
C Slowing of her heart rate when you show her a syringe
D Impairment of short-term memory
E Compulsive checking

Question 9

Clinical scenario

A 22-year-old man is brought to hospital by his family after he threatened his father with a knife. This happened when his father confronted him about the filthy state of his room. It transpires that for the past 3 years he has been collecting and keeping his own hair, nail clippings and skin. He refuses to wash. When you interview him he tells you that he has intrusive thoughts that terrible harm will come to him and his family. He spends hours each day meticulously collecting his hair and skin in a ritualised way, which he says will prevent these awful things happening. He has no other abnormal beliefs or perceptions.

Question

Which one of the following is true?

Answers

A This man is more likely to be having delusions than obsessions
B Patients typically describe obsessions as being alien thoughts inserted into their minds
C It is unlikely that his man has obsessive–compulsive disorder because the thoughts he is having and the ritualised behaviours do not have the same theme: this is more likely to be schizophrenia
D Cognitive behaviour therapy would be the treatment of choice in this case, plus a selective serotonin reuptake inhibitor
E Antipsychotic drugs are as effective in treating obsessions as delusions

Question 10

Clinical scenario

A previously well 74-year-old woman is brought to you by her daughter. Two days previously she was robbed in the street. The robber threatened her with a knife, ripped her bag off her shoulder and pushed her over as he ran away. Other than some bruising she was not physically injured. Since then she has been agitated and irritable, her concentration is poor and she has lost interest in her usual activities, and she will not leave her flat. She says she is not affected by the robbery, but feels physically unwell with the following symptoms: sweating, shakiness, rapid heart beat and insomnia. She is concerned about her heart.

Question

Which one of the following is *not* correct?

Answers

A This is most likely an acute stress reaction

B After exceptionally stressful life events some patients deny the impact of the event on them

C A low-dose antipsychotic drug may be helpful.

D These symptoms are likely to subside spontaneously with reassurance and support

E A hypnotic drug may be helpful in the very short term

Question 11

Clinical scenario

A 24-year-old policeman sees you in outpatients. He says he feels anxious and irritable all the time. Any sudden noises make him jump. He feels detached and low in his mood. His main complaint is that he is getting very little sleep because of distressing nightmares about an incident that happened 7 months previously when he and a colleague were attacked by a gang of youths and his colleague was killed. He puts off going to bed because he is frightened of having these nightmares.

Question

Which one of the following is *not* correct?

Answers

A The most likely diagnosis is post-traumatic stress disorder

B In this patient there is a risk of self-medication with alcohol

C Selective serotonin reuptake inhibitor antidepressants may be helpful

D If he had a previous history of mental illness, he would have

been more at risk of developing these symptoms

E Having survived the attack physically unscathed is a protective factor after experiences like this

Question 12

Clinical scenario

In her first pregnancy, a 23-year-old woman delivered a healthy baby boy 1 week ago. She is distressed and low in her mood. She is breast-feeding. She will not let anyone touch her baby. She is convinced that the hospital authorities want to take her baby from her. This is not true. You diagnose puerperal psychosis.

Question

Which one of the following is *not* correct?

Answers

A This patient was at greater risk of puerperal psychosis because this was her first pregnancy

B The mother and baby should be separated.

C The mother and baby should be transferred to a specialist mother and baby unit

D All antipsychotics are expressed in breast milk

E Electroconvulsive treatment is rarely used in cases like this

Question 13

Clinical scenario

A 47-year-old man with a history of recurrent depression presents with a further episode of depression that started 2 months ago. His mood is very low and he can no longer derive any pleasure from his usual activities. He feels hopeless about his future and wishes he was dead. He was last depressed 3 years previously when he responded to citalopram, a selective serotonin

reuptake inhibitor antidepressant. He had stopped taking the citalopram 6 months ago because he felt well.

Question

Which two of the following statements are *not* correct?

Answers

A He is likely to be at high risk of suicide

B He is likely to have a diminished sex drive

C Depression is less common in men

D It is unlikely that he will respond to citalopram again

E At this point he should be treated with lithium

F He is more likely to have a family history of mood disorders than the general population

G It is important to look for the presence of psychotic symptoms

H He is more likely than the general population to have had major adverse life events

I Five per cent of the general population will experience an episode of moderate to severe depression.

J Electroconvulsive treatment is still used in the treatment of severe depression

Question 14

Clinical scenario

A 30-year-old unemployed woman is brought to the Emergency Department by the police. She was arrested in a large department store for shoplifting. She was in the store for about an hour hurrying between various departments grabbing items of clothing and accessories. She was talking loudly in an overfamiliar way with other customers and the staff. She was apprehended when she tried to leave the store without paying. She was incensed, saying she did not need to pay because she owned the store and all the other shops on that street. You diagnose mania.

Question

Which one of the following is *not* correct?

Answers

A Cocaine intoxication can present like this

B She is at the mean age of onset for bipolar affective disorder

C Mania responds well to selective serotonin reuptake inhibitor antidepressants

D Benzodiazepines have a role to play in the treatment of mania

E Valproate is used in the treatment and prophylaxis of bipolar affective disorder

Question 15

Clinical scenario

You are in the Emergency Department and a 41-year-old man is brought in by his wife. He was sent home from work the previous day because he was unplugging all the computer screens in the office and became threatening and angry when his work colleagues turned them back on. His wife said that over the past 5 months he has become increasingly preoccupied about terrorists gaining information about him by using computers. He felt very threatened. He believed that they were going to kill him by setting off an explosive device near him. He is not hallucinating and his thoughts are coherent.

Question

Which one of the following is *not* correct?

Answers

A The most likely diagnosis is obsessive–compulsive disorder

B Psychological therapy may improve delusional thinking

C This is likely to develop into a chronic, lifelong problem

D He should be treated with an antipsychotic drug

E He is at high risk of self-harm

Question 16

Clinical scenario

You are at the home of a 63-year-old man who is dependent on alcohol. He has been a heavy drinker for much of his adult life. Three days previously he was sent to hospital by his GP because he had a chest infection. He discharged himself from hospital against the advice of the doctors. He is now confused, drowsy and agitated. He is also shaking and sweating. He adamantly refuses to go back to hospital. You diagnose alcohol withdrawal syndrome and a chest infection.

Question

Which one of the following is correct?

Answers

A He can be safely managed at home with a home detoxification programme and antibiotics

B He should be admitted, ideally under the Mental Health Act, but as a life-saving measure he can be admitted under common law

C This situation is best managed by admitting him to a psychiatric ward

D The Mental Health Act cannot be used in patients who abuse alcohol

E As a physician you could admit someone you know to hospital under the Mental Health Act (ie not under common law) without the concurrence of any other professional

Question 17

Clinical scenario

A 78-year-old woman had hip replacement surgery 3 days ago. She was previously mentally well. She now presents withdrawn, disorientated and drowsy. Her oral intake is poor.

Question

Which one of the following is correct?

Answers

A She is most likely to have had a stroke

B Dehydration is unlikely to cause this clinical picture

C Her sleep–wake pattern is likely to be reversed

D Alcohol dependence is not worth considering

E This is likely to resolve spontaneously

Question 18

Clinical scenario

A 42-year-old man, who is a heavy drinker, is admitted to hospital for a routine surgical procedure. He is dependent on alcohol and has been prescribed benzodiazepines for detoxification. After 2 days in hospital and prior to surgery he collapses.

Question

Which one of the following is *not* correct?

Answers

A The colloquial use of the term 'blackouts' in the context of alcohol dependence refers to amnesic episodes

B In alcohol withdrawal BP tends to be low, resulting in collapse

C It is likely that he may have had a seizure

D It is likely that he may have had hypoglycaemia

E It is possible that he has collapsed due to severe blood loss

Question 19

Clinical scenario

A 24-year-old man from Spain is admitted to your ward. He tells you that he has been a heroin user for 3 years. He says he is attending a drug-treatment unit in Spain where he is being prescribed 40 mg of methadone per day.

Question

Which one of the following is correct?

Answers

A Calculate the dose of methadone to prescribe according to the average amount of heroin he is using

B Prescribe an initial dose of methadone 10 mg twice a day if he has objective signs of withdrawal and you have confirmation from urine drug testing that he has been using opioids. Titrate the dose upwards as necessary to control withdrawal symptoms up to a maximum of 20 mg bd per 24 hours

C Quick urine drug-testing kits are unreliable and not worth using

D Naloxone will control withdrawal symptoms

E It is not necessary to treat heroin withdrawal as it will resolve spontaneously

Question 20

Clinical scenario

A 22-year-old woman in the Emergency Department waiting room is shouting abuse and kicking at the furniture. She is known to have a psychotic illness. You are the doctor on duty.

Question

Which one of the following is *not* correct?

Answers

A Call the hospital security and/or the police

B Remove other patients, visitors and staff from the area

C Take control of the situation by ordering her to calm down as she is causing a disturbance

D Delegate to someone to get background information about her

E Arrange an urgent Mental Health Act assessment

Question 21

Clinical scenario

A 30-year-old woman is referred by her GP. She was travelling to work on the Underground when she had a sudden bout of palpitations. She had had a row with her husband before setting out for work and her manager has recently given her a poor appraisal. On examination her pulse is rapid but regular and she is shaking and sweating. She sighs frequently. Her ECG is normal.

Question

Which one of the following statements is correct?

Answers

A Her liver function tests are normal so alcohol abuse can be excluded

B Hypothyroidism might be the cause

C Her BP is normal so a phaeochromocytoma can be ruled out

D Her arterial $P\text{co}_2$ is likely to be low

E Diazepam 5 mg up to three times a day for the next few weeks would be helpful until she can be reviewed

Question 22

Clinical scenario

A 30-year-old schoolteacher has been on sick leave for 7 months since she had a bout of gastroenteritis. Her diarrhoea and vomiting had stopped after 2 days, but she has felt exhausted ever since and is spending increasing amounts of time resting in bed. She sleeps badly, her concentration is poor and she is worried about swollen glands in her neck. A nutritionist has advised her to eat no dairy or wheat products, whilst her reflexologist has recommended a course of trace elements and other dietary supplements to correct an alleged postviral imbalance of her adrenal function. Extensive medical tests and investigations have failed to demonstrate any significant abnormality.

Question

Which one of the following would contribute to effective medical management in this case?

Answers

A A conservative approach of waiting until she makes a spontaneous recovery

B To encourage her to join an 'ME' self-help group on the grounds that this would improve the prognosis

C Advise her to give up her teaching career because her incapacity is likely to be permanent

D Explain tactfully that cognitive behaviour therapy/graded exercise is the only evidence-based effective treatment for this condition

E Immunotherapy is a useful adjunct to treatment

Question 23

Clinical scenario

A 22-year-old woman is brought into the Emergency Department after taking half a dozen paracetamol tablets in front of her partner, with whom she has been quarrelling. She has also threatened to cut her wrists and has a tendency to misuse alcohol.

Question

Which one of the following statements is correct?

Answers

A A past history of similar self-harming episodes reduces the risk of a future fatal outcome

B People who threaten to harm themselves do not actually do any serious damage

C The prognosis is not improved by the patient being interviewed by a mental health professional in the Emergency Department

D Her misuse of alcohol is a significant additional risk factor

E The police have to be informed because attempted suicide is a criminal offence

Question 24

Clinical scenario

A 16-year-old girl has fainted twice at school. You have excluded a medical cause and you are concerned about her emaciated appearance.

Question

Which one of the following would *not* support a diagnosis of anorexia nervosa?

Answers

A A BMI below 17.5

B The fact the she regards herself as being far too thin

C Her periods have stopped

D She thinks constantly about food

E She exercises for several hours a day

3.2 Self-assessment answers

Answer to Question 1

B

Dissociative fugue ('flight') is a psychological condition in which patients suddenly travel away from home or work. They cannot recall much of their past personal information and are confused about their personal identity. There is no identifiable underlying organic cause. The usual trigger is an exceptionally stressful personal predicament. An example is 'shell-shocked' deserters from the front line in the First World War who had unrecognised dissociative fugue.

Answer to Question 2

A

Dementia with Lewy bodies is the third most common dementia seen in older people. In addition to the cognitive impairment, which is often fluctuating, the diagnostic features also include parkinsonism, hallucinations, repeated falls due to syncopal episodes, sensitivity to antipsychotic medication and rapid eye movement sleep disorder.

Answer to Question 3

A

The symptoms described are typical of normal-pressure hydrocephalus. In addition to severe head injury the common causes of this include subarachnoid haemorrhage and previous meningitis, but often no cause is apparent. The absence of any involuntary movements make Huntington's disease and prion disease unlikely. In vascular dementia, ischaemic changes are

usually seen on CT. Dementia with Lewy bodies commonly presents with parkinsonism and hallucinations along with the cognitive impairment.

Answer to Question 4

G and I

There is now evidence that the highest risk period of inducing psychosis by smoking cannabis is in childhood and adolescence. It has been suggested that cannabis may precipitate psychotic symptoms in a person with a predisposition to developing schizophrenia. However, because cannabis is more potent in its currently available form ('skunk'), with heavy use it can produce a clinical picture indistinguishable from schizophrenia in a person without a genetic predisposition to it.

Answer to Question 5

B and C

Since antipsychotic drugs act by blocking dopamine receptors in the brain, they increase prolactin levels. This results in secondary amenorrhoea, galactorrhoea and impotence in men. A serious and often unrecognised side effect of antipsychotics is the metabolic syndrome, which includes weight gain, diabetes, hypercholesterolaemia and hypertension.

Answer to Question 6

E

This presentation is fairly typical in someone who has a borderline personality disorder. Antisocial personality disorder is characterised by a disregard and violation of the rights of others that results in frequent law-breaking. People who have a schizoid personality disorder are socially very isolated, apparently self-sufficient and have a restricted capacity to express emotion. In obsessive–compulsive personality disorder the person is excessively perfectionist and inflexible. Dependent personality disorder is characterised by extreme dependency in relationships.

Answer to Question 7

E

Pain, nausea and discomfort caused by cancer or its treatment can result in symptoms that are indistinguishable from the biological symptoms of a depressive illness, ie loss of appetite, energy and libido and sleep disturbance. The assessment therefore depends on the evaluation of mood, anhedonia, suicidal thinking and other psychological symptoms.

Answer to Question 8

C

Blood/injection/injury phobia is unusual and is counterintuitive in its autonomic nervous system response in that it is associated with bradycardia and hypotension. This can lead to fainting.

Answer to Question 9

D

In obsessive–compulsive disorder, ritualised behaviours serve to neutralise the obsessive thoughts and thus do not necessarily have the same theme, eg counting to prevent an accident to a loved one. Typically patients recognise the obsessive thoughts are a product of their own minds. Selective serotonin reuptake inhibitors can be effective especially when combined with cognitive behaviour therapy.

Answer to Question 10

C

Reassure the patient that this is a normal reaction to an abnormal event and that her symptoms should soon subside. To accelerate her recovery she should be encouraged, with the help of her daughter, to resume all her routine activities, especially those that take place outside her home, eg shopping. She should be followed up, and if her symptoms persist beyond 4 weeks she should be referred for psychological therapy.

Answer to Question 11

E

In post-traumatic stress disorder the life-threatening traumatic experience is accompanied by feelings of intense fear, helplessness and/or horror. These feelings may occur whether or not the person is physically injured, eg an underground train driver who witnesses his train striking a person on the track.

Answer to Question 12

B

This is a high-risk situation because mothers with puerperal psychosis may harm themselves and/or their babies. It is now recognised that disruption of mother and baby bonding due to early separation should be avoided as this will impair the psychological development of the infant. In a specialist mother and baby unit adequate supervision is provided ensuring the safety of both the baby and the mother.

Answer to Question 13

D and E

It is reasonable to re-prescribe the same antidepressant if someone has

responded to it in the past. Lithium is used to augment antidepressants in the treatment of resistant depression, which is defined as a failure to respond to two antidepressants from different classes that were given in therapeutic doses for adequate periods.

Answer to Question 14

C

Antidepressants can precipitate or exacerbate mania or hypomania. In the clinical situation described, the treatment of choice is an atypical antipsychotic drug, eg olanzapine, risperidone or quetiapine. This may be augmented with a benzodiazepine or a mood stabiliser, eg valproate.

Answer to Question 15

A

This is a description of persistent delusional disorder. The mean age of onset is 35–45 years. The clinical picture is dominated by delusions, which are generally persecutory in content. There may also be hallucinations, but these are not prominent. The delusions tend to be encapsulated, ie the patient can generally function fairly well in areas unaffected by the delusions.

Answer to Question 16

B

Alcohol withdrawal syndrome in people aged over 50 years carries a high morbidity and risk of mortality. The Mental Health Act 1983 cannot be used primarily to treat substance misuse problems, including alcohol, unless they are causing mental disorders in their own right, eg alcoholic hallucinosis, delirium tremens or LSD psychosis. In the situation described, the patient most likely has delirium tremens as well as a chest infection and is therefore at very high risk.

Answer to Question 17

C

Delirium (acute confusional state) can present like this, although the more common picture is one that includes agitation, paranoid ideas and perceptual disturbances. It is easy to overlook delirium in a patient who presents as withdrawn. This woman has recently had surgery so look for a metabolic disturbance, infection or dehydration. Alcohol withdrawal symptoms can also be easily missed.

Answer to Question 18

B

About 20–30% of male and 5–10% of female admissions to general hospitals are found to misuse alcohol on screening questionnaires. The complications of alcohol use are thus common. In alcohol withdrawal they tend to have a tachycardia with a fluctuating raised BP.

Answer to Question 19

B

Giving methadone to someone who is not dependent on opioids can cause death. Also, if drug users exaggerate their methadone or heroin use and you use this dose to calculate the equivalent amount of methadone, you can kill them. Look for the objective use of opioids with urine drug screens. Also look for objective evidence of signs of withdrawal, including lacrimation, runny nose, agitation, sweating, piloerection, tachycardia, vomiting, shivering, yawning and widely dilated pupils.

Answer to Question 20

C

In this situation a calm head is needed. Think of the safety of other patients, visitors, staff and the abusive patient herself. It is important to bear in mind that patients who are violent may also be at risk of self-harm. Attempt to find out what she is upset about. Do not assume that this is necessarily due to hallucinations or delusions. Consider psychiatric and non-psychiatric reasons that could explain this behaviour.

Answer to Question 21

D

This is most likely an acute anxiety state precipitated by her personal circumstances. Hyperventilation occurs in anxiety, which would be the cause of the low arterial P_{CO_2}. Symptoms caused by hyperventilation include paraesthesia, headache, dizziness, tinnitus and carpopedal spasm.

Answer to Question 22

D

This is a fairly typical presentation of chronic fatigue syndrome (myalgic encephalomyelitis or ME). A proportion of patients with chronic fatigue syndrome develop this without a preceding infection. The only treatments for which there is significant evidence of effectiveness are cognitive behaviour therapy and graded exercise treatment, and these are recommended in the National Institute for Health and Clinical Excellence (NICE) guidelines. There is no evidence that dietary supplements, exclusion diets or immunotherapy will treat chronic fatigue syndrome, although medication may be used to treat associated conditions, eg depression.

Answer to Question 23

D

Alcohol has a short-term disinhibiting effect that increases the risk of violence towards one's self and others. The above clinical picture may be very different once the effects of the alcohol have worn off.

Answer to Question 24

B

One of the diagnostic criteria of anorexia nervosa is an altered body image. The patient believes and perceives that she is overweight despite objective evidence that she is well underweight. She may challenge this evidence by, for example, questioning the accuracy of the scales.

THE MEDICAL MASTERCLASS SERIES

249

Clinical Skills

CLINICAL SKILLS FOR PACES

Introduction 3

History-taking for PACES (Station 2) 6

Communication Skills and Ethics for PACES (Station 4) 11

Examination for PACES Stations 1, 3 and 5: General Considerations 13

Station 1: Respiratory System 16

Station 1: Abdominal System 21

Station 3: Cardiovascular System 27

Station 3: Central Nervous System 36

Station 5: Skin, Locomotor System, Endocrine System and Eyes 54

PAIN RELIEF AND PALLIATIVE CARE

PACES Stations and Acute Scenarios 61

1.1 History-taking 61
- 1.1.1 Pain 61
- 1.1.2 Constipation/bowel obstruction 63

1.2 Communication skills and ethics 65
- 1.2.1 Pain 65
- 1.2.2 Breathlessness 66
- 1.2.3 Nausea and vomiting 67
- 1.2.4 Bowel obstruction 69
- 1.2.5 End of life 70

1.3 Acute scenarios 71
- 1.3.1 Pain 71
- 1.3.2 Breathlessness 74
- 1.3.3 Nausea and vomiting 76
- 1.3.4 Bowel obstruction 79

Diseases and Treatments 82

2.1 Pain 82
2.2 Breathlessness 87
2.3 Nausea and vomiting 88
2.4 Constipation 89
2.5 Bowel obstruction 90
2.6 Anxiety and depression 91
2.7 Confusion 93
2.8 End-of-life care: the dying patient 94
2.9 Specialist palliative care services 96

Self-assessment 98

MEDICINE FOR THE ELDERLY

PACES Stations and Acute Scenarios 107

1.1 History-taking 107
- 1.1.1 Frequent falls 107
- 1.1.2 Recent onset of confusion 110
- 1.1.3 Urinary incontinence and immobility 114
- 1.1.4 Collapse 116
- 1.1.5 Vague aches and pains 119
- 1.1.6 Swollen legs and back pain 121
- 1.1.7 Failure to thrive: gradual decline and weight loss 127

1.2 Clinical examination 129
- 1.2.1 Confusion (respiratory) 129
- 1.2.2 Confusion (abdominal) 130
- 1.2.3 Failure to thrive (abdominal) 131
- 1.2.4 Frequent falls (cardiovascular) 131
- 1.2.5 Confusion (cardiovascular) 132
- 1.2.6 Frequent falls (neurological) 132
- 1.2.7 Confusion (neurological) 134
- 1.2.8 Impaired mobility (neurological) 135
- 1.2.9 Confusion (skin) 135
- 1.2.10 Frequent falls (locomotor) 136
- 1.2.11 Confusion (endocrine) 136
- 1.2.12 Confusion (eye) 136

1.3 Communication skills and ethics 137
- 1.3.1 Frequent falls 137
- 1.3.2 Confusion 138
- 1.3.3 Collapse 139

1.4 Acute scenarios 141
- 1.4.1 Sudden onset of confusion 141
- 1.4.2 Collapse 143

Diseases and Treatments 147

2.1 Why elderly patients are different 147
2.2 General approach to management 149
2.3 Falls 151
2.4 Urinary and faecal incontinence 155
- 2.4.1 Urinary incontinence 155
- 2.4.2 Faecal incontinence 157

2.5 Hypothermia 158
2.6 Drugs in elderly people 161
2.7 Dementia 162
2.8 Rehabilitation 165
2.9 Aids, appliances and assistive technology 166
2.10 Hearing impairment 168
2.11 Nutrition 170

Haematology and Oncology

HAEMATOLOGY

Cardiology and Respiratory Medicine

CARDIOLOGY

RESPIRATORY MEDICINE

PACES Stations and Acute Scenarios 191

Gastroenterology and Hepatology

GASTROENTEROLOGY AND HEPATOLOGY

Neurology, Ophthalmology and Psychiatry

NEUROLOGY

Investigations and Practical Procedures 165

Self-assessment 174

Nephrology

NEPHROLOGY

PACES Stations and Acute Scenarios 3

Rheumatology and Clinical Immunology

RHEUMATOLOGY AND CLINICAL IMMUNOLOGY

INDEX

Note: page numbers in *italics* refer to figures, those in **bold** refer to tables.